# THE PHYSICIAN

# THE PHYSICIAN

## A Professional Under Stress

Edited by:

**John P. Callan, M.D.**

Medical Director
Blue Hills Hospital
Hartford, Connecticut;
Assistant Clinical Professor of Psychiatry
University of Connecticut School of Medicine
Farmington, Connecticut

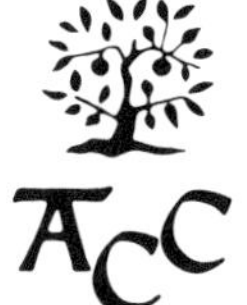

**APPLETON-CENTURY-CROFTS/Norwalk, Connecticut**

0-8385-7855-1





83 84 85 86 87 88 / 10 9 8 7 6 5 4 3 2 1

Prentice-Hall International, Inc., London
Prentice-Hall of Australia, Pty. Ltd., Sydney
Prentice-Hall Canada, Inc.
Prentice-Hall of India Private Limited, New Delhi
Prentice-Hall of Japan, Inc., Tokyo
Prentice-Hall of Southeast Asia (Pte.) Ltd., Singapore
Whitehall Books Ltd., Wellington, New Zealand
Editora Prentice-Hall do Brasil Ltda., Rio de Janeiro

Library of Congress Cataloging in Publication Data
Main entry under title:
The Physician.
Bibliography: p.
Includes index.
1. Physicians. 2. Physicians—Psychology. 3. Physicians—Mental health. 4. Women physicians. 5. Minorities in medicine. I. Callan, John P.
[DNLM: 1. Physicians—Psychology. W 62 P577]
R707.P47 1983 610.69'52 82-22602
ISBN 0-8385-7855-1

Cover and text design: Lynn M. Luchetti

PRINTED IN THE UNITED STATES OF AMERICA

# Contributors

**Susan Adelman,** M.D., F.A.C.S.
Clinical Assistant Professor
Department of Surgery
Wayne State University
Detroit, Michigan

**Perry R. Ayres,** M.D., F.A.C.P.
Clinical Professor of Medicine and Preventive Medicine
Ohio State University College of Medicine
Columbus, Ohio

**E. Ted Chandler,** M.D.
Associate Professor of Medicine
Department of Medicine
Bowman Gray School of Medicine
Wake Forest University
Winston-Salem, North Carolina

**John Donnelly,** M.D.
Senior Consultant
The Institute of Living
Hartford, Connecticut

**Julie Cotton Donnelly,** Ed.D.
Assistant Professor
Department of Research in Health Education
University of Connecticut
Farmington, Connecticut

**Patrick B. Friel,** M.D., F.A.P.A., F.A.C.P., M.R.C.PSYCH.
Director, Consultation and Liaison
Department of Psychiatry
St. Francis Hospital and Medical Center
Hartford, Connecticut;
Private Practice
West Hartford, Connecticut

**Moises Gaviria,** M.D.
Associate Professor of Clinical Psychiatry and Preventive Medicine
Department of Psychiatry
University of Illinois at the Medical Center
Chicago, Illinois

**Cheryl L. Gillespie,** R.N., M.S.
Consulting Staff
Saint Albans Psychiatric Hospital
Radford, Virginia

**Hal G. Gillespie,** M.D.
Staff Psychiatrist
Saint Albans Psychiatric Hospital
Radford, Virginia

**Thomas R. Kearney,** M.B., B.CH., M.R.C.P.(EDIN.), M.R.C.PSYCH.
Assistant Attending Physician
Department of Psychiatry
St. Francis Hospital and Medical Center
Hartford, Connecticut;
Assistant Clinical Professor of Psychiatry
University of Connecticut School of Medicine
Farmington, Connecticut

**David R. Kessler,** M.D.
Clinical Professor of Psychiatry
University of California School of Medicine
San Francisco, California

**James A. Knight,** M.D.
Professor of Psychiatry
Department of Psychiatry
LSU School of Medicine
New Orleans, Louisiana

**Spencer B. Lewis,** M.D.*
Founder
The American Society of Handicapped Physicians
Private Practice
Lewis Family Health Clinic
Grambling, Louisiana

*Deceased

**Harvey N. Mandell,** M.D.
Medical Director
The William W. Backus Hospital
Norwich, Connecticut;
Associate Clinical Professor of Medicine
Yale University School of Medicine
New Haven, Connecticut

**Austin McCawley,** M.D.
Director of Psychiatry
St. Francis Hospital and Medical Center
Hartford, Connecticut;
Professor of Psychiatry
The University of Connecticut Health Center
School of Medicine
Farmington, Connecticut

**Carol Nadelson,** M.D.
Professor and Vice Chairman of Academic Affairs
Department of Psychiatry
Tufts University School of Medicine;
Associate Psychiatrist-in-Chief
Director of Training and Education,
Department of Psychiatry,
New England Medical Center
Boston, Massachusetts

**Harvey L. Ruben,** M.D., M.P.H.
Associate Clinical Professor
Department of Psychiatry
Yale University School of Medicine
New Haven, Connecticut

**Anita D. Taylor,** M.A.ED.
Counselor
Bowman Gray School of Medicine
Wake Forest University
Winston-Salem, North Carolina

**Diana M. Taylor,** A.B.
Ph.D. Candidate
Department of Sociology
University of Pennsylvania
Philadelphia, Pennsylvania

**Robert B. Taylor,** M.D.
Professor
Family and Community Medicine
Bowman Gray School of Medicine
Wake Forest University
Winston-Salem, North Carolina

**Sharon J. Taylor**
Student
Wake Forest University
Winston-Salem, North Carolina

**Augustus A. White III,** M.D., DR. MED. SCI.
Orthopaedic Surgeon-In-Chief
Professor of Orthopaedic Surgery
Department of Orthopaedic Surgery
Beth Israel Hospital
Harvard Medical School
Boston, Massachusetts

**Ronald Wintrob,** M.D.
Visiting Professor of Psychiatry and Human Behavior
Department of Psychiatry
Butler Hospital
Brown University
Providence, Rhode Island

# Contents

# Foreword

In this volume and in an interesting manner Dr. Callan assembles a group of experts who take us backstage to understand the strategies of coping with the physician's lifestyle from his student days to retirement. Along with the occupational hazards of medical practice there are frequently family problems which clamor for attention. Due to the all engrossing demands upon physicians in practice, their family lives often become complicated.

Withal, however, there is a romance to the healer's art. The privilege of treating sick human beings is a wonderful calling and most practitioners would not want to be doing anything else. True, the complaint today is that in the selection of students too much attention is paid to proficiency in scientific subjects and not enough to humanistic qualities though, admittedly, these latter qualities are hard to measure. Nevertheless, the present method of choice may be one of the influences implicated later, as complaints arise that today's young doctors, while highly scientific and effectual, have yet to learn the curative values of warmth, of taking time to listen, and of giving evidence of real interest in and caring for the patient who consults them.

Recently there has been a renewed interest in family medicine, certainly a step in the right direction. Though there was nothing curative in that little black bag which the "old family doctor" carried, he nevertheless, Balint noted, had with him the most effective curative agent extant—one with no unpleasant side effects—it was himself and he prescribed himself in generous doses.

It is an interesting side light that the father of "Popsie" Welch, he of scientific medicine fame, was a general practitioner in Connecticut and it was said that he had only to enter a room and the patient felt better. He apparently had the presence and understanding that communicated itself to sick people and made them sure they would get well.

Though medicine as a discipline remains high in public regard, doctors have slipped a few notches in people's affection sometimes, perhaps, because of a bit of arrogance, and sometimes because of a lack of regard for the patient's sensibilities. Today there is an added disturbing factor for which the doctor bears very little if any responsibility; namely, the present economic situation. One fears that as the regulating bodies and insurance companies close in on medical practice the profession will have still more difficulties. One has only to mention the increase in the number of malpractice suits and exhorbitant jury awards to realize that trouble is in the offing. In addition, a number of hospitals require their staff members to have a million dollars worth of malpractice insurance in order to remain on the staff! All of this is deeply regreted for it penalizes sick people and discourages physicians.

As to the other problems covered in this volume, it is true that some harried physicians have fallen prey to alcohol or sedatives. This is all "out of the closet" and medical societies have become vitally interested in "impaired physicians" and the welfare of their patients. They have taken it upon themselves to see that both patients and physicians are properly cared for.

In earlier years, physicians very rarely thought of retiring and in some small towns, people would not let them retire even if they wanted to do so. The situation is changing today with all manner of reports and restrictions and demands for second opinions, recalcitrant insurance companies, and malpractice insurance costs, as mentioned above. It has taken some of the joy out of practice. Then, too, it is sad to see a once beloved old physician slip slowly out of date but "hanging on" until his practice gradually fades away.

The situation is more difficult for surgeons, for some are reluctant to give up and stoutly insist they are "as good as every they were." Hospital board members and staff officials sometimes have to get involved and the surgeon is asked to retire, often none too graciously.

Physicians' families too are subject to the exigencies of time and the doctor has to do what he can in the midst of numerous interruptions. It is hoped that when he married, someone took his bride aside and warned her that medicine is a "jealous mistress" and she would have to be number two in competition for her husband's time. Though the families are backstage as far as the public is concerned, they often become serious sources of worry. Being a doctor does not insure the family against the "slings and arrows of outrageous fortune."

The functions and art of the doctor consists of more than simply administering medications, repairing wounds or even redirecting disturbed minds. Along with the clergy, medicine has spiritual overtones. Yet the doctor's lot in the future is not going to be an easy one, no matter how competent he may be. Patients are becoming more sophisticated and asking for relationships that are more equal and less paternalistic. Along with this, medicine will have to continue to depend upon the quality of its science and an even greater promotion as a humane calling. It is in the unselfish skillful dedication to the ideals of his profession, however, that the spiritual aspect of the doctor's work continues to become manifest.

This book gives an overview of some of the physician's problems taking place in the wings, while the doctor in his professional capacity occupies center stage. It is quite worthwhile.

Francis J. Braceland, M.D.
Institute of Living
Hartford, Connecticut

# THE PHYSICIAN

# part one

# The Typical Physician

# The Normal Physician Family

Finding a "normal" physician's family is a challenge that seems as fraught with difficulty as Jason's quest to capture the Golden Fleece. The reason is simple: there are no readily identifiable standards that make it easy to establish which medical families are "normal" and which are not. Every family, medical or otherwise, has its own unique characteristics which make it distinct from other families be it in the same community or the same profession. These characteristics may deviate from the norm and yet the family may be perfectly "normal." "Normal" is defined as "conforming to an accepted standard." Physicians' families may show marked dissimiliarity from one another because physicians tend to be highly individualistic outside medicine. The "great outdoors" may be one medical family's getaway, whereas another family may delight in theater and the joys of urban living.

Bearing this in mind, Dr. and Mrs. Robert Taylor and family (Winston–Salem, NC) were asked to write a chapter on the "normal" physician family. They responded admirably to this difficult task and have come up with an intriguing contribution on medical family life. The Taylors have researched medical marriage over the years, have looked at the current state of medical unions, and have interwoven comments and experience from their own 24 years of medical marriage to provide a chapter rich with insight and knowledge.

*J.P.C.*

# 1

# Marriage, Medicine, and the Medical Family

*Anita D. Taylor*
*Robert B. Taylor*
*Diana M. Taylor*
*Sharon J. Taylor*

Most people would consider us to be a normal medical family: a physician husband; a wife active in the community; and two daughters, both in college. All four grandparents are living. Two live in the same community as we do and two live 400 miles away. We see ourselves as a close-knit family unit, mutually supportive and often spending vacations and holidays together.

The above could describe any family fortunate enough to have survived the assault on family unity prevalent during the past two decades. The physician and his wife were married while in medical school and college respectively, at a time in history when marriage and romanticism were equated. Marriage partners expected to "live happily ever after" and few doubted that two people in love would instinctively know how to maintain a mutually fulfilling relationship. Women defined their success in life through their husbands' occupations and those who married a physician were judged by society's standards to be particularly fortunate, being automatically assured of financial security, social status, and community repect. Since the ability to purchase material goods was highly valued, the physician's traditional commitment to work was considered a virtue, with the attendant absences from home a small sacrifice for the benefits promised.

However, the attitudes and values of Americans changed in the 1960s and 1970s. Interpersonal relationships and self-actualization became more important. The shift in emphasis to self-expression unsettled many who were caught up in the American work ethic; they were confused by the conflict of old vs new values. Marriage was viewed by some as an impediment to individual growth and development. The "me" philosophy of life exposed the constraints of the traditional marital union upon individuals who wanted "to do their own thing." Americans in astounding numbers filled the divorce courts. The divorce rate climbed from 2.2 per 1000 total population in 1960 to 5.3 per 1000 total population in 1980. The sharpest rise occurred during 1967–1975, with the rate increasing from 2.6 in 1967 to 4.9 in 1975. Since then the rate has continued to increase, but at a slower pace.[1,2]

Medical marriage weathered the storm quite well, at least in terms of the divorce rate. Rose and Rosow[3] analyzed 57,514 initial complaints for divorce, separate maintenance, or annulment filed in California during the first six months of 1968 and found that the rate of marital instability, as measured by these complaints, was 41% greater in the general population than among physicians. Female physicians, however, had a 48% higher risk of marital instability than their male counterparts in the Rose and Rosow study. A special 1970 census survey[4] showed that white male physicians, ages 35–40 years, were half as likely to be divorced as nonphysicians. No statistics were compiled for female physicians, who comprised 8.7% of the total physician population at that time. In late 1976 a questionnaire study was conducted in Ramsey County, Minnesota.[5] The study sample of 50 physicians, all white men between the ages of 35 and 44, had a divorce rate one-half that of the general comparable population as reported in the 1970 census data. Heins et al.[6] interviewed 95 randomly selected male physicians in the Detroit metropolitan area between July and December 1975 and found that none were divorced at the time of the survey, although 10% had been divorced previously and had remarried. Six percent of the 87 female physicians interviewed between November 1974 and March 1975 were divorced at the time of the survey and 12% had been previously divorced and had remarried. A more extensive survey[7] published in 1979 analyzed 1168 usable responses (a return rate of 30%); only 3% of the respondents were divorced at the time of the survey. However, the percentage of female physicians divorced or separated was six times that of the men.

Of those physicians whose marriages ended in divorce there are some high-risk groups in addition to female physicians. Rose and Rosow[3] report an inverse correlation between the rate of complaint and the size of city, a reversal of the liberal divorce patterns in cities and conservative trends in rural area. They found that black physicians had a 70% higher complaint rate than white physicians. There was also a variation in the complaint rate among the medical specialties. Orthopedic surgeons, psychiatrists, and dermatologists were highest, and preventive medicine/public health specialists lowest.

Experts caution, however, that statistics do not afford a complete picture of the state of medical marriage in America today. The low rate of divorce does not necessarily mean that there is a high level of marital harmony! The apparently low divorce rate may be a reflection of the general conservatism of physicians, their concern regarding their image in the community, financial considerations, or a denial that there are marital problems.[4]

In recent years, the media and popular press have scrutinized the lifestyle of medical families. The image presented had been particularly unfavorable to the physician's wife, who is often portrayed as disillusioned and frustrated regarding her relationship with an overworked, insensitive husband. Nationwide publicity accompanied the publication of the results of a survey[8] in which more than 1000 physicians' wives said they were disappointed in their expectations about their marriages. This focus on the negative aspects has brought about some positive results, however: valid research on medical family life is being initiated, medical organizations are presenting workshops and conferences on personal family issues, and individual physician families are examining their own relationships.

The purpose of this chapter is to draw a profile of the contemporary American medical family. Although the medical marriage has historically been considered as the union of the male physician and the female spouse, this chapter will also consider the marriage of the female physician. Is it possible to generalize regarding this complex of interdependent relationships? Are there aspects of marriage by and to a physician that are truly unique? What characterizes the children in the medical family, and their relationship with the physician parent? Five phases of medical family life will be outlined with a discussion of the potential problems and developmental tasks characteristic of each phase. Support systems for medical families will be suggested.

## HISTORICAL PERSPECTIVE

The physician's wife and family are depicted in historical accounts as playing an auxiliary role to the physician. It begins in courtship: John Abernethy, an 18th century surgeon, is quoted as saying to the daughter of a patient, "I have witnessed your devotion and kindness to your mother. I am in need of a wife, and I think you are the very person that would suit me. My time is incessantly occupied, and I have therefore no leisure for courting. Reflect upon this matter until Monday." It is reported that she did and subsequently became Mrs. Abernethy.[9]

A more contemporary model of physician courtship and marriage is provided by Robert S. Myers who describes himself as a "young blade (who) vigorously pursued and persuaded a charming Brookline girl until she capitulated and accepted the entirely thankless job of being a doctor's wife. One hesitates to calculate the many late dinners, cancelled parties, and lonely evenings that the former Althea Shinners has endured since her marriage in 1940."[10]

Women contemplating marriage to a physician have been forewarned: "Only strong, courageous, intelligent women, endowed with a sense of humor (should) marry doctors."[11] McClinton[12] outlined the qualities that a woman marrying a physician should possess or develop: intelligence with "accomplishments in care of antiques, the culture of flowers or the training of children . . ."; the ability to entertain "friends, cultured folk, lonely people, and those less fortunate"; tolerance for female patients; the ability to handle the telephone, especially in rural practice where the wife may answer as many as one-third of the calls; unselfishness; and, finally, love for the doctor. Terhune[11] suggests that the physician's wife must have the ability to remain anonymous, "the power behind the throne, who never lets even the king suspect it."

Dalrymple-Champneys, in writing the biographies of six physicians' wives,[13] sought to give some information on the role and activities of such a woman. He believed that a man's home life affected the quality of his work profoundly, especially in the case of the physician who, at that time, did much of his work at home. When medicine was a home-based occupation, the physician's wife usually played a large role in his practice. She welcomed the patients and often comforted them while they waited for her husband to see them. She was considered to be part of his practice, although in an auxiliary role. When a woman married a physician she married his profession as well, and was expected to be involved in the mission of caring for patients.[14] Even children were included in practice-related activities, as Hertzler recalls going on house calls: "When the roads were good and the trip not too long, I took my black-eyed little daughter with me."[15]

Changes in the practice of medicine brought about changes in medical family life. With the rise of specialization in the 1940s came the move of many physicians to hospital-based practices with offices outside of the home. In many cases the wife was left behind at home, excluded from the practice: "Father became a cardiologist in a big medical center and was away from the house about 80 hours a week. Mother was schooled by Father never to call him at the hospital except in an emergency. She was never to get involved with patients, she was to take a good message and relay it immediately. Mother felt her role as a contributor to society was by supporting Daddy in any way she knew how. She raised us by herself, took care of the house, and treated Daddy like a tired king when he was home."[14]

To compensate for the physician's increased time away from home, the family was rewarded with an enhanced standard of living. Whereas, historically, the physician's wife was cautioned that she might "know the touch of potato skin better than Wedgewood, and the texture of a mop more than ermine,"[12] the financial situation of a physician was vastly improved by the rise of technology and third-party payers. Specialists' fees were greater than those of the generalist; more medical students chose to specialize; physicians rose to the top of the financial ladder in American society.

The changes presented problems: technology brought both the promise of new, effective therapeutic methods and the fragmentation of patient care. When people realized that many illnesses were beyond the scope of scientific advances, they attempted to return to the doctor–patient relationship they remembered from their childhoods. The complexity of medicine had not only separated the physician from his wife and children, but also from his patients. The "family doctor" had been replaced by a multiplicity of specialists, each caring for a different part of the anatomy. The physician's need to be physically close to the machinery of his specialty had taken him out of his home office and away from his family. Some physicians found that this afforded a good excuse to escape an unhappy home life. More often, however, the increasing demands of patient care, facilitated by guaranteed payment from insurance companies or governmental agencies and a societal dependence on "experts," forced the physician to make choices between personal and professional activities.

At present, the physician's wife is being influenced by the women's liberation movement, whether she is an advocate or not. Her historic role as the physician's helpmate is being questioned. The once silent physician's wife is now speaking out about medical marriage and seeking her own self-fulfillment, often through paid employment. The model of the female medical student has challenged medical students' wives to assess their roles in society (and, of course, many of the female students will also be physicians' wives if past trends continue).[16] Medical student wives are being encouraged to develop a strong sense of their own self-worth and identity,[14] a radical departure from the observation of Dr. Charles J. Collins[17] in 1959: "No other group of wives had to adjust themselves to a profession or business which is so paramount in their husbands' lives as that of the medical profession. There is little doubt that these women marry our profession with us and the two merge so closely that often in their eyes they are inseparable."

## PROFILE OF THE MEDICAL FAMILY MEMBERS

### The Physician

> I am the firstborn to parents who value education highly and who sacrificed to send me to medical school. I was a good student and an Eagle Scout. My role models as a youth were the town's family doctors and I was accepted to Temple Medical School after my third year of college. The only physician in our family was the husband of a distant cousin.

Who becomes a physician? Traditionally, medical school applicants have been male, white, and either firstborn or only children. They had received encouragement from their families to excel academically, be independent, and cultivate self-discipline.[18] In the past decade there has been a dramatic increase in the number of females and members of ethnic minority groups applying to and being accepted into medical schools.[18,19]

Why does someone choose a medical career? "To follow the family tradition," "to help others," "to achieve economic security," or "to pursue the challenge of scientific learning" are all valid answers. Psychologists, however, might probe deeper. The medical school applicant is almost universally described as "achievement-oriented" and many apply the label of "obsessive–compulsive" to the future physician. Derdeyn[20] attributes this inner drive for accomplishment as possibly emanating from a desire to please others. Hence, the physician has been characterized as having unresolved dependency needs and feelings of inferiority.[21,22] Medicine offers the opportunity to respond to needs of others and, thereby, develop a feeling of self-esteem and accomplishment. Taubman[4] says that the physician's characteristic personality traits enable him to cope with the stresses of medical training, to work hard, to persevere in times of adversity, and to postpone personal gratification. On the other hand, the physician's psychological profile—single-minded, goal-oriented, and detached—may describe good physicians but, unfortunately, "relatively insufferable husbands and fathers—and I suspect mothers."[23]

### The Spouse

> I am an only child of parents who also value education. As a child I had little contact with physicians. I majored in sociology at Bryn Mawr College and became interested in medicine's humanistic aspects as a result of being a physician's wife.

Who marries physicians? Martin[24] says that physicians' spouses are equally intelligent, educated, and often have talents in nonmedical fields—the arts, music, and the humanities. Knight offers another opinion—that the physician probably spends too little time selecting a spouse and, consequently, often gravitates to a fellow health professional who will offer support in a shared field of endeavor.[25]

Many physicians are thought to marry individuals who will take care of them, especially during the medical school years when emotional and financial needs are great.[22] The young medical student may be impressed by the competence of an equally youthful floor nurse or rising young executive who also offers the security of a weekly paycheck. In turn, the young nurse or business executive may be attracted to the potential of a future physician as someone who will meet their dependency needs, idealizing the physician as a caring, compassionate, and patient person.

Deckert[26] has described the parent–child interaction as an underlying force in medical marriage. He characterizes physicians as needing, as a consequence of their psychological profile, to care for others and to be in control. Therefore, they seek to act out a caretaker role, even, in some cases, marrying spouses likely to be chronically ill.[27] Research studies on medical marriage[28–30] have identified the physicians' wives as having strong dependency needs which may presage subsequent psychiatric problems. Evans[28] reported on 50 physicians' wives who had been admitted to a psychiatric hospital during 1960–1963. In 16 cases the frequent absence of the physician husband was cited as a significant factor in the illness, with seven stating that they felt excluded from their husband's practice after being replaced by other nursing and office help. The physician husbands had only heeded their wives' dependency needs when they were expressed as demands for medical attention. Lewis[29] and Miles[30], in their studies of hospitalized physicians' wives, also found a pattern of a dependent, histrionic wife and an emotionally detached husband. To date, scant data are available on male spouses of female physicians.

The two-physician marriage may display a "parent-to-parent" interaction as two workaholics unite to solve the world's problems.[26] This might also be true of any dual-career marriage, but the potential for the medical profession to engage in this activity is reinforced by personal expectations and those of society.

## The Children

> I am Diana, age 21, and a senior at Bryn Mawr College. I plan to go to graduate school and study medical sociology. Many of my friends are premed or in medical school.

I am Sharon, age 19, and a junior at Wake Forest University. I am majoring in history with a special interest in China. My career plans are indefinite but at present do not seem to include medicine.

Fate alone decides who will be a physician's child. One doctor's daughter gives her perspective: "I was born Dr. Adler's daughter. This is how I was referred to or introduced and how I thought of myself. Such a designation brought feelings of pride, of privilege, and of responsibility."[31]

Historically, the physician's child saw parenthood as "mostly motherhood, a tiny bit of fatherhood, and practically no parenthood as a joint enterprise."[9] McClinton warns that, "The doctor's children have 50 percent more chances of being failures than others of their kind because there is only one to teach them. She must take them hurriedly to the toilet, slowly to the Sunday School and proudly to the graduation, all alone. The doctor is often busy."[12]

Much of the published data on physicians' children has emphasized the negative aspects. In return for their special status in society, physicians' children are said to be subjected to high expectations from their family, teachers, and community members. A survey of physicians concerning problems they have with their children[7] listed "poor schoolwork" and "personal appearance" as the top two items. One physician sums it up as follows: "Trying to measure up to the high educational and achievement standards we parents set makes it harder for them to find their own personalities, likes and dislikes."[7]

The lack of attention from a physician-parent is often cited as a cause of antisocial behavior among physicians' children. Martin[32] says that the physician-parent may have adequate time for his patients, but little for his family. He may placate children with material possessions as a substitute for his presence. The physician's children may often become "community rebels," engaging in drug use, promiscuous behavior, or other antisocial activity to gain a parent's attention. The alienation that may exist in a medical family is poignantly illustrated by the story of the physician's child who, when asked what he wanted to be when he grew up, said, "I want to be a patient."[33]

Despite the discouraging publicity concerning the behavior of physicians' children, statistics show that male physicians tend to have large families. In a 1979 survey,[7] 31% of the respondents had four or more children. Wilson[34] reports that female physicians marry later in life and have fewer children than women in the general population. Traditionally, many female physicians chose to stay at home with small children or work part-time. Data from the National Ambulatory Medical Care Survey[35] of 1977 shows that female physicians worked less hours and saw fewer patients than their male counterparts in two separate studies conducted in 1957 and 1969. Family responsibilities were cited as the reason for curtailment of medical activity by 57% of the married female physicians in the earlier study and by 38% in the later study. More recent data indicates, however, that this pattern is changing. In one study,[6] female physicians spend 90% as much time in professional practice as the men in addition to assuming full responsibility for home and family. Symonds[36] describes the married female physician as a "superwoman" who is trying to be a professional, a wife, and a mother simultaneously. Fletcher[37] says that if the female physicians want to be as productive as their male colleagues, it may be best for them to remain childless, or else some basic changes concerning the family roles will have to take place.

Although there are anecdotal accounts of children shouting at their fathers, "When I grow up, I'll never be a doctor,"[33] a high proportion of physicians' children do follow in their physician-parent's footsteps,[22] with one author[23] making an estimate of 25%. The commitment to help others and the example of a life of privilege based upon service may be an inspiration to children. Perhaps it can also be explained in part by the following story. A doctor's daughter remembers how one day her family ended up having their planned picnic in the car in front of the hospital because her physician father was delayed while seeing a patient: "My mother didn't drive. Even if she had, I doubt it would have occurred to us to leave him and go off. We didn't complain after the first groan 'O not again!' It was a deprivation we secretly took some pleasure in. Some of his glitter rubbed off on us."[31]

## ARE MEDICAL FAMILIES UNIQUE?

> During our two plus decades as a family we have lived in two apartments and three houses, have assumed the care and feeding of three dogs and numerous cats, and have described four different states as "home." For 14 of those years we lived in a small rural college town and were actively involved in church and community activities. We were considered to be "wealthy" by the townspeople by virtue of being a medical family although, after paying the expenses of a private solo medical practice, our net family income fell short of our neighbors' fantasies. Work hours were irregular, with little assurance that the telephone would not ring during the night or over the weekend. However, we did set aside time for vacations and as a family we continue to travel extensively, viewing these times as valuable bonding experiences.

Many aspects of medical family life are shared by other families: the irregular hours, the commitment to work, the dilemma of setting priorities. However, there are aspects of medical family life that are unique. These center around the expectations of society concerning the physician and his family, the nature of the work itself, and risks owing to stress and the increased incidence of maladaptive coping in medical families.

**The Status of the Physician**

From the day of acceptance into medical school there is a magical transformation in the way people interact with the future physician. The family rejoices, classmates are jealous, and neighbors offer congratulations. This chosen individual will learn the mysteries of life and death, and safeguard our most precious possession—human life.

In addition to receiving special rights and privileges, the physician is held up as an example of virtue in the community and leadership is bestowed simply on the basis of the profession of medicine. In an emergency the crowd will make way for "the person in the white coat." At a community meeting people will listen to the comments of the physician. In a recent Gallup Poll conducted by the American Institute of Public Opinion,[38,39] 760 people were asked: "How would you rate the honesty and ethical standards of people in these different fields?" The results showed physicians to be second only to the clergy in the opinions of the respondents. The poll rated physicians as number one in "prestige or status" and in "stress or pressure." The respondents also believed that clergymen and physicians provided the greatest contribution to society. From this data it is easy to understand how many believe that medicine is a mission, similar to the calling of a minister or priest. Osmond[40] proposes that the power of the physician in the minds of the public is derived from three ingredients: knowledge, gained from years of study and not easily available to others; moral authority, derived from expectations of service to other's rather than to self or family; and Aesculapian authority, thought by some to be God-given with charismatic features.

Pressure is also placed on the physician's family to live up to this lofty image. Particularly in a small town, the physician's family may often feel they are in the public eye. They must maintain a certain standard of living: not too ostentatious, but affluent enough to earn the respect of their neighbors. People will question the physician's ability if his family is obviously struggling financially. The physician's wife is expected to be involved in community activities, often in a leadership role. Children of physicians may find themselves the objects of peer group jealousy with the assumption by classmates that the physician's family has greater wealth and that the physician's child has a brighter future than their own. To gain acceptance by their peers, they may engage in rebellious behavior, particularly during their teenage years.

## The Nature of the Work

Demands on the physician's time by society will vary depending on the medical specialty he (or she) has chosen. If he is a radiologist or pathologist, employed full-time by a hospital or medical school, the chances are that he will not be called up to minister to medical needs of a neighbor in the middle of the night. However, if he is a family physician, he will be considered on call at all times, an asset to—and of—the community. This "on call" status was unwittingly expressed by the enthusiastic tour leader on *our* vacation one year, as she assured fellow tourists that, "We don't have to worry, Doctor Taylor will be with us on this trip to take care of any problems that may arise."

Regardless of specialty choice, there will be certain assumptions made about having a physician in the family. Relatives and friends will ask for advice on all facets of medicine, not really understanding why, as an obstetrician, one cannot explain the full details of Aunt Sue's fracture. Even the spouse and children may be expected to know medical information not commonly available in the community: "What kind of flu virus should we expect this winter?"

Traditionally, the woman in a family has been responsible for the medical care of husband and children. In a male physician/female spouse family the roles concerning medical care are often reversed. For those living with the physician there may be the false comfort of having help available in times of illness. McClinton[12] warns, "The wife must be well. She mustn't be 'ailin' all the time. She cannot have disabling hereditary diseases, stuporous psychosis and, preferably, not enuresis." He goes on to explain, "It is almost illegal for her husband to treat her. If he loves her, he's afraid to. If he doesn't, she's afraid to let him. No other doctor wants to, for there is neither fee nor praise." A physician's wife of the "older generation" explained the hierarchy which was worked out in their household in the answering of calls: children first, women next, then old men, adult males, and near the bottom, known cases of hysterical illness. Finally, the doctor's own family "who were left largely to the attentions of mother and God."[9] Another physician's wife wrote: "Woe betide the wife who inquires for medical remedies . . . ; they are doomed to be cast off as mere psychological flights of fancy. Better to keep one's thoughts of aching chilblains or children's spots deep in the crevices of the mind."[9]

A survey conducted in 1979[41] revealed that many medical wives are uncomfortable about the medical care they receive. More than half of the respondents said that they felt guilty taking up a doctor's time because they are not charged for the visits. The second reason for hesitating to obtain routine care was "embarrassment," particularly in cases where there was a social relationship with other physician families. Some felt uncomfortable when choosing a physician, fearing that this might be interpreted as criticism by others. A potentially dangerous attitude expressed by 25% of the wives was, "If something was really wrong with me, my husband would notice it."

A particularly sensitive area of health care for physicians and their families is psychiatry. Physicians have difficulty in seeking help and often present difficult management problems.[42] It is thought that physicians' wives are overrepresented in the psychiatric patient population[42] and that physicians' children receive "less than optimal" child psychiatric services.[43] The psychiatrist may face problems of overidentification, approval-seeking, or reluctance to give honest appraisals of individual or family dysfunction to a colleague.[44] The nonphysician spouse, especially if feeling responsible for the problem, may fear collusion between the physician and his colleagues.[43]

**Stress and Maladaptive Coping in Medical Families**

The nature of a physician's work—the constant pressure to respond to peoples' needs, the high level of trust from patients and society, and the absolutes of time pressures—create unavoidable stress. Vaillant[21] proposes that the amount of stress in a physician's life and how he or she copes with it are strongly related to life adjustments prior to medical school. It is, in his opinion, not so much the stress of a medical career but rather the basic personality characteristics of the physician in combination with these stresses that may create "role strain." Although not all physicians are predestined to cope poorly with the built-in stress of a medical career, physicians in general are statistically likely to have psychological needs related to dependency, pessimism, passivity, and self-doubt[45] that make them strong candidates for maladaptive coping in times of stress. Just as medical spouses and children share in the "glitter" of the physician, they also share in the job-related stresses, and the risks of coping in ways that are physically and emotionally harmful.

The medical family may cope with stress by healthful means: mutual support, open discussion, even counseling when needed. On the other hand, physicians or their family members sometimes engage in the same maladaptive behavior as other individuals: alcohol abuse, overwork, adulterous affairs, and so forth. The medical family faces one special peril, however—the ready availability of prescription and nonprescription drugs.

The abuse of drugs may stem from a pattern set in medical training to rely on medication to solve problems for patients: hence drugs may be seen as an escape from one's own problems.[4] It has been estimated that the incidence of narcotic addiction in physicians varies from 30 to 100 times that found in the general population[32] The easy availability of drugs and the subsequent impairment of a physician and/or his family members is a unique danger in the lives of medical families.

## THE STAGES OF MEDICAL FAMILY LIFE

> After graduation from medical school, I interned in the United States Public Health Service and served an additional two years. I have been in group and solo family practice, and am now a full-time academician.
>
> I gave birth to our first child while I was in college and the second, 19 months later. When they were three and four years old, I began working part-time as a nursery school teacher. Subsequently, I was elected Town Councilwoman, worked as a medical assistant in my husband's office, and am now completing a Master's Degree in Counseling Education and teaching a course in medical ethics and human values to first-year medical students.
>
> As children we both felt the effects of being "doctor's kids." One of us graduated from the home-town high school; one chose to attend boarding school beginning in the 9th grade. As we both left the local school system and as our ties with the community became less close, our father left private practice to become a medical school professor and our family moved from New York State to North Carolina. One of us is pleased by the move; one isn't.

In helping people professionally we have become increasingly aware of the significance of the phases of human relationships. We developed in a previous work[46] a couple life cycle with predictable stages and tasks. We believe that the medical family life also has well-defined stages that parallel those of the classical family and couple relationships and which are applicable to both male and female physicians. In a medical family these stages are determined by the professional activity, with accompanying developmental tasks and potential problems to address. (See Table 1.)

### Medical Training Years

During this time many couples are still in the honeymoon stage. Studies on marriage during medical school years[47–50] have revealed a high level of tolerance among the spouses who view this as a temporary stage and anticipate better times in the future. An overwhelming majority of married medical students in one study[51] not only indicated satisfaction with their marriages but also a belief that the relationship derived strength from the shared hardships. Cynics might say that this positive expression is a reflection of the relatively short duration of the relationship or perhaps the beginning of an insidious denial process in the marriage.

**TABLE 1.** STAGES OF MEDICAL FAMILY LIFE

| Stage | Potential Problem | Developmental Tasks |
|---|---|---|
| 1. Medical training | Primacy | Negotiate family values and goals |
| 2. Beginning practice | Isolation | Share interests in practice and at home |
| 3. Maximum career demands | Overcommitment | Assign priorities for use of time and energy |
| 4. Career plateau | Disillusionment | Develop renewed career interests |
| 5. Retirement | Readjustment | Renegotiate roles and responsibilities |

Even if personal satisfaction is at a high level during this stage there are interactions occurring that will set the pattern for years to come. This is a time when roles and status in the marriage are being negotiated. The nonmedical spouse may be the financial and emotional head of the household. The medical student or resident may feel the need to assert the primacy of his or her work, explaining, "I have to study," "I have to go back to the hospital," or, simply, "I have no time" when joint activities are suggested. It is important to discuss if the need to work is legitimate or rather a ploy to gain dominance in the relationship.

At the end of medical school the internship/residency matching program may create stress in a marriage. Selvin and Marini[52] cite the difficulty of finding two promising career positions in the same city for a medical–nonmedical professional couple. The disruptive effects of early job changes may harm the couple's marital relationship as one has to accommodate to the other's career plans.

The years of residency training are a time of increasing economic and emotional independence for the young medical family. The non-physician spouse may feel that the physician's patients and co-workers are strangers. Whether the spouse is embarking on a separate career path or is at home with small children, the residency years have the potential to pull the individuals apart. Nelson and Henry[53] surveyed 87 family practice residents and 58 spouses and found that this was a time of increased domestic/spouse complaints, particularly concerning irregular hours and accompanying loneliness. The problems experienced by married couples during the residency years may be an expression of the transition stage that most individuals experience during their late 20s and early 30s with an accompanying questioning of life goals and relationships.[54] However, the highest number of physician divorces occur *after* the medical training years, between the ages of 35 and 45.[55] The negotiations and communication patterns developed at this early stage are therefore of particular importance for the subsequent stability of the relationship.

### Beginning Practice

Just when the medical family believe that the worst is over, the true conflicts may begin. The excitement of beginning a practice may give way to the frustrations of the business aspects of private practice as well as the continuing dilemma of how to allocate time for both patients and family.

The spouse and children may experience increased feelings of isolation as the physician becomes immersed in work, spending less and less time at home, in order to achieve "success." Compulsive work habits, reinforced during the medical training years, are in full bloom as the physician must once again prove himself. Coombs[48] says that there is no other profession that forces one to be a neophyte so often as medicine: first as a medical student, then as a resident, and finally in the community with a practice to build.

The stresses encountered at this stage of medical family life may also include child rearing and the purchase of a first home. The developmental task of sharing interests in both the home and practice is an outgrowth of the feelings of respect for the activities of one's mate. This sharing needs to be a two-way transaction with both the physician and spouse allowing each other to fill meaningful roles in their respective arenas. It is more common to hear of the spouse and children feeling shut out of the physician's world; however, physicians also need encouragement to participate in activities at home and to develop interests outside of medicine.

### Maximum Career Demands

For many, the time comes when the physician feels overcommitted. The practice begins to demand more than one person can provide in time and energy. Society sanctions a physician's devotion to duty, even if it means neglect of family obligations. To miss a school play or birthday dinner will not be criticized; it is assumed that professional duties must come first.

Evans' study of physicians' wives[28] found that the peak age for the onset of their psychiatric illnesses occurred at the time when their physician husbands were most actively engaged in practice. It was reported that the wives felt "left out" of their husbands' lives. It is easy to understand how an overworked individual can have little emotional reserve and be unable to fill the multiple roles of physician, spouse, and parent satisfactorily. For some it is easier simply to avoid involvement with the family and devote total energy to the practice of medicine, which can often afford ego-gratification from patients and coworkers that is not forthcoming from family members.

For the physician who wishes to spend time with both patients and family, priorities must be established. Life goals should be assessed and the situation with the other members of the family appraised. In doing this, however, the physician must recognize that there are limitations to his or her abilities. Up until this time it is possible to go to medical school, complete a residency, build a successful practice, and never have to engage in self-analysis. This may be acceptable (but not optimal for one's own self-actualization) if there are no other people involved in the physician's life. But for the physician with a spouse and children, the years of maximum career demands may force such an assessment with the alternative being denial of the problems and subsequent family dysfunction: divorce, substance abuse, or the ultimate sign of distress—suicide.

**Career Plateau**

It is possible that for some physicians the practice of medicine never becomes too demanding, but rather the opposite—a failure to achieve one's career goals—may signal this stage. For the physician who had dreams of winning national recognition in his specialty by age 45, the sense of failure is accentuated as each birthday beyond that age is celebrated. Disappointment pervades the life of the faithful committee member who eventually realizes that he will never be selected to be chief of the hospital staff or president of the county medical society, the associate professor who knows he will never be promoted to full professor. The female physician who chose to combine children and medicine might feel a twinge of envy as she sees unmarried or childless colleagues with successful private practices while she is working in a part-time salaried position.

Other physicians may have passed through the maximum career demand stage, somehow finding satisfaction in the high stress level as they juggled their multiple roles. At some point, however, they will become aware that they have reached the peak of their ability and that life will force changes upon them, either through physical aging or emotional exhaustion. An illness may occur either to the physician or a close family member or colleague, forcing a reexamination of life. The gratifications from patient care may diminish as competing physicians move into the neighborhood or if there is a sudden threat of malpractice from a long-cared-for patient.

At this stage it is important to be able to express one's feelings honestly. If the physician assumes the "martyr" role, the family will bear the burden of this silence and become even more alienated. Disillusionment with career achievement may afford the physician "permission" to renew interests in home and family. One highly successful physician said, "Most men don't realize what's happening to their marriages until they get into their forties, and by that time they've lost contact with their families. Upon seeing that the road to glory is going to end and that they are achieving the thing they have striven for, their disappointment is bitter to find that this success is really cotton candy; there's no substance to it. The thing that's really important—their interpersonal relationship—has gone down the drain."[48]

Positive steps can be taken at any age to change the direction of family interactions. A change in focus in the medical career may be the key. Those in private practice can become affiliated with a medical school part-time; the academician can develop a subspecialty interest or skills in writing or research; a geographic change may inject new spark into professional life (as long as the family members are supportive of such a move). Alternatively, during this phase the physician may begin to decline new responsibilities and cut back his or her practice in anticipation of retirement.

### Retirement

Traditionally, physicians do not retire; instead, they age along with their patients. The sense of power and control has become part of the physician's self-image, a part that is difficult for many to relinquish. One recently retired physician wrote that there were a number of reasons his colleagues gave for not retiring: "I can't affort to quit. I still have kids in college. I like what I'm doing too much to quit. I would have to deprive my patients of the knowledge and skills I have accumulated over the years in my practice." He thought that the real reason was that they did not have interest in or knowledge of anything other than medicine.[56]

The physician who has planned for the later years of life by nurturing family relationships and nonmedical activities will not feel threatened by the slowing down, and eventual cessation, of medical practice. Retirement can be thought of as the beginning of a "third career," the first being 25–30 years in education and the second, 30–40 years in practice.[56] The options pursued during this third career will depend on individual interests and talents.

Vincent[56] predicts that there will be an increase in the number of physicians who retire owing to various factors: the growing number of physicians, the need to keep up with technical advances, peer review, the expense of malpractice insurance, and general dissatisfaction with the red tape of third-party payers and governmental edicts. Society has a stake in the adaptation of physicians to retirement since the knowledge they possess can be a valuable resource to physicians of the future.

## SUPPORT FOR THE MEDICAL FAMILY

> Through the years our need for support has fluctuated in response to the stresses in our lives. We spent the early years of marriage uniting our individual support systems of family and friends and forming new joint affiliations. Medical training years offered struc-

> tured wives' groups and colleague organizations as well as informal social activities. Upon entering private practice we found support from couples in our new community who also had young children and whose interests paralleled ours. As our family has aged, we have found ourselves spending more time together, seeking mutual support from within the family structure, with friends and professional colleagues assuming a secondary role.

The family, like the individual, receives support from others, shoring up the group's collective value systems, lifestyle, and interpersonal relationships. Who supports medical families? The prototypical medical family—physician, spouse, one or more children, and a household pet—receive support from three sources: extended family members, the community, and the medical profession. In both ongoing and crisis situations these groups will either sustain or undermine the medical family. The impact of such support, whether offered or denied, can be profound.

**Extended Family Support**

The extended family—parents, siblings, aunts, uncles, and cousins—will usually consider the physician's personal welfare, physically and emotionally, above that of the patients and will generally support decisions to reduce professional duties in favor of family activities. If they live close to the medical couple, they can offer ongoing companionship to the physician, spouse, and children. When difficulties arise, extended family members who observe poor coping patterns and express their concern can help prevent impairment by prompting the medical family to acknowledge that there are problems such as drug or alcohol abuse or overwork.

The extended family, in an expression of concern, may be counterproductive at times. One physician tells of how a relative would say, "Don't worry, it is bad being married during medical school, but it is going to get worse! Interns are never home and when they are home, they are sleeping." He felt that such discouraging remarks added to the stress of his family life.[57]

On the positive side, the extended family can provide support during times of stress or separation; e.g., when an individual family member faces a personal crisis, when the physician must overwork (as when a professional partner is ill or absent), or when one spouse or the other must be away from home.

**Community Support**

The medical family has often been isolated from other families in the community. An early 20th century doctor is described by Hertzler: "He lived for his patients like all country doctors. He had few social contacts. He joined the lodge but seldom attended."[15] Another author says, "Medical couples don't make many close friends. No matter how busy they are socially, they remain essentially lonely people. . . ."[5] In the past, the physician seemed to be almost superhuman and his family often was endowed with the same qualities. It was understandable that the medical family might have seemed unapproachable as friends.

Today there are several factors that might allow the physician to receive more community support. The increasing numbers of physicians nationwide, with projections of an oversupply by 1990,[58] may help relieve practice pressures and allow physicians and their families more free time to cultivate friendships in the community. The children of the 1960s are now entering medical school with increasing value ascribed to personal and family life. There is also the belief that the influx of women into the profession will change practice patterns and priorities concerning family vs patients. Fletcher[37] says that the trend towards egalitarianism and personal concerns started even before the large number of women entered medical schools, but that the increase of women will hasten the inevitable change.

**Support from the Medical Profession**

Historically, many in the medical profession discouraged the physician from having an active family life. William Osler, an influential physician model in the late 19th century, said to a group of medical students: "What about your wives and babies if you have them? Leave them. Heavy as the responsibilities are to those nearest and dearest, they are outweighted by your public. Your wife will be glad to bear her share of the sacrifice you might make."[14] Medical students 30 or 40 years ago might not be accepted into a top internship or residency if they were married.[59] A third-generation physician's wife tells how it was when her parents were married while her father was in residency at Johns Hopkins: "Father was unable to tell anyone of his marriage for fear of losing his residency. Wives at that time were considered a hindrance to medical education."[14]

Support for the medical family is in an embryonic stage in medical schools today. Studies have indicated a need for counseling services, particularly to teach couples communication skills.[48,50] At one institution a couples workshop for medical students conducted in 15 1½ hour weekly sessions helped the participants better understand their personal lives and relationships.[60] In a study of medical student wives,[47] loneliness was the most frequently cited problem, even among those who are employed outside the home. A spouse support group during the medical training years will be of assistance in meeting others who share similar stresses. However, personal adjustment problems and concern over the performance of a medical student spouse will not be adequately addressed in a group format, so individual intervention may also be necessary.

In many residency programs there are attempts to include spouses and children in orientation programs.[14] The 1978 National Conference of Family Practice Residents recommended that a spouse organization be formed to offer support and information, that spouses be encouraged to attend and participate at medical meetings, and that there be more interaction at local, state, and national levels between spouses and physicians.[61]

The American Medical Association Residents Section in late 1976 began to study the problems of impaired residents, citing the patterns that develop during medical training as a possible cause of future impairment. They soon included in their considerations the prevention of personal and family dysfunction.[62] The American Medical Association and the Auxiliary have sponsored workshops at state and national meetings on the impaired physician and the Auxiliary has published a booklet, "The Family of the Impaired Physician."[63]

## CONCLUSION

What is a "normal medical family?" We prefer to interpret the word "normal" as a state of effective functioning. Each family must define this for itself. If we set a standard for normalcy in medical families, we might be setting unrealistic goals for some and surpassed expectations for others. The status of any family's functioning depends on the stresses its members encounter and the methods they employ to cope with the stresses during the phases of medical family life. A strong influence will be the amount of support the medical family receives, both from one another and from outside sources in the community and in the medical profession.

## REFERENCES


1. National Center for Health Statistics. Advance Report of Final Divorce Statistics, 1979. Monthly Vital Statistics Report. Washington, D.C., United States Department of Health and Human Services, Public Health Service, Office of Health Research, Statistics and Technology 30 (2), Supplement, May 29, 1981.
2. National Center for Health Statistics. Births, Marriages, Divorces and Deaths for 1980. Monthly Vital Statistics Report. Washington, D.C., United States Department of Health and Human Services, Public Health Service,

Office of Health Research, Statistics, and Technology 29 (12), March 18, 1981.
3. Rose KD, Rosow I: Marital stability among physicians. Calif Med 1972, 116(3):95–99.
4. Doctors and marriage: The special pressures. Medical World News 1977, 18(2):38–50.
5. Garvey M., Tuason VB: Physician marriages. J Clin Psychiatry 1979, 40(3):129–131.
6. Heins M, Smock S, Martindale L, Jackson J, Stein M: Comparison of the productivity of women and male physicians. JAMA 1977, 237:2514–2517.
7. Mattera MD (ed): After hours. Medical Economics 1979, 56(10):9–96.
8. Seligmann J, Simons PE: The doctor's wife. Newsweek 1979(6):99–100.
9. Scarlett EP: The doctor's wife. Arch Intern Med 1965, 115:351–357.
10. Beta Chapter, Nu Sigma Nu Fraternity, (ed.). Profiles, Vol II, The Clinical Years. Cambridge, Mass., Beta Chapter, Nu Sigma Nu, Harvard Medical School, 1948, p 85.
11. Terhune WB: The doctor's wife: the acolyte of medicine. Connecticut State Medical Journal 1947, 11(7): 576–581.
12. McClinton JB: The doctor's own wife. Can Med Assoc J 1942, 47(11):472–476.
13. Dalrymple-Champneys W: Wives of some famous doctors. Proceedings of the Royal Society of Medicine 1959, 52(11):937–946.
14. Cavanaugh S: Medical School and beyond. Facets 1979 (Spring), 40:24–26.
15. Hertzler AE: The horse and buggy doctor. New York, Harper and Brothers 1938, pp 36, 126.
16. Wilson MP, Jones AB: Career patterns of women in medicine. *In* Spieler C, (ed.) Collins CJ: Quoted in: Women in medicine-1976. New York, Josiah Macy, Jr. Foundation, 1977, pp 89–104.
17. Harrison W: Characteristics of physicians and their families. J Fla Med Assoc 1978, 65(5):351–353.
18. Coombs RH, St John J: Making it in medical school. New York: SP Medical and Scientific Books 1979.
19. Thomae-Forgues ME, Tonesk X: Datagram: 1979–80 Enrollment in U.S. Medical Schools. J Med Educ 1980, 55(12):1042–1044.
20. Derdeyn AP: The physician's work and marriage. Int J Psychiatry Med 1978–79, 9(3&4):297–306.
21. Vaillant GE, Sobowale NC, McArthur C: Some psychologic vulnerabilities of physicians. N Engl J Med 1972, 287:372–375.
22. Kales JD, Martin ED, Soldatos CR: Emotional problems of physicians and their families. Pa Med 1978, 81(12): 14–16.
23. Trainer JB: Is the medical marriage hazardous to your health? J Fla Med Assoc 1981, 68(4):261–264.
24. Martin P: Introduction: the physician's marriage. Facets 1978 (Fall), 39:15.
25. Knight JA: Doctor-to-be: Coping with the Trials and Triumphs of Medical School. New York, Appleton-Century-Crofts 1981, pp 67–81.
26. Deckert GH: Destructive role-playing in the M.D. marriage. Sexual Medicine Today 1981 (Feb), p 33.

27. Mackie RE: Family problems in medical and nursing families. Br J Med Psychol 1967, 40:333–340.
28. Evans JL: Psychiatric illness in the physician's wife. Am J Psychiatry 1965, 122 (8):159–163.
29. Lewis JM: The doctor and his marriage. Texas State Journal of Medicine 1965, 61(8):615–619.
30. Miles JE, Krell R, Lin T: The doctor's wife: mental illness and marital pattern. Int J Psychiatry Med 1975, 6:481–487.
31. Perr M: Social and cultural influence on the doctor's family. Am J Psychoanal 1979 (Spring), 39(1):71–80.
32. Martin MJ: Psychiatric problems of physicians and their families. Mayo Clinic Proc 1981, 56:35–44.
33. Cray C, Cray M: Stresses and rewards within the psychiatrist's family. Am J Psychoanal 1977, 37:337–341.
34. Wilson MP: The status of women in medicine; background data. J Am Med Wom Assoc 1981, 36(3):62–79.
35. National Center for Health Statistics: Characteristics of Visits to Female and Male Physicians, The National Ambulatory Medical Care Survey, United States, 1977. Hyattsville, Maryland: National Center for Health Statistics, 1980. (Vital and health statistics. Series 13: Data from the National Health Survey, no. 49) (DHHS publication no. (PHS) 80-1710).
36. Symonds A: The wife as the professional. Am J Psychoanal 1979, 39(1):55–63.
37. Fletcher SW: Women physicians: old times or a new era? The Pharos 1982 (Winter), 45(1):2–9
38. Taylor DM: The medical wife: her life and her marriage. Unpublished paper.
39. AMA News 1981 Dec 4, p 9.
40. Osmond H: God and the doctor. N Engl J Med 1980, 302:555–558.
41. Schamadan W: Being a physician's spouse may be hazardous to your health. Facets 1979 (Fall), 40:22–23.
42. Waring EM: Psychiatric illness in physicians: a review. Compr Psychiatry 1974, 15(6):519–530.
43. Mattsson A, Derdeyn A: The child psychiatrist treating physicians' families. J Am Acad Child Psychiatry 1977, 16:728–738.
44. Chessick RD: Intensive psychotherapy for the psychiatrist's family. Am J Psychother 1977, 31:516–524.
45. Maddison D: Stress on the doctor and his wife. Med J Aust 1974, 2:315–318.
46. Taylor AD, Taylor RB: Couples: the art of staying together. Washington, D.C., Acropolis Books 1978.
47. Bruhn JG, du Plessis A: Wives of medical students: their attitudes and adjustments. J Med Educ 1964, 41:381–385.
48. Coombs RH: The medical marriage. *In* Coombs RH, Vincent CE, (eds.): Psychological aspects of medical training. Springfield, Ill, Charles C. Thomas 1971, p 133–167.
49. Eagle JR, Smith BM: Stresses of the medical student wife. J Med Educ 1968, 43:840–845.

50. Perlow AD, Mullins SC: Marital satisfaction as perceived by the medical student spouse. J Med Educ 1976, 61:726–734.
51. Newkirk DD: The medical student and his marriage. Bull Tulane Medical Faculty 1967, 26:209–222.
52. Selvin M, Marini MM: Can Ph.D.-M.D. intermarriage work? (Letter) N Engl J of Med 1979, 301:278.
53. Nelson EG, Henry WF: Psychosocial factors seen as problems by family practice residents and their spouses. J Fam Pract 1978, 6:581–589.
54. Berman EM: Life transition points. Facets 1979 (Winter), 40:25–28.
55. Clements WM, Paine R: The family physician's family. J Fam Pract 1981, 13:105–112.
56. Vincent MO: The physician's retirement. Ontario Med Review 1977, 44:322–325.
57. Van Dyke J, Van Dyke G: A medical student marriage. J Fla Med Assoc 1979, (May), 66:537–538.
58. Report of the Graduate Medical Education National Advisory Committee to the Secretary. Vol. 1. Summary Report. Washington, D.C., Government Printing Office 1981.
59. Owens A, Reynolds JA (eds.): Experts view the doctor as a family man. Medical Economics 1966, 43(10):115–122.
60. Porter K, Ziegler P, Charles E, Roman M: A couple group for medical students. J Med Educ 1976, 51:418–419.
61. AAFP Reporter. 1978 (Winter), p 5.
62. Horizons. 1981 (May), 4(1).
63. American Medical Association Auxiliary: The family of the impaired physician. Chicago, American Medical Auxiliary, Inc. 1981.

# The Medical Student

"A career in medicine is anchored in responsibility, not freedom," points out Dr. James A. Knight in this chapter on medical students. That considered judgment comes from a person who has had wide experience both in the fields of medicine and medical education. In his contribution Dr. Knight explores underlying reasons why a person might be attracted toward a career of contented yet challenging medical bondage. The apprentice years in medicine are not easy and their attrition rate is significant. As many have attested it is a road that continuously tests the mettle of even the most qualified individual. Despite hardship, less than 2% of students who start the long course fail to finish and graduate. Yet, despite the formidable obstacles to becoming a doctor, more than 40,000 men and women annually decide it is a road they want to travel and apply for admission to medical school. Less than half of those who apply are accepted.

In this chapter medical students will pick up clues as to why they want to become doctors. The clues can be pieced together like a jigsaw enabling them to gain insight into their own motivations. Established physicians will recognize their own uncertain vicissitudes in Dr. Knight's crisp description of personality and pressure. The established physician may even experience a bittersweet nostalgia and anger for an earlier time when he blundered through medical school like a blind person, unled. Time was, students had to travel through medical school without the benefit of emotional and practical supports such as those outlined by Dr. Knight. Both students and physicians can learn much from his incisive observations.

*J.P.C.*

# 2

# Medical Students

*James A. Knight*

The transformation of a medical student into a physician is a rugged and remarkable endeavor. The student's education in medical school is probably the most intense and emotion-laden of all educational experiences. In each stage of training, the sick person's presence is real or implied; this brings a special human dimension to every aspect of the student's learning.

The medical student can be understood best if the importance of "identity" as a principal motivation in one's life is recognized. The concept of identity acknowledges that much of what one does, whether rational or illogical, really has to do with what one strives to be. In professional development, identity means the acquisition of character and skills through being, feeling, and achieving. It distinguishes each medical student from all others. In this personal individuation, there are also qualities of teachers and peers that are assimilated. Thus, the student's identity has two facets: one looking inward for a sense of uniqueness; the other looking outward for a sense of community with colleagues and patients.

Students' formal medical education begins when they enter medical school and continues throughout their lives. This in part accounts for the often-quoted statement that when the sun sets on the first day of school for beginning medical students, they will be behind in their work and will never catch up during their lifetimes. Such a statement is true. It is not meant to discourage, but rather to add challenge and anticipation to the lives of aspiring doctors.

A career in medicine is anchored in responsibility, not freedom. In fact, the M.D. degree is rooted in such enormous responsibility that new doctors may feel that bondage, rather than freedom, characterizes their lives. Yet it is that kind of responsibility that truly brings freedom. When one's commitment is to others, when one's work comforts and heals, one finds meaning in life, and with meaning comes the only freedom worth cherishing.

Persons who choose medicine seek throughout life to gain a clearer understanding of what led them to medicine in the first place and what sustains them in its practice. Changes in curriculum or medical school organization do not modify the student's need to learn to cope with a more total responsibility and unrelenting authority over the lives of others than is borne by any other profession. Nor do such changes spare them from learning to face, without anxiety, the most tabooed issues of society. Much of the daily work for which they prepare is a transgression of the ordinary prohibitions and taboos of the community. From wrestling with ethical decisions to working with their own feelings about death, medical students are occupied daily with many personal tasks beyond the acquisition of technical skill.

## MOTIVATION

As persons apply to medical school, understanding their motivation for studying medicine influences their acceptance and indicates, in part, the chances of future success in medicine. A number of motives may be identified which can be seen in better perspective if projected upon a broad pattern of motivational factors. These factors can be grouped into three categories: (1) motives stemming from inner needs; (2) motives stemming from vocational appeal; and (3) motives stemming from conceived purposes.

Motives stemming from *inner needs* are many and varied. Positive or negative relationships with parents may play a decisive role in a person's choice of a career in medicine. A reason for the choice of medicine as a career may be to control one's own excessive fear of death. By becoming a physician, the person secures him or herself against the jeopardy of death and obtains dominion over mortal anxiety by having the power to cure. Another motive is the need to rescue, and the opportunity for the expression of this need is great in medicine. The need to be needed is a multifaceted motivating factor. Feeling needed is at the core of every person's sense of worth. Further, there is the triad of intellectual curiosity, professional pride, and ambition that is believed by many to be the three basic motives of professional life. One cannot overlook the quest for security as a motive related to inner needs; financial success in our society often becomes a form of self-validation.

Motives stemming from *vocational appeal* include the influence of great models, the image of physician, medicine as a challenging and versatile vocation, and job freedom. The family physician often serves as a great model and may be seen by even the young child as a hero and a person that one would like to emulate. As for the physician's image, it is surrounded by great drama and romance; stories related to medical practice possess lasting appeal. Further, endless opportunities exist in medicine for a wide variety of careers, and a doctor is eligible for a multitude of jobs. Thus, versatility and challenge are ever present in the career options that medicine offers. In medical practice, physicians are free agents and enjoy work that permits considerable self-direction with relatively little structure.

The third category involves motives stemming from *conceived purposes.* Students attracted to medicine frequently have had a long-standing need for, enjoyment of, and capacity to tolerate being in a caring, providing, dispensing, nurturing relationship to other people. Also, intimate personal contact with physical or psychological suffering, in themselves or others, seems to have disposed certain students toward a vocation in which their lives will be devoted to combat suffering. Further, it is not uncommon for a student to decide to become a doctor after the death of a family member or close friend, sometimes with the conscious desire to learn how to fight wasteful death. About one-third of the applicants to medical school whom I have interviewed through the years mentioned altruism as a part of their motivation for wanting to enter the medical profession, although often they apologized for introducing a motive that today seems suspect. Still other students are attracted to medicine because it can be a vehicle for social reform. They may be more interested in healing society than healing individuals.

In summary, students are motivated by interacting conscious and unconscious factors. Motives for entering the field of medicine, as well as adaptations necessary in the transitional period before graduation, are influenced by personal development and past experiences of the student. Highly respected motives such as noble ideals and service to humanity are only one segment of the influences that may lead the student into medicine.

The problem of determining which unconscious personality factors promote the development of an effective physician and which interfere with competent medical practice is difficult. The way particular factors are handled by the student's conscious and unconscious mind may make the difference. For example, the student whose unconscious motivation is to save the life of a sick parent or to bring a deceased parent back to life may function differently as a physician from the student whose unconscious motivation is atonement by reaction formation for death wishes against a sick or deceased sibling. Thus, there are even alternatives in the psychological handling of the same motivation.

## ADMISSION TO MEDICAL SCHOOL

The admissions process varies considerably from school to school, but certain shared guidelines are commonly followed. The submission of an application to medical school, usually through the centralized application service of the Association of American Medical Colleges, is probably the most significant action ever taken by a student in his or her life up to that time. In turn, the admission of a student is the most critical step a school takes in the education of a physician.

There is widespread interest in selection committees and how a school sets its policies for admitting new students. Usually the faculty of a school of medicine establishes operating policies and methods of selection for the admissions committee, and these guidelines are followed carefully and diligently. The committee must rely heavily on objective criteria, such as grade averages (overall, as well as in science coursework), Medical College Admissions Test (MCAT) scores, appraisal by faculty from the applicant's college, special accomplishments and talents, the substance and level of courses taken in college, whether the academic performance has continually improved or suffered reverses, and physical and emotional health. If the students' academic records and faculty evaluations meet a prescribed standard, the students are usually invited to visit the school for interviews.

The task of the admissions committee is formidable, and service on the committee is not cherished by every faculty member. Medical students now serve on most of the selection committees in this country, and also help with interviewing and other tasks related to evaluation and selection of candidates.

In the provocative book *Zen and the Art of Motorcycle Maintenance,* Robert Pirsig tells of the gifted scholar Phaedrus who lost his mind trying to define "quality."[19] Each year, such a definition is required of the admissions committee in every medical school. Professor Morowitz addresses the urgency of the task: "The issue is not an abstract one, but an immediate, pressing, tangible, existential reality, for each committee must select a small number of matriculants from a large number of applicants."[15] Generally, admissions committees do a remarkably good job. Still, many committee members express nagging doubts about their work, and wonder frequently if they didn't reject, for example "better candidates than the ones accepted." Further, many within and without the medical school are at times critics of those selected.

Pearl Rosenberg, in discussing academic excellence along with noncognitive factors as criteria for admission to medical school, emphasizes creativity and the capacity for independent work.[21] Yes, each medical school looks for the typical traits or qualities in the students it selects but almost always seeks to identify other qualities. Whether these qualities are new, different, or the same, they deserve further amplification. Five of them are discussed here.

The first relates to the maturity that comes with a sense of *accomplishment* in some particular field. Before applying to medical school did the student accomplish something significant in any other field, such as music, writing, sports, or special studies, (etc.)? Some admissions directors of medical schools have identified this special accomplishment as a reliable indicator of success in medical school. A British study emphasized that such students with accomplishment in other fields, including experience in working with older colleagues, generally were easily able to establish the satisfactory interpersonal relations so necessary for the successful practice of medicine.[13]

The second trait relates to personal *energy*. The student who is capable of doing an exceptional amount of hard work and also has time and energy to spend in activities other than studies possesses a trait in common with most successful physicians. In a study of a group of physicians who made distinguished contributions to neurology, Nathan found that the only characteristic or trait common to the 133 physicians studied was the unusual amount of energy each possessed.[9,17]

The third quality relates to *social consciousness*. Today's students must be humanity oriented in the finest sense of those words. Not infrequently in the past, students and their physician-teachers focused sharply on the individual patient and neglected the complex social and psychological factors that influence sickness and health. A new set of demands confronts today's students. A deep social consciousness is essential if they are to prepare themselves to deal adequately with the change and ferment in medical education, the unavailability of medical services to many groups in our population, changing patterns of delivery of health care, and involvement in the social problems of humankind.

The fourth trait is *"reasonable adventurousness."* Heath, in a study of Princeton undergraduates, identifies six attributes that characterize the "reasonable adventurer": intellectuality, close friendships, independence in value judgments, tolerance of ambiguity, breadth of interests, and sense of humor.[10] Such attributes would make for a fully functioning human being, one who is open to new experiences in the changing world, and would serve the person well in both the study and practice of medicine.

The fifth trait is *creativity*, a trait not easily defined or identified. In the light of what is known about creativity, however, the student possessing this quality brings to medicine a precious gift. Because of the increasing concern with identifying and nurturing the creative potential in students, some of the relevant dimensions of the topic are introduced here.

Nobody will deny that medicine needs the creative person. Very little in medicine is routine, for each patient and each situation bring new challenges, as well as demands for problem-solving skills. Creative thinking may be the physician's most important weapon in coping with emergencies and crises encountered daily in the practice of medicine.

Psychologist Paul Torrance sees creative talent as a cluster of traits, ones that admissions directors usually try to identify and evaluate: high sensitivity, capacity to be disturbed by problems, ability to see relationships in a flash, divergent rather than conformist thinking, and a powerful drive to take intellectual risks and push ability to the limit.[24]

In observing medical students whom their teachers identify as original and creative thinkers, one can easily note a few common denominators. These students are self-teachers, quick to raise questions about "facts" and "theories" in medicine that most people consider well established. They are better able than other students to live with uncertainty. They are profoundly aware of the brevity of life and the gravity of their purpose and feel impelled to strive. They yearn to change, to grow, to be different, and to escape from many of their human limitations. They possess personal courage which helps them stand aside from the social collectivity and often in conflict with it. Their courage is related to being themselves in the fullest sense.

Admissions committees are frequently urged to keep in mind the predictors of physicians' performance suggested by the Price-Taylor study.[20] These predictors include realistic self-appraisal, coping ability, ethical behavior, evidence of staying behavior, evidence of orientation to lifelong learning, decision-making ability, and compassion and sensitivity in interpersonal relations.

The medical profession attracts to its ranks students with a diversity of talents and interests. Some difficulty comes in trying to describe the exact qualities these students should possess. The word "ideal" has often been used to emphasize excellence as the standard of measurement. Mistakes are made in the selection of some students, but the majority of those who become physicians prove themselves to be exceptionally fine persons.

## TO WEAR THE HEALER'S MANTLE

The educational life of medical students has been described as a constantly changing environment to be navigated for four perilous years.

The unique purpose of the medical school is the transformation of laymen into physicians. Students have the right to expect that their education will equip them with the rudiments necessary for ultimate professional competence. Thus, the school must teach students the specific skills of medicine as well as the more general techniques for coping with the vocational anxieties that inevitably confront the healer.[8]

In medical school, students have many important learning or maturing experiences that cannot be duplicated elsewhere. They observe the entire range of human behavior in times of sickness and trouble and learn by participation the defined role of the physician in dealing with these problems. This is the process of acculturation often called "professional socialization" or "rites of passage." Despite studies suggesting that socialization in medical school often results in acquisition of the culture of the medical student rather than that of the physician, I believe the crucial part of the student's identity as a healer is established in medical school.[1]

The medical educational process poses a succession of developmental and adaptive tasks with which students must deal as they progress through medical school. Sometimes factors within students interfere with successful adaptation. When those who help students in their professional growth emphasize reality components of student stress, they help them recognize the issues with which they are struggling. Usually students are helped simply by realizing that the difficulties in adjustment which they are experiencing are common to other students.[8]

The medical student world comprises more than academics. Students are presented with a broad, often bewildering, array of demands to be met and opportunities to be used. While studying and being taught, they interact in myriad ways with the life of an elaborate, intricately formed, and curiously specialized world.[4,11,16,22]

Students must deal with many problem issues over the course of school. These constitute tasks to which the students must respond as a result of both external pressures and inner need. Problems include: ambiguity and uncertainty in a profession that prides itself on rationality and competence; the fact that students' technical knowledge cannot be as detailed and extensive as the faculty demands or as they themselves would like; forming a student subculture for purposes of mutual protection and assistance or for providing a measure of autonomy from authoritative demands; and choosing a specialty.

The medical school strongly influences the student's approach to these tasks. It helps the student find a balance between cold detachment and anxious concern for patients. Ample training is offered for decision making in the presence of uncertainty, as well as numerous opportunities for exploring what is involved in various specialties. Students' efforts to resolve these issues, although influenced by environmental demands and opportunities, are ultimately their own. Students selectively assimilate and integrate pressures that impinge upon them from all sides. In the process, their inner fantasies, character traits, talents, and personal commitments are also involved. Thus, students' professional growth is a function both of the external socializing system or environment and of personality.[2]

Most of the literature on medical student maturation emphasizes the high degree of anxiety encountered. The availability of appropriate counseling and treatment facilities is one approach toward assisting them in mastering their anxiety. Probably more important is appropriate recognition of the readily understandable anxieties of students.

An overriding source of anxiety lies in the students' concern over their ability to perform as physicians taking care of the sick. They must face difficulties encountered in clinical situations where doctors must act with insufficient data and meet the challenge of difficult patients. Students usually bring to medical school an expansive view of the physician as an omnipotent and omniscient healer. Their own self-image, once they are assigned to care for patients, stands in sharp contrast to their view of what a physician should be. Thus, they readily become anxious, guilty, and depressed.

The students' concerns regarding what doctors do and how they do it are further compounded in some medical schools by postponing meaningful clinical exposure until after the second year, when students have mastered the basic science material to the satisfaction of the faculty. Students are challenged more easily and adapt more successfully if they participate in carefully planned clinical programs at the outset of medical training, along with basic science work. Fortunately, this is what is happening in most medical schools today. A planned sequence of clinical exercises throughout the four years, with gradually increasing responsibility, brings into sharp focus the problems of being a physician. Students do not develop professional identity as physicians until they deal with patients. Ascribed, assigned, and perceived roles are congruent only when students actually relate to patients.

Part of the identity of a physician is in knowing who one is and bringing that self-awareness to the care of patients. As physician and ethicist Edmund D. Pellegrino has beautifully stated: "To be a physician is freely to commit oneself to the moral center of the relationship with the patient and to do so with one's whole person. . . . It is a daring and a transforming experience to heal another person. To do so is to penetrate in some way the mystery of that person's being, and that becomes disastrous unless we are clear about our own being.[18]

Stress management is an important part of professional development. As Keniston has lucidly described, three ways of adapting to stress seem especially prominent among medical students in their professional development.[12] First, many medical students react to anxiety-provoking situations not by trying to live with them or escape them, but by strenuous efforts to master, overcome, or counteract them. When confronted with a problem, medical students usually head straight into it and try to eliminate it. Second, medical students, in general, are oriented primarily toward changing their environment rather than themselves. Compared with graduate students in other fields, medical students are notable for the speed and zeal with which they attempt to devise practical, well-organized plans for changing things. They are not strongly inclined to examine their own feelings, fantasies, and motives or explore techniques of self-reform. Third, medical students, like other students with developed scientific ability, generally possess a considerable capacity to translate feelings into ideas, manipulate these ideas, and at times forget the feelings that originally prompted them. In summary, when medical students confront a personal anxiety or a stressful situation, they are less likely to be interested in or aware of their own feelings than to be preoccupied with understanding intellectually what is happening, planning a rational course of action, or studying the theoretical implications of the problem.

Course requirements of medical school serve a dual function: to teach technical competence and prepare students for the psychological hazards of their vocation. From the first incision in the cadaver to the care of their first terminal patient, they tend to respond in a similar way: an initial phase of anxiety or dread gives way to an effort to learn about the object of anxiety. They try to develop the intellectual knowledge and psychomotor skills to do a competent job, and to master the task at hand. Emotions are gradually detached from the work of medicine, and what remains in consciousness is the knowledge and skills of the physician. The process of learning how not to react emotionally to the confrontations of medicine gives added impetus to learning its subject matter. Thus, acquiring medical knowledge is not only a way of helping patients, but also a necessary defense against the personal anxieties that might otherwise be aroused in the medical student.

## PSYCHOLOGICAL PROBLEMS OF MEDICAL STUDENTS

Each step in educating a medical student, of producing a physician, carries with it the potential of threatening his or her equanimity, depending on personal history and personality structure.

The deepest concerns of new students are their performance in medicine and competence in interpersonal affairs. They want to establish a niche in their class and to know what their fellow students expect of them and what they can expect of their fellows in return. They are constantly assessing how they fit in the class and what kind of role their classmates are assigning them or they are assigning themselves: will it be a rivalrous sibling, clown, scapegoat, leader, teacher's pet, lover, helpful colleague, or nonentity?

The stressful process of preparation for medical school may become the anlage for later incapacitating anxieties during medical school. Because competition for admission is keen, and places are available for only some of the well-qualified applicants, selection policies of admissions committees give rise to a great deal of speculation and the perpetuation of the superstitions, myths, and legends that are indigenous to most undergraduate campuses. Particular science courses are emphasized to the exclusion of important courses in other fields. Grades acquire a disproportionate and frightening degree of importance and become the ultimate goal, rather than learning and preparation for later professional training. Those students whose natural bent is not along the lines of the physical sciences find it necessary to work doubly hard to attain the necessary grades. The preexisting substratum of anxiety that these students carry into medical school is easily aroused by the heavy scientific curriculum in the early years of medical training.

College students need time to work through the adolescent problems that are part of the life of this age group. Busy premedical students, using all their time and energy to qualify and compete for admission to medical school, neglect psychological maturation. Thus, they bring to medical school a host of unresolved adolescent conflicts to blend with the numerous problems awaiting them there. The developmental tasks of late adolescence have been postponed. The total engulfment of their premedical studies usurped the usual and necessary period of late adolescence needed to resolve internal conflicts.

Students may develop a variety of hypochondriacal complaints when they study disease processes. Fears of physical illness appear in conjunction with the study of anatomic pathology and pathophysiology. Later, students may develop fears of mental illness when they have close contact with mentally ill patients. The nature of the symptoms, precipitated by the subject matter under consideration, is most often related to the life experiences of the student and frequently may be traced to a personal or family history of disease.

As students advance in their training from minimal exposure to patients to intensive clinical work, new adjustments are required. Students' primary problems in patient care emanate from their feelings of insecurity and anxiety in attempting to apply the theory they have learned, and from the loss of the structure that had previously been provided by lecture and laboratory courses. These feelings reveal themselves in the clinical situation as overt anxiety, indifference, hostility, and destructive argumentativeness, or inability to carry out practical responsibilities. Students may experience guilt and a sense of helplessness when confronted with seriously ill or dying patients, or worry about being faced with an urgent medical situation wherein their failure to have some information or skill at their fingertips might result in the death of a patient. How to protect themselves from too deep an emotional involvement with patients is a formidable task. Before developing enough detachment to function effectively, they may swing between exaggerated sensitivity and callousness.

Among the psychological problems seen in medical students, depression is probably the most serious, causing acute and chronic impairment of the students' social and academic functioning. It also may result in withdrawal or dismissal from medical school. The threat of suicide is present in depressed students, and they are often ready to speak of their suicidal ruminations.

Depressed students are often referred not for depression but for declining grades with concomitant difficulty in study and concentration. They report that they cannot absorb their reading and gradually lose interest in their studies. They feel guilty over their supposed laziness and for wasting time and their parents' money. Fatigue and lethargy are constant symptoms. They convey a sense of helplessness and hopelessness. They often ask about withdrawing from school. An overtly depressed state is easily recognized, and often by the student. Less easily recognized is the latent depressive state, which often escapes notice by patient or physician. A student with a latent depression will show minimal obvious signs and symptoms but complain of boredom, lethargy, preoccupation, and difficulty in studying.

Overtly or latently depressed students often find that their underlying emotional difficulty either escapes recognition or is ascribed to the pressure of the work load. Medical school officials then assume that such students are lazy or have poor work habits. Depressed students may hide their real emotional difficulty behind their studies. The academic work load, however, is only the major situational stress of the moment; it contributes to the burdens of depressed students but usually plays no actual part in the precipitation of the depression. The precipitating factor tends to consist in an actual or fantasized rejection, resulting from a direct conflict with a parent or parent surrogate. The findings with depressed students generally corroborate the essentially Freudian theory of the depressive reaction as a reawakening of unconscious childhood feelings of rejection, triggered by current stimuli.[7] It is remarkable how in so many cases the depression is associated with the premature loss or absence of one or both parents in childhood or the conviction of rejection by a parent. The feeling of being unworthy of love is associated with the feeling of rejection.

Depressed students usually respond well to brief, psychoanalytically oriented psychotherapy. Unfortunately, the latent depression in many students tends to be overlooked and, therefore, psychotherapy may not be considered for these chronic underachievers who often have high intellectual ability. For such students, depression is their way of life, and they usually view the world as cold, prohibitive, and depriving. In avoiding close personal relationships out of fear of dependency, they seem isolated and regressed. This avoidance perpetuates their emotional deprivation. Brief treatment is often sufficient to help such students stem the depressive regression, acquire useful insights, and make some successful readjustments in work and interpersonal relationships.

Probably the two most anxiety-provoking situations for a medical student are situations that imply academic failure and those that have to do with death. The fear of failure concerns us here.

At times the wish to be in medical school (and at a *particular* school) springs more from the parents' motivation than the students'. Parental pressure for a particular life direction may alienate students from their own ambition. Hungry, however, for their parents' affection and appreciation, they strive for good grades. Thus, in this competitive milieu, even the receiving of love is tied to extraneous standards of performance. Probably students today are prepared more for the competitive world of an affluent society than they are for the opportunities for companionship, competence, and the sharing of ideas.

Married students often feel guilty about not having the time or energy to be a good marriage partner. They find themselves relegating the spouse to a secondary place in life, for medicine is demanding and consuming. They are troubled by the spouse's loneliness, desire to have children without further delay, and their own financial dependence with its accompanying loss of self-esteem. They are never sure that the spouse understands the magnitude of the stresses, anxieties, and insecurities imposed upon them by the nature of their studies.

The spouse is troubled by an inability to compete for affection with his or her partner's studies. Often the spouse spends evening after evening watching the partner occupied with studies to the point of almost total exclusion of any appreciation of the spouse's presence or desire for attention. Later, during the clinical clerkship the spouse is alone at home while the student is on duty at the hospital. Further, the spouse feels excluded from the challenging work of medicine since he or she can share only vicariously in bits of the experience. In reality, the spouse may feel rejected and negatively compare the relative inattention and inactivity in the marriage to the romantically affectionate attentiveness of both before the wedding when they were suitors.

Major stresses for the spouse of the student are loneliness, limited finances, adjustment to irregular hours, the partner being home too little, as well as being under definite tension and pressure. Adjustment to these stresses is facilitated by patience and understanding, as well as evolving personal ways of handling stresses.[5] Developing mutual support between wife and husband is crucial. Communication in depth must be maintained and nurtured with partner, family, and friends.

Helping students anticipate what lies ahead is central in the maintenance of their equilibrium. Medical fraternities or similar student organizations function effectively in the field of anticipatory guidance. Thorough orientation programs by the deans at the opening of school and at critical transitional points in training do a great deal to reduce anxiety and frustration.

Some deans regularly call class meetings at periods when the stresses are severe to discuss frankly the fears and gripes of the students, always guiding the interaction in constructive problem-solving channels. Usually, there is a clown, who may be used to help introduce some humor at the hard points. If only to comfort the distraught, such meetings are worth holding. A wise educator once said that one of a dean's duties is "to comfort the afflicted and afflict the comfortable."

Attention to the educational climate of a medical school will readily illuminate the areas where students typically experience difficulty: integrating the personal and professional dimensions of one's life; handling the frustration, anxiety, and consequent learning difficulties arising from the weighty requirements of medical school; and developing and maintaining social and emotional sensitivity.

## RELATIONSHIPS WITH THE FACULTY

The impact of the institutional atmosphere on students is a major factor in their successes and failures in learning the science and art of medicine.[14] The ideas and actions of the faculty and house staff (residents and interns) affect the students by setting the conditions under which problems arise and learning is enhanced or hampered. Faculty expectations of students, rules of the road, and the way the faculty interprets and defines the rules constitute facets of the environment in which students learn and act.

Medical schools are organized in an "authoritarian" manner. The faculty and administration have enormous power over the students. Students learn shortly after their enrollment that if they are dropped, their chance of being reinstated in that medical school or another one is slim. Until the M.D. degree is conferred, their budding medical careers could be permanently terminated. The faculty and administration, in principle, can tightly control a variety of student activities. If such control and power are exercised, students will have little opportunity to build their own perspectives and will simply take on ideas forced on them.

Students, moreover, face a series of school situations in which they are obliged to perform academically for the faculty. The faculty assess students' ability and the amount learned largely on the basis of these performances. Students realize that survival in medical school is dependent on making the right kind of impression on the faculty—to present them with either the substance or the appearance of learning. The question arises immediately, however, as to what will impress the faculty as real learning, for students testify that faculty reactions often cannot be predicted in any logical or uncomplicated way. Simple methods of making a good impression may not suffice. Thus, students must be sensitive to faculty demands and modify their behavior accordingly even when these demands seem unrelated to the real purposes of medical school.

While students must be sensitive to faculty demands, what kind of relationship to faculty do students really want, or think is most helpful? Stritter and associates asked medical students to identify characteristics of teachers which they thought were most useful in facilitating learning. In a factor analysis of these data they found that the most important factor was making students active participants in the learning process.[23] This included teacher behavior such as encouraging students to raise questions, providing students opportunities to practice both technical and problem-solving skills, and explaining to students the basis for the teachers' own actions and decisions. Thus, what the students want and see as important is different from what often happens; i.e., teachers do the preponderance of talking, provide mostly factual information, and rarely challenge students to think through a response.[6]

## COMING TO TERMS WITH FEELINGS ABOUT DEATH

The medical student confronts death almost daily. This confrontation awakens an ancient impulse deep within the person—to move away from the dying. Moving away from the dying is not caring for the dying, which is a major professional and human responsibility. The task then is to work with one's feelings about death so that one will be free to care for patients and not be controlled by fears and defensive behavior.

The ability to endure the presence of death in life is of paramount importance in human living. To open oneself to death is to accept the aspect of becoming, that is, of transformation, which is the very essence of life. Because, however, medical students are suddenly flooded with an "excess of death" in anatomy laboratories, autopsy rooms, and dying patients in hospital wards, they may quickly shut themselves off from this aspect of life by putting aside all thought of death. This inhibits their own psychological growth and creates in its place an appearance of security which is, in fact, continually threatened by unconscious anxieties.

How does one relate to, and come to terms with, death, which seems to stand in irreconcilable contrast to life and to all one's experience of living things? The concern is not with one's intellectual response to physical defenselessness, but with the way in which the person, in the center of one's being, feels touched by the inevitability of death. Is one able to bring this fact into harmony with one's feelings for life?

Medical students, through their experience with dying patients, are forced to recognize at some level of their consciousness the interrelation of the anticipation of death and the conduct of life. Although seldom emphasized in medical school, this interrelation has been recognized and commented upon by generations of philosophers and theologians.

Again, how can one accept one's finitude and come to terms with one's feelings about death? There is no easy answer to be given by others, for the solution lies in a deep personal struggle to understand something of one's own nature and destiny. In this search, the medical student has often found the dying patient an excellent teacher. Keeping company with the dying can be a fulfilling and rewarding experience for one who demonstrates concern by caring for patients in the full sense of the word. With the help of such patients one can begin one's own preparation for death. It is interesting that the great physician William Osler always thought of himself as a student of the art and act of dying; patients saw Osler as one who had looked deeply into the eyes of death and understood something of its impenetrable mystery.

A further step is to read great literature and see how those portrayed there faced death and sought its meaning. For example, Leo Tolstoy's *Death of Ivan Ilyich* is probably the greatest masterpiece on death that has been written in either ancient or modern times. Other writings include Alexander Solzhenitsyn's *Cancer Ward*, John Gunther's *Death Be Not Proud*, Albert Camus' *The Plague*, and Helmut Gollwitzer's *Dying We Live*.

Also, we should seek in history how others have handled death or maintained a mortal perspective. We can learn much from the ancient Greeks' tragic sense of life, and much from the Romans who repeatedly reminded themselves that all glory is fleeting and that all must die.

One of the most ancient of all admonitions declares that since there is no remedy for death we should then prepare for it. Preparation and acceptance go hand in hand. May we be guided by the words with which the 17th century physician Sir Thomas Browne closed his book of self-revelation, *Religio Medici:*

> Bless me in this life with but the peace of my conscience, command of my affections, the love of thyself and my dearest friends, and I shall be happy enough to pity Caesar. These are, O Lord, the humble desires of my most reasonable ambition, and all I dare call happiness on earth: wherein I set no rule or limit to thy hand or providence. Dispose of me according to the wisdom of thy pleasure. Thy will be done, though in my own undoing.[3]

It is only in daring to accept one's death as a companion that a person may really possess life. Medical students are no exception. They, like their patients, will guard their Thermopylae, and they deserve honor if they are able to forsee that Ephialtes will finally appear, and in the end the Medes will go through.

## REFERENCES

1. Becker HS, et al.: Boys in White: Student Culture in Medical School. Chicago, University of Chicago Press, 1961.
2. Bloom SW: Socialization for the physician's role—a review of some contributions of research to theory. *In* Shapiro EC, Lowenstein LM (eds): Becoming a Physician—Development of Values and Attitudes in Medicine. Cambridge, Massachusetts, Ballinger, 1979, pp 3–53.
3. Browne T: Religio Medici. Winny J, (annot-ed). Cambridge University Press, 1963, p 96.
4. Coombs RH: Mastering Medicine—Professional Socialization in Medical School. New York, Macmillan, 1978.
5. Derdeyn AP: The physician's work and marriage. Int J Psychiatry Med 1979, 9:297.
6. Foley R, Smilansky J, Yanke A: Teacher student interaction in a medical clerkship. J Med Educ 1979, 54:622.
7. Freud S: Mourning and melancholia (1917). *In* Riviere J (trans): Collected Papers. London, Hogarth Press, vol 4, 1925, pp 152–170.
8. Gaensbauer TJ, Mizner GL: Developmental stresses in medical education. Psychiatry 1980, 43:60.
9. Haymaker W: The Founders of Neurology. Springfield, Illinois, Charles C Thomas, 1953.

10. Heath R: The Reasonable Adventurer. Pittsburgh, University of Pittsburgh Press, 1964.
11. Jonas S: Medical Mystery—The Training of Doctors in the United States. New York, Norton, 1978.
12. Keniston, K: The medical student. Yale J Biol Med 1967, 39:346.
13. Lister J: Selection of medical students. N Engl J Med 1978, 298:1182.
14. Marshall RE: Measuring the medical school learning environment. J Med Educ 1978, 53:98.
15. Morowitz HJ: Zen and the art of getting into medical school. Hosp Pract 1976, 11:132.
16. Mullan F: White Coat, Clenched Fist—The Political Education of an American Physician. New York, Macmillan, 1976.
17. Nathan PW: Selection of future doctors—lessons from the past. Lancet 1954, 267:407.
18. Pellegrino, ED: To be a physician. Texas A&M College of Medicine Convocation Address, October 14, 1977.
19. Pirsig RM: Zen and the Art of Motorcycle Maintenance—An Inquiry into Values. New York, William Morrow, 1974.
20. Price PE, Taylor CW, et al.: Measures and Predictors of Physicians' Performances. Salt Lake City, University of Utah Press, 1971.
21. Rosenberg PP: Catch 22—the medical model. *In* Shapiro EC, Lowenstein LM (eds): Becoming a Physician—Development of Values and Attitudes in Medicine. Cambridge, Massachusetts, Ballinger, 1979, pp 81–91.
22. Shapiro EC, Lowenstein, LM (eds): Becoming a Physician—Development of Values and Attitudes in Medicine. Cambridge, Massachusetts, Ballinger, 1979.
23. Stritter FT, Hain JD, Grimes DA: Clinical teaching re-examined. J Med Educ 1979, 50:876.
24. Torrance EP: Creativity and its implications for the gifted. Gifted Child 1968, (Summer): 67.

# Internship

Internship, or the first post-graduate year as it is now known, is seen frequently as a time of trial and tribulation. Like in a medieval hazing, interns traditionally have been subjected to diverse stress before they can enter the ranks of fully fledged physicians. It has been axiomatic that there should be constant pressure on them from all quarters during this year. The demands of seriously ill patients, constant criticism from supervisors, and ultimatums from nurses and other hospital staff make the intern's life less than heaven on earth. To top this off there is the nagging self-doubt that somehow the intern is not equal to caring for the lives of others. In addition, a dearth of free time during the year means that the intern has little opportunity to reflect on what is happening to him or her as a person.

In this chapter Dr. Julie Donnelly focuses on the metamorphosis of internship. Not infrequently the long hours spent attending to patients result in short tempers, frayed nerves, and compromised personal and professional functioning. For her material Dr. Donnelly followed a group of interns through their first post-graduate year, studying their reactions, recording their thoughts, and analyzing the ways in which they cope.

From this wealth of data Dr. Donnelly has been able to plot a course of progress from the earliest days of internship to its completion. The anger, frustration, resentment, exhaustion, gratification, and satisfaction are all here in the pithy words of drained interns, from whom she quotes liberally. Many physicians will recognize from the interns remarks the strain they underwent during their own internship.

The transformation from cocooned medical student to winged physician progresses subtly; it is difficult to discern when one ends and the other begins. Yet somehow during internship that transformation does occur as students learn to don the mantle of healing. Dr. Donnelly outlines how such change takes place and offers suggestions for how this change can be facilitated.

*J.P.C.*

# 3

# Coping and Development During Internship

*Julie C. Donnelly*

> No one can understand the life of an intern—except another intern.
> As an intern you feel constantly beseiged, like one man fighting alone against all the Indians [*sic*] at the Alamo.
> As an intern you have to learn to act like an adult whether you feel like it or not. You gain strength of character and a tremendous amount of discipline.
> As the year goes on you get very tired of patients. You don't want to see another patient for the rest of your life.
> You really feel insecure because you know what you really are. You're an intern, not a doctor.
> When you're depressed, you mind everything.
> Internship structures my reality. It creeps in and captures my thoughts.

## INTRODUCTION

For young men and women in medicine four salient themes emerge as especially critical to their personal and professional development:

- *Change:* Major simultaneous shifts in identity and roles, both personal and professional, e.g., adolescent to adult, student to professional, single to part of a couple, nonparent to parent.
- *Challenge:* Intellectual and academic pressures, career uncertainties, discovering appropriate level of involvement with patients. Can I take care of others and myself?

- *Competence:* Can I do it? Can I learn it all? Cognitive and technical competence may be achieved at the expense of interpersonal and affective competence.
- *Conflict:* Confusion and conflict between personal and professional identity—I am (only) what I do; conflict between competency and intimacy, often expressed as tension between time for work and time for self and partners/families; conflict between dependence and independence and between impotence and omnipotence often expressed as lack of personal freedom and fear of acknowledging any need for attention or care.

Within medical training internship has been viewed as critical in the professional development of a physician. Of equal significance is the effect that internship may have on the physician's personal development as well. Coping mechanisms that are relied upon to deal with the conflicts of this year may be a key factor in the physician's future development and well-being, both personal and professional. The type of care that is ultimately delivered to patients may also be related to these same coping mechanisms. If a physician has never learned to deal effectively with stress and the feelings generated by stress, his or her ability to help patients deal with their stresses may be impaired. Difficulties that arise during internship may persist throughout an individual's medical career and lead to serious difficulties for individuals and families. In turn, they may affect training programs and to some degree the whole medical care system as well.

Internship is critical in a number of ways. It is the bridge between student and full-fledged professional and can thus be seen from the point of view of role change.[1] Of substantial significance is the corollary self-concept change accompanying the student to physician change, i.e., from adolescent to adult. One of the paradoxes of medical training is that the typical intern just out of medical school, although 25 or 26 years old, has experienced a prolonged adolescence in that schooling has continued for 20 uninterrupted years. Because formal training in medicine continues for an average of 3–5 years beyond graduation from medical school, this quasi-adolescent status may last until an individual is close to 30 years old. The first year of postgraduate training is significant in that the individual is now an actual M.D., may legitimately be addressed as "Doctor," is earning a salary for the first time, is in a supervisory position over medical students, and has primary patient responsibility. At the same time, the intern is at the bottom of the medical hierarchy, accountable to and evaluated by those in higher-strata, and bears a work load of 70–100 hours per week which typically includes an on-call schedule of every third night and weekend and going without sleep for as much as 36 hours. To refer to these 12 months as maximally stressful and challenging is merited in most instances.

Internship and residency have been the subject of a great deal of research. Within this brief period of time for most young physicians there is enormous growth in several separate but related areas, including skill acquisition, competence in diagnosis and patient management, level of self-confidence, and consolidation of professional identity as a physician. What is also clear from a review of the research on residency is that it can be a time of enormous personal distress. Incidents of depression,[2] marital problems,[3] emotional instability,[4] disillusionment about medicine,[5] and resentment toward patients and the medical system[6] are more the rule than the exception. Although much less frequent, suicidal thoughts and alcohol and drug abuse are by no means unknown. Since 1978 the AMA has recognized that residents represent a group at high risk of developing emotional problems.[4]

Although to some degree these and other professional stresses of internship have been documented, their effects have been discussed almost solely in terms of jeopardizing patient care. Even with clear evidence that the intern's judgment, reaction time, and interest in patients is affected, little has been done to alter the situation.[7] In addition, almost no attention has been given to the effects of this kind of work schedule on the intern, spouse, and children. For those who find they can cope with the situation, internship is a tremendous opportunity for feeling good about themselves; for those who have more difficulty, it can provide a unique means of coming to know their own limits and making appropriate choices thereafter. Internship is critical not only in terms of the stress of the year itself, but also for the expectation it sets that this is the way medicine works, and how the life of a physician must be.

This chapter is based upon studies by the author which provided a descriptive account of medical internship.[8,9] Through an in depth inquiry into personal and professional development in young physicians, they examined the degree to which interns experienced the same life event (internship) differently. Twenty young men, each completing his internship in Internal Medicine, Family Medicine, or Pediatrics in a program affiliated with a university-based teaching hospital in the Northeast were studied.

Loevinger's stages of ego development were utilized to discern individual differences in patterns of experience. These stages describe a progression of levels of maturity and a developmental sequence for tracing changes in an individual's frame of reference for interpreting and responding to daily experience.[10] Since each stage comprises a theory of how to deal with one's world, people at different stages undergoing what appears to be an extraordinarily similar life experience may attach very different meaning to this experience. Loevinger's stages can be described briefly as follows:

- *Self-Protective/Opportunistic:* Events and people are seen in terms of exploitation and expedience; life is a zero-sum game.
- *Conformist:* Rules are partially internalized; mutual trust exists only between in-groups; preoccupation with appearances.
- *Self-Aware:* Beginning of self-reflection and recognition of alternative possibilities.
- *Conscientious:* Evaluates rules and allegiances; internalized morality; capacity for self-criticism; preoccupied with obligations.
- *Individualistic:* Increased concern with individuality, emotional dependence, and complexity of experience.
- *Autonomous:* Appreciation of paradox and ambiguity; copes with inner conflict; recognizes others' autonomy.
- *Integrated:* Reconciles conflicting demands; renounces the unattainable; cherishes individual differences.

All subjects were given Loevinger's Sentence Completion Test and assigned to either a lower-(Self-Protective—Self-Aware) or higher-(Conscientious–Integrated) stage group on the basis of their scores. Extensive, semi-structured interviews with the interns were examined for stage-related differences in functioning both at work and home, including anticipated future repercussions. Interview data was analyzed to elicit the issues and dilemmas which were of most concern and to gain understanding of how ego development and coping influenced experience. The primary difference between the two groups was an overall tendency for the higher-stage interns to be more aware of complexity and emotional impact, whether in the situational, interpersonal, or psychological realm. Compared to the lower-stage group they reported a greater gap between the ideal and the real, and were consequently less content with internship. (For a more extensive discussion of developmental stage differences see Donnelly.[8,9])

The interview material was further analyzed for individuals' self-reported coping mechanisms. Two major patterns of coping were identified and were found to be highly related to ego development level. The lower stage interns exhibited predominantly nonpalliative (direct problem-solving) coping whereas the higher-stage interns were more likely to rely on both nonpalliative and palliative (emotionally oriented) coping. Interns who used both palliative and nonpalliative coping and who were in the higher-stage group received the highest supervisory ratings of their clinical performance. Further discussion of the significance of coping style is included toward the end of this chapter.

This research focused on individuals rather than on a group, and on personal feelings rather than a description of daily life events. In-depth, clinically oriented, semi-structured interviews were conducted to elicit the intern's concerns. In order to maximize the richness of individuals telling their own stories, the first part of this chapter includes selections from these interviews which were chosen to illustrate both the commonalities and the individual variations of the experience. The primary emphasis here will be reporting on these issues and dilemmas and describing how these were experienced by various individuals.

Whereas most accounts of internship depersonalize the experience, the intent of this chapter is to bring internship to life as vividly as possible on paper. These young physicians are quoted verbatim (italics added) with names and details changed only when necessary to ensure anonymity. The power of these young physicians' words help bring to life the richness and intimacy of their experience.

## CHARACTERIZATIONS OF INTERNSHIP

In the initial interview each subject was asked to characterize his experience to date. Frank volunteered that he was feeling better as he became more competent. He described his awareness of the effect on other aspects of life, particularly his relationship with his wife:

> I've thought a lot about this, especially the effect on my personal life. *As the year passes I'm getting more and more resentful.* I feel the problems are more acute for those of us who are older and for those of us who are married. I need to keep medicine in perspective with the other things in my life, my other interests have become telescopic. I've lost friends, I have little time with my wife.

Mitch noted changes in himself, the recognition that responsibility contributed to an increased sense of competency and maturity:

> *It's been a little like growing up.* I've been in school steadily for all my life, one year right after another and this is the first time I had a job where I earn money. This is the first time I really felt productive in some sense. It's nice handling responsibility, things are mine to decide and so I like that aspect of it, and that's a growing experience for me. *Responsibility is the whole thing of being an intern.* It's tough, but it's worthwhile. I guess that's basically the reason for a whole year of struggling. . . . *It's also been extremely, extremely lonely.* I live alone,

my girlfriend is many hours away. *Everyone is plus or minus a stranger. There's very little feeling of esprit de corps among the house officers.* I haven't gone out socially with any of the interns.

Nat was primarily in touch with his anger:

*Feeling angry sticks out because I never get angry.* If you're a normal person and you had a fight with your wife or somebody, you get angry once in a while. Someone hits your car, you get angry. But I never get angry. But there were times here that I got so angry. I hate to feel angry because you really feel you're burning up. You think, "I'm going to get a heart attack in ten years from going through this. What am I doing this for?" And you wonder what you are being angry about. I felt myself being angry about things like something wasn't done. I'm saying to myself, "Why am I being so angry? It's not me, it's the patient. Do I really care that much about the patient?" I guess obviously at times I do.

Nat also spoke of being afraid to begin internship:

I was very, very uptight. Looking back at it I was, *I was afraid to start, I was afraid that I would flop.* I never did it before. In a way they prepare you in medical school, but in a way it's not the same thing; it is a totally different experience. In medical school, you are on with your resident, but you never have any responsibility. You never even have to show up if you really don't want to. It's not the same thing. *This was the first time that it would be my responsibility. . . .* You feel beseiged, like one man fighting alone against all the Indians [*sic*] of the Alamo. Like one resident told me, "Internship is the worst year of your life, it stinks. There's no way around it." I was afraid that I was not going to be able to do the job.

Robin, who indicated that he expected to learn nothing, stated:

*It has done its best to make me hate patients and hate medicine to some extent.* You see the worst part of medicine. You feel like a clerk, a very tired clerk and you don't learn medicine. You learn how to keep charts well. Nights on keep coming, a 32-hour shift—*you want to say, "Stop, I have had enough."* The following day you're back again. At least the year goes fast. You get very tired of patients, very, very tired. You don't want to see another patient for the rest of your life.

Perry referred to his wide variety of experiences and stated that if he did not like what he was doing at any point in time, like the New Englander mulling over today's weather, he simply had to "wait and it would change automatically." He added that the other side of that for him was that he always felt like he was:

> . . . learning a new game with a whole new routine and a new lingo, requiring a radical amount of reprogramming. . . . Every time you start a new situation you have to decide where your boundaries are. When will you call back up people? Where does your responsibility end and someone else's begin? Most rotations try to communicate those things to you. Sometimes it would help if people would be more specific in what they want. Sometimes people say, "Why didn't you do that?" and you don't know anything about it because no one ever told you.

Brian and Jeff both seemed to have an early sense that the year would be difficult for them. Brian stated candidly,

> *I expected to feel inadequate*—I guess that's the best word to describe it. I had fears that I hadn't learned enough in medical school and I couldn't apply what I had learned.

Jeff, whose last two years of school had been fairly easy-going, was not terribly eager to begin. In fact, he would have preferred anything other than to start an internship. Still, he had some hopes at the beginning:

> My expectations were very low and my attitude was bad coming here. As incredible as it may seem, *it was actually worse than I expected. . . . I certainly hoped that it would be something that I'd enjoy,* that I would enjoy getting up to do it every day and that I would like the people that I was working with, that I would have found some people to like. My wife and I gave a lot of thought as to where we would settle. One program compared to another is difficult to evaluate. You could get a big name that would probably serve you as far as credentials, but as far as training I think that they're all about the same. I think it's just where you want to be. So we picked this state because we like it. We could have gone down South or West or any place. So we were almost looking at this place as "this can be home." *That was my wish, that to find a place . . . that would be home.*

Asked if his wishes had materialized, he ruefully said they had not.

***Summary.*** These comments give an introduction to this group of young men and express their concerns as they were initially presented. For many, these first comments were a good indication of some of the major themes throughout the interview; for others who took more time to open up, later statements were far more indicative of what was on their minds. Major themes included ambivalence toward growing up, particularly the dramatic increases in professional responsibility; the degree of resentment, anger, and emotional blunting which can result from chronic tiredness; and the family distress and personal loneliness that arise from long hours in the hospital.

## DEGREE AND SOURCE OF STRESS

The next area about which the interns were questioned was the degree of stress they experienced during the year. The first question listed several specific stress areas (long hours, night call, sleep loss, patient responsibility and decision making, lack of time for self, friends, family, outside interests) and asked which were most difficult. Stressful circumstances and situations varied widely from person to person, with emergencies and many simultaneous demands as the most common work-related stresses and the decrease in time for self as a major source of personal distress.

For Owen, having only 1½ days off every third week produced a feeling of constant pressure both at work and at home. This interfered with learning since "I'm not that efficient when the emotional stress is great and I'm exhausted." Regarding his home life, he said,

> I just don't have much. On a good day I'm home by 6:30, on a bad day, God knows when. I have so few waking hours at home. *I didn't have time with either my wife or my newborn son who was born early in my internship.* I used to do photography, bike riding, I managed to keep up with my gardening. With so little time I find it hard to work up enthusiasm for the things I've always liked to do. I essentially gave up everything.

Another factor for Owen was the responsibility of caring for sick people:

> You're dealing all year with sick people who are not representative of the real world. It takes a while to get used to that. It's hard to relate to people and get your job done while you're tired. Basically all the demands on us are a whole order of magnitude beyond any other professions—the hours, the responsibilities. You come to accept the responsibility that whatever does or doesn't get done is up to you, whether the blood doesn't get drawn or the phones don't work.

For Alan, the stress was related to having to put off enjoying the things he most liked to do:

> All your friends are out, graduated from college, and they're working, have a lot of free time, and they're making money. You're just

> too busy to go out on a picnic or go to a movie at night. You just feel that you're wasting away, working your tail-end off so that when you're an older guy you'll have time to do everything you wanted when you were younger. So that bothers you, that gets to you a lot. Even when you do have time you're so tired that you don't feel like doing what you want to do.

Barry, who felt there had been little personal growth during the year, commented, *"You change from your work but I feel I've mostly put my life on a shelf."* He then described a specific instance of how internship affected a friendship and the pain this caused:

> I have several friends who are very important to me and I've had very little time for them, which has been a great loss. One good friend needed to be hospitalized this year for mental illness, someone I've been very close to for many years. I had to limit my involvement with him, both because of my time and my emotional energy. *I felt so marginal in what I had in my own life that I didn't feel I could give to him.* It damaged the relationship which I'll now have to try to repair. That was enormously painful and I feel very guilty, but I don't see what I could have done.

These two themes—waiting for a time which never seems to come, and watching others participate in life in a way that feels denied to them, were major for these young physicians.

As far as stresses within the hospital, Nat provided the most dramatic examples:

> There were times when . . . I was afraid to come to the hospital. I was afraid I'd be confronted with, "You didn't do this, you didn't do that." Your supervisors come down exceedingly hard on you, and sometimes unjustly. *There was always the fear, "Am I doing the right thing? What's going to happen?"* If there is some patient that didn't get better or did get worse I was afraid, "Did I do the right thing? What's going to happen?" There were fears, real fears. . . . You manage and you go along but whenever I got paged, whenever I got a phone call I said, "What happened now?" Because so many things were always happening and I was afraid to hear what they'd say on the other end. Imagine that! Fortunately, nothing serious really ever happened. . . . When I was in medical school, I used to wish I could hear my name over the loud speaker or get beeped. I never thought that the day would come when I'd hate it. I cringe when I hear this thing go off. It's my worse enemy.

Whenver a child dies, someone, often an intern, has to tell the parents. Alan remembered his first time:

> I think the one thing that really produced a lot of stress was the first time I had to inform parents of their child's death. I think that was a tremendously stressful thing which I don't know if I was quite prepared for. You hope that it doesn't happen, and you never like to see it happen, but it's part of your learning experience. It's something you're going to have to do eventually in your career, so you have to learn how to handle it, how to cope with it. It was a very stressful event and I think I really felt distress. I was very afraid of how I was performing.

Robin identified the physical and emotional demands as being most difficult for him, especially when dealing with dying patients who were close to his own age:

> You get very involved with patients sometimes, like talking with patients about what their death will be like. You have a lot of mental tension. I have a 21-year-old who's about to lose her colon, a 24-year-old leukemic who's about to die, a 23-year-old who just had a heart attack with end-stage liver disease. That's very depressing because they're about my age.

Ben spoke in similar terms of "a law of diminishing returns." He believed one of the purposes of internship was to "see how you function under stress" and added,

> It's just too stressful. There have been times when I've felt this is just crazy. Working continually is absurd, 36 hours is a hassle. The other elements in my life suffer and I get frustrated. After you do it for so long, you just accept it. The sleep interruption is a big one, and it all affects your personal life. There's no one else that's expected to work so hard or so long. *We're in a humanistic business, but the number of hours we're expected to work is inhumane.*

Ben felt the effect of these hours most acutely in lack of time with his wife. He described their relationship as one based on a lot of verbal communication:

> When I'm not around for two or three days, there's a lot that doesn't get attended to, a lot of catching up to do. I'm not as spontaneous, it's not the same as dealing with each other on a day-to-day basis. I also never have time for myself, time at home. I'm always saying, "Well, when I get enough time next year . . ."

Jon saw time for himself as one of the major deprivations:

> Sometimes it feels like being a soldier. I've felt all the stresses, especially the sleep deprivation and the night call. Those who were on

> every other night think we have it soft. *It's crazy that doctors are considered superhuman.* For everyone else, their prime time lasts about 8 hours, then their powers wane. We're on 36 hours every third night—that's crazy.

With insufficient sleep, one worries about slipping up or missing something. Brian recalled a vivid, unfortunate example of this:

> Well, I think of the occasion of when I was called to what goes by the name of Rush Pace in this hospital which means someone has arrested and this was a night I was on call back in the fall. I arrived on the floor and realized that it was one of my patients. I learned later on that I had not seen his potassium value during the day. (That's one of the critical substances in serum as far as cardiac function is concerned.) If I had seen that the potassium was low, I probably would have administered some potassium into this particular patient at some point during the day. He arrested and he died. There was no way that I could prove that his low serum potassium was the precipitating factor for his arrest and his death. He had other things working against him but I felt very badly and I felt very much on the line. I felt guilty and I felt very angry with myself for not having done a better job.

For Frank the primary result of the stresses of internship were changes in himself: *"I've become stultified in my interests and my vision has become very telescopic. I've lost interest in a lot of things I used to be interested in."* The conflict between going home and staying in the hospital was the most stressful for him. In his words, "I always feel a conflict about where I am supposed to be."

Alan saw the desire to do *anything* well as likely to produce anxiety for him, but viewed medicine as especially stressful:

> *I think that stress is something that is put on yourself.* You want to do a good job roasting peanuts and they're not coming out well. Well, that's going to be a tremendous stress on you. You feel that it reflects on you. But then again I think there are some natural stresses that medicine does put on you that you don't get from another job. I think when you are really responsible for a person's well-being that's a big responsibility. If you're selling suits and the suit rips, well, you're responsible for that and you make amends for it but you can always go over it again. But if you have an asthmatic in the emergency room who's really tight and you don't do it right, you might not get a second time to do it. There's a certain finality to the things that you do . . . there is more stress because of that.

Although many interns reported some stress from patient care, that did not seem to be the primary source of pressure; more significant for most interns were the effects on their lives outside the hospital. What was most important about their responses was not so much whether medicine, and particularly internship, was in actuality more stressful than any other job, but that so many interns felt that it was. The bitterness, the feeling sorry for oneself, the weight of dealing with responsibilities of enormous proportions and doing so alone, were rarely acknowledged openly to anyone, although experienced by almost all of those interviewed.

### Sleep Loss

No discussion of the stresses of medical training would be complete without specific attention to sleep loss. Hayden summed up the feelings of almost all subjects when he said, "When I think of internship, I think of one thing. I never got any sleep for a whole year." Alan, with his customary humor, commented, "There are times when everything looks like a bed to you," and Glenn responded, "In the hospital *you find your endurance is phenomenal. But on occasion you feel a bit demented."* As mentioned earlier, the research on sleep loss of interns has been directed primarily to various objective indicators of on-the-job performance. The following describes the interns' subjective sense of how sleep loss has affected them, both on and off the job. Once again the interns speak for themselves, first regarding how they functioned in the hospital:

Bruce: You get used to it. *Sometimes it feels as though you're not within yourself.* Your mind isn't with you. In 36 hours I may drink 20 cups of coffee. It slows me down everywhere. Sometimes I can't get my brain started. *I'm very tired, irritable, have a short attention span, not very concerned or compassionate at all.* You can draw your own conclusions about the effects on work from that. When I go home, I go to sleep.

Mitch: When I am extremely fatigued, I don't work as well, for sure. When I was in the clinic I generally didn't get any sleep and that really hurt because especially as stressful as that place was and as busy as that place was, you need all the sleep you can get. I felt I was not working at full capacity because of the sleep loss. When I saw a patient I knew I wasn't doing the right thing.

Michael: The lack of sleep and the ridiculous hours are outrageous. There's no reason for it, it's an economic reason, an initiation rite. Maybe there's something to say for dealing with stress over those long hours of time that makes you a better person, but you don't learn more, *there's a point of diminishing returns in delivering care.* I just think that's outrageous.

The following comments describe the effects of insufficient sleep on their outside life.

Brian: It makes me a dull and uninteresting person. When I get home after a night on call, if it's been a busy night, *I'm sort of a blob.* I want to be fed, I want to take a shower and I want to go to bed. *Creature comforts are uppermost in my life usually.* It takes a real effort and sometimes some coaxing by my wife to get me to come out of my shell and relate to her. Fatigue dulls your sensitivities and your ability to relate to other people and to enjoy life. It makes you irritable, angry, more susceptible to being ticked off by minor inconveniences. You're more likely to be an unattractive person to relate to.

Alan: There are times when you are up at 3:00 in the morning and you just can't wait to lie down. I never felt that affected my performance. When you wake up and you get called out of sleep, it's really hard to get going, but once I get going I never found it difficult to do anything, so *I don't think that it affects my job that much.* I've had weeks where I've been on every other night and I think *when it hits you the most is when you get home.* Boy, it just all adds up and you just collapse.

Ben: I'm tired and I don't feel like doing very much. I get cranky and irritable. . . . A lot of the learning does occur at night but 24 hours on, 24 hours off, or 12 on 12 off would be a much better system. Everything is easier when you're rested. It gets to be a constant drag.

***Summary.*** All interns regarded their internship as highly stressful. Stresses existed both from within the training experience—the extraordinary number of hours worked, the sleep deprivation, and the overwhelming patient care responsibilities—and from severe inroads into personal and family time. Over and over again, these interns asked, "Must it be this way? Must the process of becoming a physician take such a personal toll? What will this mean for me over the long-term?"

Major themes included the effects of chronic overwork, exhaustion, depression, loss of outside interests, and chronic tension. On the personal side, these men made frequent reference to their lack of time for loved ones and their partners' resentment of their time at work. On the professional side, they referred to the anxiety attached to their level of responsibility, their fears of making mistakes and dread of being paged, and the understandable but regrettable focus on illness to the neglect of health. A frequently mentioned theme was having so little opportunity to process their experiences: life at work became a relentless series of events, some fascinating and dramatic, some routine, some traumatic, but very few receiving adequate personal reflection.

## SELF-ASSESSED FUNCTIONING AT WORK

When asked about their performance at work the interns said that both positive and negative feedback were lacking, leaving them needing to guess how their performance was being viewed. This in turn contributed to increased feelings of vulnerability and anxiety, at a time when the opposite was needed to ensure personal and professional self-esteem.

For Alan the feedback from patients, nurses, and fellow interns counted most:

> I think that the feedback that for me has been really rewarding is when the patient says, "Well, I like this doctor because he's a really good doctor". . . . When the nursing staff and the other interns . . . tell you that you're doing a good job, that means even more because that is the professional opinion. . . . If you can walk out of the hospital at night and feel that other people think that you're doing a good job, you don't mind getting up again the next morning.

Jeff provided a graphic example of the potential danger to the patient and the anguish of the intern when job requirements are not clearly perceived. He described one particular night during his first month when he went to sleep before getting the results of some lab data on a particular child:

> I had gone to sleep. I thought the kid was all right. We started antibiotics and it really wasn't my concern whether there were three white cells in the spinal fluid or 50 or 500. It wouldn't have changed what we were doing. But that wasn't the attitude of the others when I woke up the next morning. "I didn't know the lab results? How was that possible?" In retrospect it seems entirely reasonable that perhaps there could have been something there. Maybe there was a gross bleed, two million red blood cells. Yes, that would have changed things. But it was highly unlikely. I haven't gone to bed since without knowing lab data or at least had it telephoned to me after I had gone to bed. *Initially I certainly do think I didn't know exactly what was expected of me: now I'm not sure if I do. I think there is a possibility that I still don't know what is expected of me.*

Clearly this was one of the many sources of anxiety that Jeff dealt with throughout his year. Ten months into his internship he was admitting there was still a very good chance he did not know what was expected of him. For purposes of this discussion, it is not critical whether Jeff's perception of the facts was accurate; what is relevant is that he felt he had nowhere to go to get the expectations of his work clarified.

Since many interns did indicate they received some positive feedback, one explanation for Jeff's lack of such may be that feedback was given infrequently, with little positive to be said. Jeff was undoubtedly in need of a great deal of help which he did not receive. His own inadequacies, personal and professional, were magnified with the stresses of internship. In situations such as this, everyone loses.

## COMPASSION FOR PATIENTS

Perry saw his compassion toward patients decrease as a result of his frustrations:

> Low patient motivation often makes you wonder why you're there. I stopped at the A & P on the way home from work, and I swear every woman in there was a patient at the Ob-Gyn Clinic, pregnant with several other kids, and all of them had a grocery cart full of potato chips and cake, paying for this with food stamps.

Alan admitted he had never really thought much about compassion. He focused on feeling competent at work:

> When I first started out I really wasn't thinking too much about being compassionate as much as I was worried about getting the job done. As you become more comfortable with your competence you start thinking more about the patient and being compassionate. I don't think it's something I think about. I think it's something either you are or aren't, and some people are overly compassionate and I think that can interfere with your work. I think it takes a certain amount of balance. You can't become involved emotionally to the extent that you can't be objective. I think it is easy to let it happen.

Brian expressed a common theme for interns: the degree to which the conflict between the demands of time and the sheer number of patients and procedures short-circuited relating to patients as fellow human beings:

> When you're pushed, when you have too little time to do the number of things you have to get accomplished, you take shortcuts, and those shortcuts often affect your interpersonal relationships with the staff, within the ward, with nurses, and with your patients. You

> don't want to stand there and talk about the nurse that infuriated them last night, or who came to visit them last night, or who won the football game on TV, things they like to talk about. You don't have time to relate to them as persons. The demands of hours and responsibilities tend to make you compress relationships and skip things.

Jon relished the personal involvement and recognized the growth that dealing with death provided for him:

> I just finished working with a family of a boy, Bobby, who died after seven weeks in the hospital. He is the only patient I handled that died. . . . I took care of him for six weeks and I had many conversations with the mother. He was a four-year-old boy so I didn't talk much with him. He didn't want to talk with me, for a lot of time he was angry and isolated. He talked to his mother only. I felt very strongly attached to the mother, the boy, and the father. It sounds like a travesty of a dying child to say it was the highlight of your internship. It was important . . . that's the kind of thing that makes you grow. To go through the stresses, cope with the family, knowing that you can't go in with a formula. You must listen to what they say and react to it. It is so different from an organic illness. You shouldn't use a formula for organic illness either, but that is what the year often does to you.

Michael chastised himself for the way he handled relating to some patients:

> There have been times in the hospital when I didn't have compassion. It's been beaten out of me, usually by fatigue. The other thing is that there is a socializing process whereby people are categorized as good patients or bad patients. Bad patients are labeled as crocks, dirtballs, hystrionics, whatever, and the labeling system kind of makes you see people that way. . . . I've done it, too. I have fallen into that to some extent.

As an intern, the pressures to get the job done and not dwell on personal, emotional reactions is enormous, but those like Michael were very troubled by the tendency to lose sight of the emotional significance of the events surrounding them and sometimes to lose compassion for their patients as well.

## STUDENT TO PHYSICIAN TRANSITION

Many subjects reported a fairly smooth transition from student to physician. Perry wondered if he were capable of making it:

> After graduation you suddenly realize that although you don't feel any different inside, when you start internship you have a piece of paper that says you're a doctor. You begin to wonder about your *weaknesses and if you are going to be capable of doing the job.* It's gradual, but it gets worse just before internship. Nothing magic happens at graduation. . . . The overwhelming effect is a move toward adulthood, although you are still sheltered.

Alan expressed the belief that the only problems were the expectations of others:

> *You graduate from medical school, all your friends think that you're going to get a Mercedes now,* that you're really a doctor. . . . They call you up, "I got this rash on my hands, I think it's poison ivy what should I do?" And you don't want to say anything because you feel really insecure because you know what you are, you're an intern and not a doctor. *Doctors say I'm a doctor but you don't feel any different than a medical student,* except you can write your prescriptions, you don't have to run around and get somebody to sign them for you.

Alan's comment that being treated as a doctor made him feel important illustrated the relationship of the role and self-concept transition. Rather than the role change enabling him to act like a physician, it worked the other way around. By being placed in situations where he was treated like a physician, he could then feel like one.

Michael reported that the transition lasted throughout the year and that ten months into his internship, he was just beginning to feel like a doctor:

> I feel like I know what I'm doing and that's just started to happen. The first few months of internship I was certainly only a scut boy, examining body secretions, doing very compulsive histories and physicals, but not sitting back and examining what was going on, not making choices. You're just a student, actually a little less than a student, because as a student you're not so burdened down with the task that it gets in the way of learning. That's not the highest priority. Learning gets lost. I guess it's a matter of becoming efficient. *The point when I started to feel more like a doctor was when I got efficient enough at taking care of that scut* that I was able to save some energy for making decisions and thinking about what I was doing, reading a little bit.

Brian recognized pushes and pulls in both directions:

> Like most people I enjoy being looked up to by laymen on the outside who don't know what it's all about. People have some idea of what it means to be an intern, *but I am a physician, I do have two letters, "M.D." after my name. People give me a certain honor for that.* That

> certainly is in opposition to the sort of role I assume and the treatment I receive while I work in the hospital.

Jeff indicated a substantial degree of uncertainty regarding his status in the eyes of others:

> Everytime I talk to my father he always asks me some inane questions like, "You really look at the X-rays yourself?" What am I supposed to say? "No, I go ask my doctor!" I'll always be just Jeff to them. *When I was a kid, I looked up to doctors as knowing everything. Now I know doctors know what they come into contact with.* I consider myself just Jeff. . . .

Both Jeff and Brian reported a painful transition in large part due to the number of simultaneous changes occurring in their lives. Both of these men had moved a great distance, and found that feeling at home in a new location was not easily accomplished. Both also became fathers during this time, one just before internship, and one several months later. After moving one thousand miles with his pregnant wife, Brian reported a huge sense of relief that he finally had left medical school behind to begin his internship:

> A lot of energy was spent in the physical act of moving up here. We also experienced the birth of our daughter this year. I didn't know when my wife would go into labor, whether I would be on call. It was an especially difficult time. She tried to cope with the new child, she learned she had to be by herself, she didn't have me at home to support her.

Jeff reported the aftereffects of having moved here just two weeks before beginning his internship, including social isolation and drastically decreased personal freedom:

> We didn't have much of a social life, I didn't feel at all at ease with the people I was working with, we didn't have any family, we had a kid who was three months old. . . . I remember crying and crying literally because I was just so upset that I didn't know what to do.

***Summary.*** Two major factors, then, appeared to contribute to the degree of difficulty in the student–physician transition. The first of these was the amount of experience gained in one's clinical years in medical school and the accompanying level of responsibility. Where this was high, the transition to internship was not perceived as major. The second was far more personal and related to the degree of simultaneous additional changes in one's life, e.g., geographical move, marriage, and/or new parenthood. Table 1 shows how these young physicians'

**TABLE 1.** YOUNG PHYSICIANS' DESCRIPTIVE TITLES FOR THEIR LIFE PERIODS

| Period Just Left (Medical School) | Present Life Period (Internship) | Next Period (Posttraining) |
|---|---|---|
| The Making of a Physician | The New Haven to Boston via Hartford Schizophrenic Commuting Pediatric Pre-Psychiatric Premarriage Blues (and Highs) | Settling In |
| Marriage Abroad | Financial Freedom at Last | Adventure |
| The Conquest Over | My Internship, or How I Arrived (Occupationally) | The Fertile Years |
| Continued Drizzle with only Slight Chance of Clearing | Here Comes the Sun | Generally Fair with only Slight Chance of Showers |
| Obedient Student | Young Doctor Explores His Limitations | Practicing MD Defies Stereotypes |
| The Intern | The Resident | — |
| I'm Still Young and Idealistic—Aren't I? | Crash Course in Competence, or An End to Adolescence | Internal vs External Stability—Do I Need Both? |
| Insecurity | Transition | Insecurity |
| Leaving Childhood | The Leap | The Unknown |
| Striving | Transition | Personal Development |
| Last Fling on an Upward Slope | Uncertain Transition | Transition with Consolidation |
| How to Work Your Ass Off in One Easy Lesson | Who I Really Am and What I Want to Do | This Is Your (My) Life |
| Europe | Internship (Unfortunately) | Challenge |
| The Terrible Difficulties and Sacrifices Required to Get Where I Am | Now That the Fruits of My Efforts Have Been Realized There Are Some Sobering Realizations | Adjusting the Conflicting Interests and Maximizing My Lifestyle |
| 2 + 2 = 5 | How to Serve Two Masters Without Really Succeeding | Finito |
| Schooling | Adjustment | Settling Down |
| Group Study | Contemplation—"Where to Now St. Peter?" | Is This Where It's At? |
| Education and Frustration | Preparation and Fulfillment | Early Practice and Family Life |

view their own adult development through their descriptive titles for medical school, internship, and posttraining. Internship is depicted as a clear transitional time between life as a student and life as a "real doctor." There appears to be obvious awareness of both change and conflict, with the future envisioned as primarily a period of consolidation and, hopefully, of easier times.

## SELF-ASSESSED FUNCTIONING IN PERSONAL AND FAMILY LIFE

This section discusses the interns' self-assessments of the effects of internship on themselves as young adults, including their own personal growth and intimate relationships. Several questions were posed in both these areas. For Alan, the concept of growth unrelated to his profession did not carry much meaning; the two were inextricably linked. He therefore responded in solely professional terms:

> I think there is very little to do . . . outside of medicine. If what you mean is your maturity overall, I think that an internship is a very maturing experience. I think medical school is to some degree. *I think anything that puts you in a position of great responsibility tends to be a maturing experience.*

Alan was probably right that his professional growth affected him personally, but also of significance was that he had no conception of personal growth other than as a by-product of his work.

In Nat's view, internship "promotes your psychological growth because you see so many different kinds of people, so many tragedies, . . . so many problems with people." For Jon internship was unquestionably a time for growth in competency and self-esteem, but he also acknowledged feeling depressed, angry, and frustrated frequently, even though, "You're on the go so much it sometimes takes a few weeks to realize you're feeling lousy." When he did, he reminded himself, "This is just one year. It's a continuity of what's happened before and what's going to happen again. This is better than getting so bogged down with it that you can't see your way out." This sense that everything will be all right was an important source of strength for Jon throughout the year.

Brian expressed a similar, although more negative point of view. His response was lengthy, seemingly in direct proportion to the amount of time he had spent thinking about his issue. Inquiring about the effect on his own growth clearly struck a responsive chord:

> You gain strength of character from being an intern. You gain a *tremendous amount of discipline* which is a very helpful entity. You

> have to discipline your mind. You can't sit home five hours a night drinking beer and watching TV, it just doesn't fit in with your profession. *There's a sense of superiority and pride that creeps in.* You feel that sometimes you're worth more than the guy next door who's a barber and *there's a sense in which you look at other people as inferior.* Someone who is telling you about the number he picked for the daily lottery some afternoon after work when you've been trying to save someone's life in the Cardiac Care Unit.As a physician you are supposed to relate to people in a very deep and very therapeutic fashion. Yet the demands of medicine probably tend to force you to draw into your shell psychologically, to cut you off from other people. It tends to make you less compassionate, less empathetic and sympathetic. *You also tend to develop a certain disregard for the value and sanctity of life.* You see so many people who are so very ill and some who are dying. *Life and death become commonplace.* You're not touched anymore by the birth of a baby, you've seen too many. You've been called to see too many sick babies at 4:00 A.M.

***Summary.*** Most of these interns viewed internship as growth-producing in terms of their work. They spoke of themselves as different than when they began, and for the most part they were comfortable and even pleased with these changes. Most of the positive change was associated with the responsibility of caring for people. Personal growth apart from one's work was a salient issue for many of the subjects, but a large number felt their internship had allowed no personal growth at all and were clearly distressed by this. Although feeling remarkable growth in skill, competence, and confidence with patients, this was often experienced in dramatic contrast to the sense of treading water in their personal lives. Thus, these young men were probably far more mature and responsible in their professional lives than their peers outside of medicine, yet often quite inexperienced in any other realm. By having to channel so much of themselves into their work, they experienced vicariously through their patients many of life's most profound moments. They felt their personal lives were at a standstill. Many viewed their lives as a continual race to catch up with everyone else.

## PERSONAL AND PROFESSIONAL ROLE CONFLICT

The development of intimacy is a major task of young adulthood—just as important as the consolidation of identity as an adult, based in part on professional role. As the next series of quotes on personal/professional role conflicts make clear, most young physicians who are in a committed relationship feel strongly that their own needs for intimacy, as well as their partners', are largely unmet. Much of the research on medical marriages[11,12] is very critical of the training years as a time when the seeds are sown for substantial mutual discontent and resentment. In his article on medical marriages, Taubman[13] devotes the following paragraph to the particularly devastating effects of internship on family relationships:

> What is known to every physician who has experienced internship training has only recently been documented. The tremendous demands on the intern, with the accompanying sleep deprivation; the massive assault on the interns' intellectual and technical resources; the drain on his personal–emotional resources—the effects of these impositions have been clearly assessed. The loss in cognitive and affective functioning caused by these excessive demands on the intern decreases the quality of patient care; it also tends to destroy the personal effectiveness of the intern's life at home. When the intern does go home to wife and family, there are no reserves of emotional energy left; the intern is likely to be so drained that his sole concerns are directed toward sleep and rebuilding his own strength. *Wife and children may be regarded only as impediments to sleep and recuperation from the exhausting responsibilities of the 100-hour week.* But the measure of the residual energy in the intern is only partially described by the number of hours served on duty, the emotional drain is not easily quantified. [Italics added]

Ray exhibited a great deal of tension as he spoke of his marriage of ten years, then faring poorly:

> Before we got married, I told my wife I wanted to be a doctor and she said fine. But neither of us had a realistic sense of what that meant. If I'd talked with some people about what it was really like it would have helped. I probably would have done it anyhow, since you always think you can do it—even if other people can't. . . .

Had Frank and *his* wife thought about the impact of medicine on their personal life ahead of time?

> I don't think there's any way to know until you're into it. I wasn't thinking of medicine when I decided to get married. Medicine became a goal in and of itself. I never even thought about how much time it would take just to reach the goal. *Being married probably detracts from my being a physician. Being a physician probably detracts from being married.*

In regard to personal/professional strain, most interns placed the emphasis quite squarely on *time*. This varied from an emphasis on time for oneself, to time for starting relationships, to a preoccupation with time for work versus time for wife and family. Sandy's comment that "Almost everything conflicts with everything," is reflective of this.

The two unattached men, Bill and Hayden, certainly felt less personal/professional conflict than the others. Bill stated, "My personal life is just me." However, Hayden did express how difficult it was to start a relationship within the time constraints of an internship. "You either have to have had a preexisting relationship or an extraordinary amount of instantaneous rapport."

Among others there was more emphasis on the emotional tensions which resulted from the simultaneous pressures from work and home. Brian expressed these pressures as follows:

> It takes energy and it takes time to maintain a relationship. The person on earth I most want to relate to is my wife and I haven't had time, I haven't had energy, those two central factors to give to her.

To Frank, this conflict expressed itself concretely as "I do everything less. My wife does everything more."

As Bates and Carroll[3] have written about marriages during internship:

> There is a certain amount of stress on any new marriage; there is a stress on any new marriage in which one partner is absent for long periods of time, and there is a stress on a marriage when one partner's career is a very absorbing one. The marriages we saw were subject to all these stresses simultaneously; we regarded these people as having serious problems.

## ANTICIPATED IMPACT OF MEDICINE ON FAMILY LIFE AND NEED FOR LIMITS ON PROFESSIONAL INVOLVEMENT

Too often in professional careers individuals come to be defined by what they do; their work can become the sum total of their identity. These interns expressed lifestyle preferences which suggest a substantial change from viewing total dedication to one's work as the way it must be physicians must live.

Sandy perceived the only alternatives as mutually exclusive: "There are two extremes. You either work 9:00 to 5:00 or your patients have unlimited access to you. *There is no way of being a good doctor and a good family man at the same time.*" In contrast to this pessimistic point of view, two others, Ray and Perry, both recognized the need to set definite limits. Ray framed the issue in the following terms:

> Some people regard themselves as only physicians. *For me being a physician is only a small part.* I know I could be a better physician if I

> spent more time at that, but I refuse to do it. I have to be adequate. I know the endpoints. I'll pick them and not go beyond that. I'll spend the rest of my time sailing or just doing what I want to do.

Similarly, for Perry,

> It's important to start out from the beginning with the sense that you're not going to sacrifice your whole life to medicine. You have to become involved in a practice that gives you room to live.

For Robin,

> If you're one of the guys who's going to work 100 hours a week, then marriage is for the birds. . . . When you are your own boss you determine the way it goes. I won't have the greatest income in the world, but I'll determine it.

Owen realized he had not yet worked out a viable solution and was not even sure how he would manage to do the necessary medical reading:

> You can't take a half day off to read and not see patients. . . . I see a lot of physicians who are awfully hard on their marriages. They come home and work out a lot of problems there. They're very demanding and picky at home.

For Alan, it was inevitable that "you do become what your career is" and that was acceptable to him. Nevertheless, he recognized the importance of "leaving your job behind in order to make time for yourself":

> At any cocktail party you can see the guys that are in lumber are talking about lumber. "I made a great deal and bought a billion trees." Every time you go to a party people are talking, asking you questions because you are a doctor and you end up talking about medicine all the time. There's nothing I hate more than that. It seems you never have enough time to do the other things that you want to do. I think that you just have to have that in mind and try to make time for yourself. You have to make it so that when you leave your job you can leave it there and you don't have to think about it. I think that if you can't do that you're robbing yourself. I think that there are things you can do to prevent yourself from getting so wrapped up in work. *I think that a doctor who has his office at home is crazy, because you never escape it that way.* You are always in your office, you can't escape it, people always know where to get you.

Brian was clear about his priorities:

> I don't intend to let medicine eat up my whole life. If it does, I will not continue in medicine. Medicine to me is an occupation, a very special occupation, but I don't intend that I should be considered a physician only.

Frank was well aware of the tendency for a lot of people to define themselves solely in professional terms:

> A lot of people feel that they are a doctor, they are a lawyer. But that's only their job. When they go home, they're human beings. Some jobs become 24-hour-a-day jobs, they're on call all the time. When are they other than a doctor? It slays me when they come in on Saturdays wearing a tie. Here I am, almost an adult, and I still can't put a suit on. Thank goodness we wear whites.

Frank had also reached the following conclusion:

> If someone functions crackerjack in the hospital, they don't have a together family life. If they're here at 8:00 at night, then they're not at home. *You have to be mediocre to be good in family.* If you want to star in family, then you've got to say I'm going to be a mediocre doc. I'm never going to be a Nobel prize winner if I want to have a good family life. If I want to go to the theatre, to the ballet, to concerts, take trips to Europe, I can't be a great doc.

Frank appeared to be content with his decision to "be mediocre." For him it represented the best possible solution to his dilemma, at least for now. While his use of the term "mediocre" may sound offensive, of more significance was his conscious decision to limit his aspirations in order to have what he considered a more balanced life. Delivering quality patient care remained a priority, but he would not aspire to be a star.

Mitch gave the following concrete illustration of the way in which he set his own specific limits:

> When I am not needed on a floor anymore for that day, when I have written my notes and carried out those tasks which need to be carried out for the day, *I try to get my ass out of there.* I go home and do all sorts of different things. Some will be medical things but in addition I run, I ride my bicycle around the block. I'll do this, I'll do that. *I set very definite limits on time. If I can get out, I do it.* I intend to always be this way.

Although Bruce was single and had no definite plans for marriage he too believed in limiting one's medical practice:

> I've seen what happens when it becomes your whole life and I think it's obscene. Often wives suppress a lot of anger and become submissive. They feel cheated and frustrated and it has to come out. I avoid one of my friends because his wife is so angry. *Wives have to have a full sense of what they're getting into. The men have to realize that they're married.* They will have to refuse to stay late at certain times. Both have to know what they're getting into.

***Summary.*** There is no question that this group of interns was concerned about the impact of medicine on their family lives, present and anticipated. Maintaining a constant vigil on one's work and personal boundaries, as well as "knowing what you're getting into" were the most commonly cited remedies, although no one seemed to kid himself that these alone were sufficient.

These young physicians also exhibited awareness of the impact of their medical training on personal growth. Many contrasted their personal growth with professional growth, describing the former as a kind of psychological time-out, a personal moratorium. Intimate relationships were generally perceived as a part of this moratorium, with concerns expressed for the emotional trade-offs and the negative impact on one's partner. Many provided vivid descriptions of role conflicts between their personal and professional lives and spoke poignantly about the need to set limits on their future professional involvements in order to preserve a compatible personal life and not to "become one's career." Although some believed that the passage of time would erase some of the emotional scars of their internship, many others believed that time would not alter their perceptions.

## STYLES OF COPING

In a highly humorous yet extremely telling Class Day speech to Harvard Medical Students entitled "Internship, Liberty, Death and other Choices," Cassem[14] listed the ten risks associated with internship (which includes all of those stresses discussed earlier in this chapter) and added that the benefits consist of an unsurpassed opportunity for learning, skill mastery, and growth in self-confidence. He then proceeded to give a brief list of ways to cope with internship which emphasized recognizing one's own limits, shutting off feelings in order to get the work done, taking advantage of time off, utilizing one's peer group to share feelings, and by implication, using humor whenever possible.

In their study of pediatric interns in Los Angeles, Werner et al.,[6,15] placed a great deal of emphasis on the significance of effective coping mechanisms. They documented a decrease in appreciation of psychosocial factors in the doctor-patient relationship, in positive feelings about internship, and in the interns' own quality of life, as well as in the number of coping mechanisms used over the course of the year. They also indicated that those interns who reported the highest degree of stress also exhibited the lowest self-confidence and received the poorest performance ratings, although they hastened to add that the direction of causality here was not obvious. This group of researchers emphasized the interns' comments regarding their dissatisfaction with their ability to process and learn from the stresses they experienced. They concluded that putting doctors in a situation in which they must suppress feelings may increase the risk of poor attitudes and poor adaptation. They also cited Stevens, who hypothesized that one reason many doctors experienced personal dissatisfaction in their careers is that they have not learned to examine their feelings and share them with supportive colleagues.[6]

In an article entitled "The Residency as a Developmental Process" Brent[16] discussed five developmental tasks which residents need to master:

- *Vulnerability/Invulnerability:* the ability to accept feelings of vulnerability in oneself while still maintaining a self-image of competence;
- *Active/Passive:* the desire to cure and control versus care and nurture;
- *Helplessness/Problem-Solving:* working with the medical system rather than against it;
- *Boundary Maintenance:* discovering the appropriate balance between closeness and separateness, objectivity and empathy with one's patients; and
- *Developing a Professional Identity,* based on both ideal standards, operational utility, and accurate self-assessments.

In all five of the developmental tasks listed by Brent there is an apparent conflict between an active, instrumental, external orientation with a focus on *doing* and a more passive, process-oriented, and internal approach with a focus on *feeling*—the latter requiring the kind of opportunity which the interns in both this and the Los Angeles studies reported not having. In the group of interns studied by this author, while it appeared clear that the level of maturity was a powerful contributor to differential responses to internship, it was also clear that these levels could describe only broad patterns of individual differences; in order to investigate specific differences in mastery of internship, other methods of analysis would be necessary. Further investigation of the ways in which individuals respond to stress led to the utilization of a taxonomy of coping developed by Lazarus[17,18] which emphasizes two major functional domains: nonpalliative and palliative modes. *Nonpalliative* modes include coping by direct problem solving and responding directly to the source of the stress. *Palliative* coping, in contrast, refers to thought or actions whose goal is to relieve the stress or the emotional impact of stress (i.e., bodily or psychological disturbances). The term palliative implies that these methods do not alter the threatening or damaging events so much as make the person feel better. According to this classification, most people employ complex combinations of both nonpalliative and palliative methods to cope with stress.

Table 2 lists these coping categories reported by the interns in this study and used in this analysis. For this group of interns a coping style comprising both palliative and nonpalliative modes was found more likely to be associated with high performance than one which relied on only one or the other. Furthermore, it was the combination of both types of coping, together with a higher level of ego development, which was the most predictive of a higher performance rating. Flexibility in coping was found to be the most important characteristic. In the high-performance group, this flexibility was demonstrated by the presence of many different, specific coping mechanisms including both palliative and nonpalliative modes. Such a coping repertoire made possible a wider range of responses to stress, higher satisfaction, and, when combined with a high level of ego development, high performance as well. While a flexible and broad coping repertoire appears to be most adaptive, both palliative and nonpalliative coping have advantages and disadvantages. Reliance on one to the total neglect of the other, over the long term, would be most likely to affect both external performance and internal well-being.

## INTERNSHIP TRAINING IMPLICATIONS

Some of those who have written about internship have concentrated their criticisms on the structural aspects of the situation, while others have been more concerned with affective and interpersonal issues. If the findings of this study are indicative of anything, it is that consistent with a varied coping repertoire, modifications of the internship should include attention to both the structural and the affective and interpersonal realms.

**TABLE 2.** INTERNS' SELF-REPORTED COPING MECHANISMS (COPING CLASSIFICATION SCHEME)

I. **Nonpalliative modes:** Behaviors which are designed to alter a troubled relationship with one's social or physical environment.

A. *Direct Problem-Solving Actions at Work*

1. I leave the hospital
2. I order things by priority
3. I set my own expectations
4. I do what I need to do
5. I do the best I can
6. I have given up other interests
7. I am organized and efficient
8. I logically think things out
9. I make decisions quickly
10. I look it up
11. I avoid problems
12. I anticipate problems
13. I get help/know my limits
14. I weather it, once solved, forget about it
15. I count the days
16. I become compulsive, hyper
17. I hang in there and keep plugging away
18. I accommodate/make compromises
19. I assert power/manipulate
20. I wake up/fall asleep quickly
21. I have learned to hang loose
22. I step back and try to evaluate how I am doing
23. I respond to positive feedback
24. I shift part of the responsibility to someone else
25. I consciously chose a program where I could be one of the best
26. I try to be easy to get along with
27. I try to understand what people are saying to me
28. I think out loud with my patients
29. I get involved with my patients
30. I assume a professional role/act like an adult

B. *Addressing Personal/Professional Role Conflict*

31. I anticipated the difficulties
32. I can leave my work behind
33. I have established clear priorities
34. I will set concrete limits on my work life (limiting career time and aspirations)

II. **Palliative modes:** Thoughts or actions whose goal is to relieve the emotional impact of stress, not by altering the situation, but by making the person feel better. Defense mechanisms are one type.

A. *Developing a New Self-Image as Adequate to the Situation*

1. I feel more competent
2. I believe I have something to offer
3. I feel more mature
4. I feel good when I can do something I did not think I could

B. *Managing the Emotional Consequences of Stress*

5. I pay attention to my feelings
6. I cry
7. I keep to myself
8. I do something constructive about my feelings
9. I grumble and complain
10. I talk with others
11. I fight with others
12. I react less viscerally
13. I close off, withdraw
14. I try to ignore what is bothering me (selective perception)
15. I try not to identify with the patients
16. I rationalize
17. I have learned to accept certain things
18. I intellectualize
19. I have become paranoid
20. I use/keep my sense of humor
21. My feelings are muted by other situations or time
22. I keep perspective
23. I look forward to next year

C. *Relying on Comforting Belief System*

24. What's done is done
25. What I cannot do now, I will do later
26. I enjoy it and want to be here
27. My belief in religion helps me
28. I believe it can change
29. If I can teach others, it means I have learned something
30. I believe in myself

D. *Tension-Reducing Behaviors*

31. I rely on physical activity
32. I listen to music
33. I read
34. I watch television
35. I drive
36. I smoke
37. I drink
38. I use drugs
39. I meditate
40. I sleep

**Direct Stuctural Changes**

Some redesign of the work schedule of an intern to provide for fewer continuous working hours, less sleep loss, and more personal time is an obvious consideration. A more radical change is suggested by Howell,[19] and Shapiro and Driscoll[20] in their recommendation of the availability and acceptability of flexible-time residencies. Although all residency programs are now required to offer these, informal barriers often prevent their utilization by other than a very few, most often women with a young child or children. Most such flexible-time positions require two people to share the position of one intern, earning half a salary, and working two-thirds time, which still amounts to 60–70 hours/week.

**Increasing Individual Coping Abilities**

It is clearly desirable to enhance an individual's ability to cope with internship. Once the training years are long behind them, the effects of the stress of this period may endure. There is the distinct possibility that many physicians become so accustomed to the kind of schedule required during their training that they continue to impose the same kinds of requirements and restrictions on themselves once these are no longer necessary. It is almost as if they have forgotten there was an alternative; for many, depending on how long this pattern existed prior to medical training, perhaps there never was.

Drawing upon the data from this study, suggestions include offering a preinternship orientation to highlight the significance of the student–intern transition, to allow for exploration of mutual expectations, wishes, and fears, and to compare these with the expectations of program directors and other faculty. In addition, there is a definite need for clearly stated job requirements in the areas of patient care, learning, and teaching, as well as for feedback and for specific training in how to teach. Interns have to know whether they are meeting requirements and satisfying expectations; they need to know what they are doing well and where they need further work. They need assistance in how to change, and they need this early enough in the year to be able to do something about it. Being informed of one's inadequacies in time to allow for midcourse correction is critical. Relying on "no news is good news" as a barometer of performance is at best inadequate—at worst, potentially dangerous to patient care. The availability of various mechanisms of support including individual and couple counseling, structured interviews, retreats and workshops on coping with various aspects of a medical career, and support groups would each provide opportunities for assimilating and reflecting on one's experience and for venting feelings.

As a final question in the interview, all subjects were given an opportunity to talk about anything that may have been brought up in the interview, but not adequately covered. In addition, each person was asked whether the process of participating in the interview was useful. The interns expressed the feeling that being interviewed about their year's experience was extremely valuable. It had provided them a much valued opportunity to reflect on their year, to share their feelings with someone who appeared to be interested, and possibly even to effect some change by "letting other people know what it's really like." Internship was seen as a time in which so much happens so quickly that there is little if any time to assimilate, absorb, or reflect on one's experience and one's feelings. Paticipating in this type of interview seemed to satisfy some of the need for this processing.

It is remarkable how infrequently these young men have thought about why they chose medicine and what being a physician is really like. At the same time they appeared to be struggling to identify what they already know about themselves (or they could learn) that would help them choose a direction, how their characteristics relate to what is known about physicians and their families, what their long-term goals are (both personal and professional), and whether or not these goals are compatible with their questions. By developing components of medical education which could address some of these issues, training programs would legitimize them as serious concerns.

### Strengthening Interpersonal Bonds

Siegel and Donnelly[21] reported on their experience leading a support group for interns designed to encourage reflection and provide and strengthen interpersonal support. This group appeared to meet a variety of needs and the authors concluded that, "While the effects for participants and their families, patients, training programs and staff need to be elucidated and evaluated more completely over time, the fact that group members reported feeling more at ease with themselves and one another, both on and off the job, represented substantial justification for its existence." Such groups should be seen as one means of primary prevention within medical education, with full integration into the overall training program to allow for maximum participation and impact. Groups that include family members, program directors and other faculty who have an interest in serving as role models, are other important mechanisms for building a sense of community and strengthening interpersonal bonds during internship. Other research which has reported on the value of support groups for residents includes that by Berg and Garrard[22], and Bergman.[23]

## CONCLUSION

We have seen that internship contributes to the confounding of personal and professional identity by leaving very little room for the personal side of life. In the study on which this chapter was based,[8,9] many subjects referred to internship as having a significant impact on future plans. One of the most frequently cited ways was the decision to stay away from primary care and to consider a variety of subspecialties which appeared to offer more personal freedom. If in fact internship does encourage many young physicians to begin to think this way, while at the same time there are many external pressures to urge more physicians into primary care, this could be a very real source of tension and a further reason for internship to be changed. Funkenstein's 1978 study of factors affecting the career choices of young physicians also found that the overwhelming majority planned to practice in groups primarily as a means to limiting their hours of work.[24] Reporting on a generation of medical student, he describes the enormous change in students' concerns and plans about their lifestyle with nearly all wishing to work fewer hours in order to have more time for families and outside activities. These findings prompted Shapiro and Driscoll to argue that, in light of the changing expectations of physicians in training, to the extent that a purpose of graduate medical education is to instill in physicians an appropriate level of professional commitment, one can argue that the training should conform to medical care as it will be practiced: "It may be counter-productive to attempt to inculcate a level of commitment in which medicine has absolute primacy in physicians who have determined to give high priority to other aspects of their lives."[20]

The study on which this chapter is based strongly suggests that individuals' experience internship, their perceptions of critical incidents, salient features of the learning environment, the nature of stresses, and the adaptive mechanisms available to them differ in ways that are related to their level of development. As Sheehan has indicated,[25] this same developmental spectrum is often a critical determinant of an often unarticulated educational philosophy, shaping assumptions, goals, interpersonal behavior, and methodologies. Faculty and program directors who take to heart the basic assumptions that psychological distress often arises out of developmental transitions can find a new level of appreciation and empathy for the degree of stress accompanying these changes, and understand the need to design into training programs clear and effective means of reducing the stress.

Transitions both in roles (personal and professional) and in life philosophies dramatize the degree to which a previously consolidated identity must be left behind in order for an emerging identity to take its place. For the young men in this study, and others like them, such transitions too often occurred without their having the time or opportunity to reflect and learn from their own experience. Giving recognition to the capacity for self-reflection as a critical component of adult growth, and encouraging the importance of attention to one's feelings by structuring in a variety of experiences which encourage such expression, should improve young physicians' adaptation during their internship and posttraining years as well.

Rorty has written of the need we each share for "time for sheer musing, for reading novels, playing music, wandering about the rivers."[26] She calls attention to the degree to which this is precisely the kind of time efficient, scholarly men and women do not have. "We become harried, impatient, harsh, less in touch with the wilderness in the world and in ourselves." The medical training system must assess the degree to which it unwittingly produces physicians who may be highly competent medically, yet are quite without the ability to "muse and wander" and often feel distressed by (but unable to influence) the human problems in their own lives. The data presented in this study demonstrates that young physicians should not think in terms of either competency or sensitivity. Physicians will be more able to care for themselves, their patients, their families and one another if the system which trains them devotes serious attention to both personal and professional development, to knowing how to express feelings, and how to care for *oneself*.

## REFERENCES


1. Mumford E: Interns, From Students to Physicians. Cambridge, Massachusetts, Harvard University Press, 1970.
2. Valko R, Clayton P: Depression in the internship. Dis Nerv Syst 1975, 36:26–29.
3. Bates E, Carroll P: Stress in hospitals, the married intern: Vintage 1973. Med J Aust 1975, 2:763–765.
4. Tokarz JP: Beyond Survival. Chicago, AMA, 1979.
5. Bates E, Hinton J, Wood T: Unhappiness and discontent: A study of junior resident medical officers. Med J Aust 1973, 2:606–612.
6. Werner E, Korsch B: Professionalization during pediatric internship: Attitudes, adaptation and interpersonal skills. *In* Shapiro E, Lowenstein L (eds): Becoming a Physician, Cambridge, Massachusetts, Ballinger, 1979, pp 133–138.
7. Friedman RC, Kornfeld DS, Bigger JT: Psychological problems associated with sleep deprivation in interns. J Med Educ 1971, 48:436–441.
8. Donnelly J: The Internship Experience: Coping and Ego Development in Young Physicians. Doctoral Dissertation, Harvard University, Cambridge, Massachusetts, University Microfilms, 1979, No. 7927912.
9. Donnelly J: Coping and Ego Development in Internship. Proceedings of the 90th Annual Meeting of Research in Medical Education Symposium, Association of American Medical Colleges, Washington, DC, November, 1979.

10. Loevinger J: Ego Development. San Francisco, Jossey-Bass, 1976.
11. Coombs R: Medical marriage. *In* Coombs R, Vincent C (eds): Psychosocial Aspects of Medical Training. Springfield, Illinois, C.C. Thomas, 1971.
12. Smith C: Doctor's Wives: The Truth About Medical Marriages. New York, Seaview Books, 1980.
13. Taubman R. Medical marriages. *In* Abase D, Nash E, Lauden L. (eds): Marital and Sexual Counseling in Medical Practice. Maryland, Harper and Row, 1964, p. 499.
14. Cassem E: Internship, Liberty, Death and Other Choices. Unpublished manuscript, Harvard Medical School, May 1979.
15. Werner E, et al.: Attitudes and interpersonal skills during pediatric internship. Pediatrics 1979, 63:491–499.
16. Brent D: The residency as a developmental process. J Med Educ 1981,56:417–422.
17. Lazarus R: Psychological Stress and the Coping Process. New York, McGraw-Hill, 1966.
18. Lazarus R: A cognitively oriented psychologist looks at biofeedback. Am Psychol 1975, 30: 553–556.
19. Howell M: Stop the treadmill: we want to get off. The New Physician, November 1974, pp 27–30.
20. Shapiro E, Driscoll S: Training for commitment: Effects of time-intensive nature of graduate medical education. *In* Shapiro E, Lowenstein L (eds): Becoming a Physician, Cambridge, Massachusetts, Ballinger, 1979, pp 187–198.
21. Siegel B, Donnelly J: Enriching personal and professional development: the experience of a support group for interns. J Med Educ 1978, 53:908–914
22. Berg J, Garrard J: Psychosocial support in residency training programs. J Med Educ 1980, 55:851–857.
23. Bergman A. Marital stress and medical training: An experience with a support group for medical house staff wives. Pediatrics 1980, 65: 944–947.
24. Funkenstein DH: Medical Students, Medical Schools and Society During Five Eras: Factors Affecting the Career Choices of Physicians 1958–76. Cambridge, Massachusetts, Ballinger, 1978.
25. Sheehan TJ: Economics of curriculum change. Proceedings of 7th Annual Symposium on Veterinary Medical Education, Purdue University, West Lafayette, Indiana, May 22–24, 1978, pp 58–63.
26. Rorty AO: Dependency, individuality and work. *In* Ruddick S, Daniels P (eds): Working It Out, New York, Pantheon Books, 1977, pp 38–54.

# The Creative Physician

Hildebran, the foreman, towering above me, glared, and turned his head to direct a stream of tobacco juice that splattered against a bridge piling a few feet away. "What kind of work you been doing?" he inquired. Relieved that I hadn't been his target, I replied, "I've been in school." "This ain't no damn schoolhouse" he exclaimed savagely motioning me to the tool house. At the end of the summer Hildebran watched me go as he remarked sagely, "You ain't gonna have no trouble understanding the working man when you doctor." That blunt exchange imprinted an indelible mark on the memory of a freshfaced premedical student working his way through college by working in construction. That impecunious student is now a successful physician and the author of this chapter, E. Ted Chandler. Dr. Chandler's experiences underscore that not all the knowledge physicians utilize in the everyday practice of medicine is obtained in medical school. Knowledge is everywhere and it is gleaned through experience with life. Medicine is a perennial challenge and each stage of the physician life cycle brings its own particular challenges. The young physician is tested by his raw inexperience and insecurity. The mature doctor faces challenges of a different sort, fighting battles with the temptation of affluence, indifference, and cynicism, as well as the "tyranny of the urgent"—which often turns out to be less than pressing. Dr. Chandler offers his own particular perceptions of what bogs down physicians and suggests a formula by which a physician can *create* an environment where medicine remains stimulating and an enjoyable challenge indefinitely.

*J.P.C.*

# 4

# The Creative Physician

*E. Ted Chandler*

## MEDICAL HUMANISM

### An Enduring Tradition

Most doctors enter and pursue the profession with a goodly mind. Their motives are honorable, their personal ethics reflect judgments, values, and beliefs used in everyday life, and their goal is the relief of the misery that plagues and becomes a part of the human condition.

Furthermore, as doctors become educated they usually fulfill the characteristics of the educated man and woman as suggested by Dr. Henry Rosovsky, former Dean of the Faculty of Arts and Sciences of Harvard University.[1] Rosovsky emphasized two principles toward ethical and moral concepts: first, that a university graduate must develop "some understanding of and experience in thinking about ethical and moral problems"; second, that "he should have high aesthetic and moral standards." Additionally, Dr. Rosovsky stated that the most significant quality in educated persons is the informed judgment that enables them to make discriminating moral choices.

Medicine is a tradition founded on the principle of helping those less fortunate; its ideals are sound enough, its work intellectually stimulating enough, and its results adequate to place it at the top of the professions, as well as at the top of the list of those services most trusted and admired by the public. The statement by Robert Louis Stevenson[2] in which he described the ideal physician says it well: "there are men and classes of men that stand above the common herd: the soldier, the sailor, and the shepherd not infrequently; the artist rarely; rarelier still the clergyman; the physician almost as a rule. He is the flower (such as it is) of our civilization; and when that stage of man is done with, and only to be marvelled at in history, he will be thought to have shared as little as any in the defects of the period, and most notably exhibited the virtues of the race. Generosity he has, such as is possible to those who practice in art, never to those who drive a trade; discretion, tested by a hundred secrets; tact, tried in a thousand embarrassments; and what are more important, Heraclean cheerfulness and courage. So that he brings air and cheer into the sick room, and often enough, though not so often as he wishes, brings healing."

Generosity, discretion, tact, courage, cheerfulness; are these but high sounding, though abstract ideas or attributes that mark a life as outstanding? Are such attributes inborn and manifest during our early years? Or are they acquired at the bedside of those sick with diseases that smother hope, to yield comfort and hope as the doctor works in the company of gifted teachers?

In all honest work there must be ultimate good, but in medicine the rewards of skill, of devotion, of forgetting self for the good of others, are more immediate; the harvest is gathered on the field. The sense of saving life or relieving pain, as when pulling an unconscious man from a flaming building, is immediately joyful, no matter the grateful expression of the one saved.

Yet, in my search for the joy that is manifest in the good done for my patients, I cannot ignore or forget those other desires that pull at me. I desire the time to seek knowledge about the world in which I live; a world of books to be read, music to be heard, conversations to be enjoyed, friends to be made, and family to be loved and provided for. We are robbed of the richness of life if, in the pursuit of excellence in medicine, we are unable to control the commitment. Patients too are robbed if doctors allow no time for exposure to the world of working people outside the hospital. Such exposure broadens the base of knowledge.

The summer before beginning medical school I signed on with a crew building a bridge on Interstate 40. Hildebran, the foreman, towering above me, glared, and turned his head to direct a stream of tobacco juice that splattered against a bridge piling a few feet away. "What kind of work you been doing?" he inquired. Relieved that I hadn't been his target, I replied, "I've been in school." "This ain't no damn schoolhouse," he exclaimed, motioning me to the tool house. At the end of the summer Hildebran watched me go as he remarked sagely, "You ain't gonna have no trouble understanding the working man when you doctor."

That experience now evokes a clear picture if someone tells me he builds bridges. I know what it is to roll a georgia buggy full of concrete to pour a span of bridge, to unload a rail boxcar full of cement, to tie steel rods, and to build forms. I signed on because I needed the money, but this and other experiences became an indelible part of my education. I learned not only the work of a bridge builder, but also that to live in Hildebran's world exposes one to lying, cheating, and stealing, in addition to honesty, courage, and fair dealing. It's a world of choices not unlike those of other worlds, including medicine.

**Portrait of the Doctor**

Kipling, in *A Book of Words,*[3] described "A Doctor's Work".

> The world has long ago decided that you have no working hours which anybody is bound to respect, and nothing except your extreme bodily illness will excuse you in its eyes from refusing to help a man, who thinks he may need your help, at any hour of the day or night. Nobody will care whether you are in your bed, or in your bath, or at the theatre. If any one of the children of men has a pain or a hurt in him you will be summoned; and, as you know, what little vitality you may have accumulated in your leisure will be dragged out of you again.
>
> In all time of flood, fire, famine, plague, pestilence, battle, murder, and sudden death it will be required of you that you report for duty at once, and go on duty at once, and that you stay on duty until your strength fails you or your conscience relieves you; whichever may be the longer period. . . . Have you heard of any Bill for an eight hours' day for doctors?
>
> You belong to the privileged classes. May I remind you of some of your privilege? You and Kings are the only people whose explanation the Police will accept if you exceed the legal limit in your car. On presentation of your visiting-card you can pass through the most turbulent crowd unmolested and even with applause. If you fly a yellow flag over a centre of population you can turn it into a desert. If you choose to fly a Red Cross flag over a desert you can turn it into a centre of population towards which, as I have seen, men will crawl on hands and knees. You can forbid any ship to enter any port in the world. If you think it necessary to the success of any operation in which you are interested, you can stop a 20,000-ton liner with mails in mid-ocean till the operation is concluded. You can order whole quarters of a city to be pulled down or burnt up; and you can trust to the armed co-operation of the nearest troops to see that your prescriptions are properly carried out.

How do we respond to the greater complexity of the stresses that confront the doctor in this modern era? Innocent at first, insidious in its threat, devastating at its worst, is the use of drugs and alcohol to relax us. Resentment builds in the mind of the doctor because of the amount or the gravity of his or her work. Furthermore, the spouse does not understand, and another web of resentment is being spun at home. This, based on too little time, lack of control or diminished interest, leads to a coolness, perhaps an open constant hostility. The doctor's reaction—accede to every whim of the spouse and children, buy them more; spend more time at the hospital where you are appreciated, or at least respected. Close at hand, in the office or hospital, is a sympathetic ear, ready to listen to a tale of unhappiness, ready to provide a shoulder to cry on, to tender a caress that soon becomes a passion. The stage is set for an ugly scene, a marriage break-up, suicide, alcoholism, drug addiction, or a flight from the profession. Prevention of such drama is unquestionably far more satisfactory than treatment.

**Hostage Unawares**

The incomparable Dr. Osler once gave the following premonition:

> While nothing disturbs our mental placidity more sadly than straitened means, and the lack of those things after which the Gentiles seek, I would warn you against the trials of the day soon to come to some of you—the day of large and successful practice. Engrossed late and soon in professional cares, getting and spending, you may so lay waste your powers that you may find, too late, with hearts given away, that there is no place in your habit-stricken souls for those gentler influences which make life worth living.[4]

As one advances in medicine, financial security becomes a reality. This area of life then becomes a training ground for ethical principles. If the acquisition and control of wealth for one's own use becomes the chief reason for rising from bed each morning to venture forth, not only are the doctor and patients robbed, but the doctor becomes hostage to his or her lifestyle and desires.

When my wife and I were younger, both the desirable and undesirable attributes of the financial security enjoyed by doctors' families gave us concern. We didn't want to negate the advantages of that blessing, but neither did we want it to become a curse—a stumbling block to teaching our children frugal ways. We found it especially difficult to be objective in distinguishing between the needs and wants of our children.

In this day and time our hallmark seems to be lots of psychological chatter, lots of self-consciousness, lots of "interpretation." As the saying goes, "Let it all hang out," and then we will talk about it. A crude kind of popularized psychology has become the moral standard upon which many, many people rely. Coupled with this is the sleek god of affluence whose worship is now proclaimed the purpose of life, replacing the high-minded view of the world our culture seems to have lost. Bombarded with ads hawking a profusion of available goodies, it is no wonder we have difficulty distinguishing between needs and wants. We become victims of affluence, spending much of our time like Narcissus, considering ourselves.

## TIME MANAGEMENT PRINCIPLES FOR THE PHYSICIAN

### Less Stress, Better Control, More Time

Stress becomes a constant companion for doctors. The public recognizes it—a recent poll listed the doctor's work as the most stressful—but doctors may not recognize as clearly the role of stress, the pressures and demands that are made on them by the nature of medical decision making. The youth wishing to pursue and capture the prize of an M.D. degree develops so that uncertainty is no stranger, competition is hardly ever absent, and one end becomes the means to another goal. The queasy feeling of the gross anatomy lab passes, histology patterns become as familiar as roadways, and the other way stations through microbiology, pathology, and biochemistry are left behind for the excitement of the real thing—the clinical years. The diploma then becomes a means to another end. So it goes, and the professional path becomes a matter of choices.

We work toward each goal, making those choices that seemed better because they were easier, quicker, and more likely to succeed. Such thoughtful purposeful action presupposes that doctors act in a practical manner after thinking in a practical way about an end to be attained. The end is more obscure once the practicing days begin; obscure by virtue of the plurality that life assumes. The family's needs are to be met, community activities beg for attention, teaching becomes an alternative, office management a necessity, financial strategy vital—by this time there is no time left for one's self. Time management is undoubtably a primary way for doctors to avoid the frustration of not feeling in control of their lives.

Socrates, Plato's teacher, as Plato was Aristotle's, said that an unexamined life is not worth living. Aristotle went further and said that an unplanned life is not worth examining, for it is one in which we know neither what we are trying to do nor why, nor where we are trying to go or how to get there. Clearly the first step in developing a strategy or tactic to gain the most from our time and control our stress is to identify and expand discretionary time.

The life of the doctor can be a continuous struggle to overcome the "tyranny of the urgent"—staff meetings, patients' appointments, telephone calls, personnel problems, and emergencies. A common problem is the inability to find time for planning, goal-setting, and accomplishing long-range projects. Today's activist ethic encourages constant, short-range activity, fosters guilt feelings if you're not busy, and discourages the use of time for reflection. Furthermore, the future is ambiguous, comfortably avoided for the more satisfying clear-cut, short-term problems. "Time is money" was Benjamin Franklin's phrase, but time is more than money—time is life itself. More effective management of time not only allows us to make more money, but to pursue our personal aspirations for a fuller life. Just as well and perhaps more importantly we must have time to plan in order to resist the erosive action of the world. Oliver Wendell Holmes shared his feelings about life in *The Professor at the Breakfast Table*[5]:

> The longer I live, the more I am satisfied of two things: first, that the truest lives are those that are cut rose-diamond fashion, with many facets answering to the many-planed aspects of the world about them, secondly, that society is always trying in some way or other to grind us down to a single flat surface. It is hard work to resist this grinding-down action.

## Nullifying the Tyranny of the Present

The nature of the practice of medicine, with few exceptions, is one of frequent addenda: add on a few more phone calls, another patient or two, another drug representative, another conflict in the office. Yet these and a hundred other kinds of interruption are not the real villains. According to Ross A. Webber, a time-management consultant for industry and a professor of management in the Wharton School of the University of Pennsylvania, the three fundamental time wasters are fractionated days, short-run perspectives, and fear of ambiguity.[6]

***Fractionated Days.*** The workday of medicine is dominated by "response" behavior—putting out fires, handling emergencies, and performing programmed tasks in preference to less defined and long-ranged objectives. Thus, the future shrinks in importance. Few spans of time are available for concentrated thought, reading, planning, and reflection. As a result we become time-harried people with restricted interests and perspectives. We may lose track of our values and downgrade our aspirations. Transitions from short- to long-term considerations become increasingly difficult; fundamental changes are rarely initiated. The future is never confronted.

***Short New Time Perspective.*** Doctors are trapped in their early practice years by indebtedness, growing families, and low net worth. Concentration on the present is mandated by the circumstances of that entrapment and the rewards clearly favor intense work which generates profits and growth. It is clearly not a time of planning for the future.

***Fear of Ambiguity.*** In medicine, as in business, many of us focus on the present because the future is too ambiguous, too threatening. We prefer the known—attending those patients on today's appointment sheet, making rounds on hospitalized patients, sewing up lacerations, setting bones, removing appendices. These activities with measurable results are well-defined tasks with limited objectives that insulate us from the need for contemplation, data gathering, and planning.

So each day passes, seemingly filled, unquestionably busy, but little has been accomplished that will spur us to define our objectives. Time has been used, each second, minute, hour; some wasted, all expended. We need some workable approaches—benchmarks—for managing time and making it work productively for us. The concept is vital for stress reduction; for life control, for releasing us from the entrapment of the "tyranny of the urgent," for maintaining our professional skills, for keeping us interested in our work and, should that interest wane, for pointing us toward another career. It brings an orderliness to life, spawned through contemplation and organization.

Before considering methods of time management it is well to heed the words of Osler in 1906:

> Sooner or later—insensibly, unconsciously—the iron yoke of conformity is upon our necks: and in our minds, as in our bodies, the force of habit becomes irresistible. From our teachers and associates, from our reading, from the social atmosphere about us, we catch the beliefs of the day, and they become ingrained—part of our nature. For most this happens in the haphazard process we call education, and it goes on just as long as we retain any mental receptivity. It was never better expressed than in the famous lines that occurred to Henry Sidgwick in his sleep:
>
> > We think so because all other people think so;
> > Or because—or because—after all, we do think so;
> > Or because we were told so, and think we must think so;
> > Or because we once thought so, and think we still think so;
> > Or because, having thought so, we think we will think so.
>
> . . . Walter Begehot tells us that the pain of a new idea is one of the greatest pains to human nature. "It is, as people say, so upsetting; it makes you think that, after all, your favorite notions may be wrong, your firmest beliefs ill-founded; it is certain that till now there was no place allotted in your mind to the new and startling inhabitant; and now that it has conquered an entrance, you do not at once see which of your old ideas it will not turn out, with which of them it can be reconciled, and with which it is at essential enmity."

## Keeping Logs and Diaries

Peter Drucker, a management consultant of enormous talent, advocates the collection of actual data on how you spend your time over a period of several weeks to a post facto analysis of activity drawn from memory.[6] He claims that the data recorded can be used to alter behavior after it is subjected to three questions:

1. What does not have to be done?
2. What could be done by someone else?
3. What do I do that wastes the time of others?

Your decision as to what activities can be ignored without detriment to your practice is at the core of the definition of an effective manager. It is indeed rare to be able to transcend current issues and events, visualize the past, present, and future, and distinguish the important from the trivial. You are not called upon to be a seer with a crystal ball, only to exercise your best judgment on the data collected.

Drucker's guidelines for delegation of authority and responsibility are appropriate for the doctor's office. First, he suggests, follow the classic "management by exception" principle. Keep the unique; delegate the routine to allow yourself time to concentrate on truly important items. Second, since you cannot do everything, keep the activities in which you enjoy the greatest differential advantage. Delegate activities which you handle less effectively.

It is presupposed that effective systems have been selected for the medical office; the right type of desk, an efficient record-keeping system, a billing system, work-saving devices and methods. Furthermore, crises can be averted in some instances by the establishment of standard, previously established policies and procedures to broad categories of possible events. Not every problem is unique.

Unquestionably, the work of diagnosis and treatment is the doctor's, but even this area has attained flexibility with the advent of physician's assistants and nurse practitioners. In the delegation of specific tasks there is a weakness because tasks not specifically assigned elsewhere, fundamental or trivial, may have to be handled by you. For a period of time the performance potential of subordinates may be difficult to assess and, similarly, your own capacity may be hard to gauge. It may take some time before you develop the courage to delegate trivia that you do well and focus on crucial jobs for which you have the differential advantage, even though your talents lie elsewhere. This approach will nullify one fundamental block to effective time management—habit—and allows you to identify and expand discretionary time.

**Expanding Discretionary Time**

The central message of most time-management literature is to separate controllable from uncontrollable time and consolidate discretionary activities—major projects requiring concentrated effort—in controllable time units. Time that can be controlled is estimated by various experts to run from 20 to 50%; all agree it should be higher than it is.

The minimum usable time span for focusing on a complex issue, plan, or project is 1½–2 hours; yet discretionary time is usually so minced as to be virtually useless. There are ways to develop it, however.

***Insulation.*** This technique, used in business, buffers the manager from organizational demands and "response" time by assigning responsibility for control of calls, conferences, and meetings to a special subordinate. This technique is used in some medical offices but has the danger of isolating the doctor from the mainstream of his or her professional life—patients and colleagues.

***Physical Isolation from the Normal Workplace.*** Working at home, closing your consultation room door, using travel time, and eating alone may help to consolidate discretionary time. Decisions about the frequency and length of withdrawal will depend on the demands of your practice, magnitude of potential emergencies, and faith in your subordinates. Withdrawal sometimes creates personal animosity: people are easily offended by "no entry" commands.

More fundamental than insulation and isolation is an awareness of the need for an entire unit or organization to plan on a weekly basis for periods of uninterrupted time for longer-range discretionary concerns. Forward-looking companies are now experimenting with "quiet hours" that reduce external and internal communication throughout the managerial component. They do this by closing doors and placing signs that announce to the world that the one inside is having a "quiet hour."

***Concentration on the Task.*** The practice of medicine categorizes doctors as "simultaneous people," sufficiently flexible to respond continuously to various people and problems requiring simultaneous attention. There is another category, "sequential people." To make the best use of discretionary time, you must be sequential, focusing undistracted on relatively few major projects. Transition from topic to topic will only fractionate your time.

***Scheduling Personal Prime Time.*** Specially valuable in time management is an awareness of the time of day when you are most alive, effective, and creative. Such time should be reserved for solving difficult and ambiguous projects and, conversely, routine work should be avoided during this time. I have found that I can have several periods such as this—not by drinking coffee, but by leaning back in my chair or lying down on an exam table for an 8–10 minute nap.

## Eliminating Time Waste

***Tidbits of Time.*** Unanticipated free time should never be frustrating. Prepare for broken appointment or other unexpected periods of empty time by having handy a book to read, or a folder with an ongoing project.

***Single-Handling of Paper.*** Alex Mackenzie[8] is particularly critical of multiple handling of drafts, rough copies, and other papers that are a part of the back and forth process between boss and secretary. He suggests using the original letter to respond, using prepared forms for response to routine inquiries, minimizing taped dictation, and analyzing your bulging briefcase: it may be a procrastination file.

Many decisions, it is true, must be handled slowly and only after much data collection—hiring, firing, promoting, evaluating, buying, or trading; but the main point is that most paper can be handled with a single pass across your desk.

***Overcoming Procrastination.*** Much time is wasted because of procrastination. We may fear failure, the project may lack clarity, there may be no interest or motivation, or we may be just plain lazy. On the other hand the project may sound so "impossible" that we are unwilling to attempt it. Simple tactics should help fight this time waster.

Begin a project by setting a deadline. Generate momentum with some easy, programmed tasks; then confront the ambiguous. Reward yourself for progress as you complete significant segments of a complex job. Meet artificial deadlines by confronting difficult and unpleasant aspects of a job sooner rather than later.

***The Place of Responsiveness.*** Urgent requests and activities should not determine all personal contacts. It is sensible to be responsive to colleagues, office help, hospital personnel, and patients. Time for office politics (good human relations) is a wise investment in the future. A doctor cannot and should not control all of his time. After all, more efficient management of personal time and a lifestyle satisfying self at the expense of being in touch with the reality of the demands, information, advice, and problems of your patients and your staff weakens the performance of your organization. In the long run, it is self-defeating.

## Setting Specific Goals

Habit, preoccupation with the past, and sleepwalking through our careers are central causes of wasted time. Yet, how many good ideas have we all had that would have stimulated our lives and brought our dreams to realization, if we had only followed through and achieved them. Undoubtably, all doctors have had some really nice bits of success in their lives—bright spots that gleam with real consequence, even if most of life has been somewhat drab. Good luck sometimes gives a bigger push than at other times but the things that really count toward success are ideas that eventually set in motion a whole chain of useful and profitable events.

Recently I met a doctor who had achieved financial independence outside of his medical practice by buying small businesses in conjunction with another person. In each case the other person, known beforehand to be of good moral character, was a partner with ownership of 20% of the business. Though there was considerable diversity in the businesses, the doctor had learned basic business principles well enough to make good judgments about each. He rarely invests more than $10,000–$15,000 in any one business but, through earnings and tax savings, each property will be paid for in 10–12 years and be worth two to three times its original value.

For some years I have carried a small notebook for collecting ideas and for use as a time management tool. Knowing that each new development or bit of creation starts from something else, I am alert to interesting ideas that I read or that come to me anew. Each new idea is integrated with those I have already accumulated. Most pieces of creation as they stand today do not represent just one jump but many successive jumps. Thousands of scientists and inventors, for example, contributed a small bit to get the field of computer science where it is today. Sometimes the little bit that one contributed was of such importance that the scientific world bestowed the reward of recognition. Ideas are piled one on top of another, and thereby make history.

Setting personal goals and objectives and, in the long run, effective time management means dealing with yourself at the most intimate level. As we grow older we tend to behave without thinking. One method of increasing our awareness and ability to concentrate is to focus on personal objectives every three months. These are divided into subunits:

- *Innovation objectives.* Each quarter put one major aspect of your practice on trial and examine it to justify its existance. Can it be eliminated? Improved? Modified? Delegated?

- *Growth objectives.* These include planned professional reading and daily pursuit of a new skill requiring intensive practice, a new language, new musical instrument, new hobby.
- *Maintenance objectives.* The final target is to make one improvement in your well-being at the most personal behavioral level: physical conditioning, diet, or recreation. Such control will permeate your life, spill over into your job, and improve your general sense of mastery.

***Formats for Weekly and Daily Time Control.*** These have been adapted in my own usage by having a rubber stamp made for each. The notebook I use is a spiral 5″ × 7½″. Each stamp fills about half a page.

| A. Today's Activities | B. Today's Communications |
|---|---|
| 1. Most Dominant, do today<br>__________<br>__________<br>__________<br>__________<br>__________ | 1. Scheduled Meetings<br>__________<br>__________<br>__________<br>__________<br>__________ |
| 2. More Deferrable<br>__________<br>__________<br>__________<br>__________<br>__________<br>__________ | 2. Other People to See/Phone<br>__________<br>__________<br>__________<br>__________<br>__________<br>__________ |
| 3. Personal<br>__________<br>__________<br>__________<br>__________<br>__________<br>__________ | 3. People to Write to<br>__________<br>__________<br>__________<br>__________<br>__________<br>__________ |

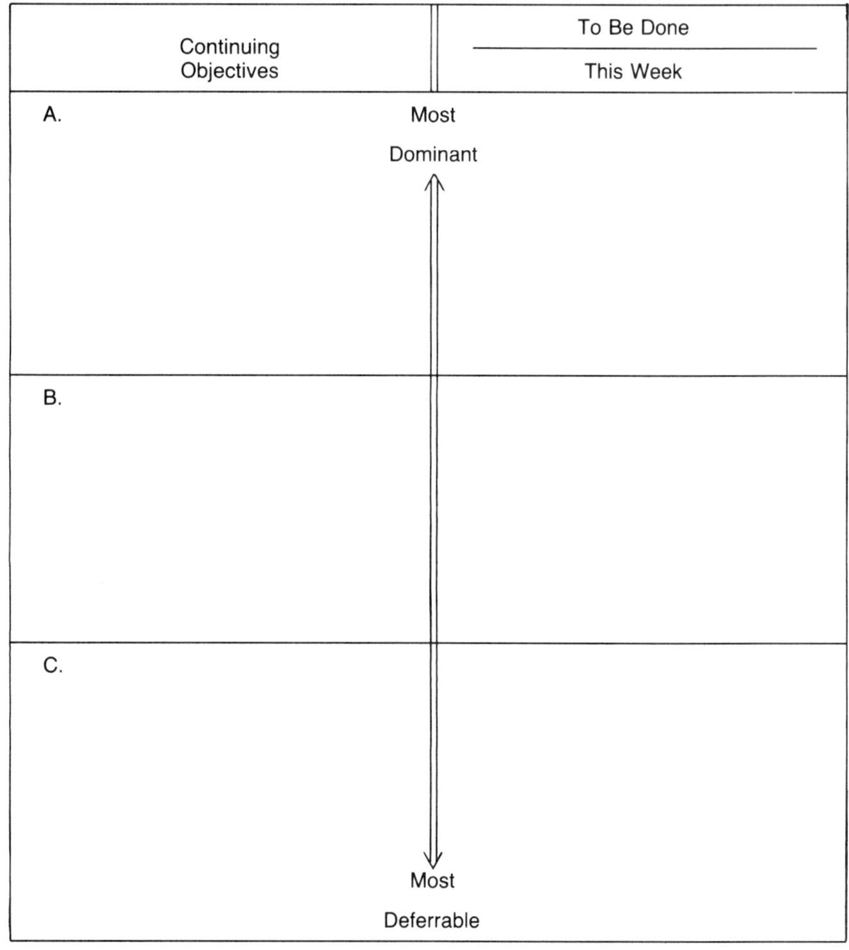


## HOSTAGE NO LONGER

*Always a learner.* "Each one of us, however old, is still an undergraduate in the school of experience. When a man thinks he has graduated, he becomes a public menace."[9]

A recent article[10] in *Physician's Management* promoted the view that doctors should dress in Brooks Brothers suits and wear imported shoes at prices that seemed quite steep to me. I do not categorically reject the idea that a doctor should wear Brooks Brothers suits or imported shoes, but I do reject the principle that someone else should set the standard for me. After all, the person considering such clothing is, as we all know, faced with a world of choices and his choice is made from a multiplicity of factors, all personal to him. It's quite a personal thing to decide what I should wear, what kind of car I should drive, where I should live, who my friends should be, and where I should invest my money.

Personally, I scrutinize and study such decisions much more carefully than I did during my first few years in practice. I make a much greater effort to have my decisions be more than educated guesses. My friends are chosen because they like me and can be trusted to stand as a bulwark to help me when I need it. My future financial goals are to increase my income to whatever bounds I can, but to use it wisely. By wise use, I mean that my motive for the dispersal of my income is not to provide for myself every whim, convenience, or luxury, but to provide for my family's needs and use the remainder to help others. For this to work my family and I have to work toward an accord, reducing the chance of conflict to a debatable and negotiable level.

The chance of accord within my family is high, for we have spent time together traveling and working in cultures other than our own. We have a common unity on this point. We have professional friends who have given up the chance of lucrative positions in American medicine for service in developing countries. I not only applaud their courage, but wish to support them financially as well as join them from time to time. Such work is not only intellectually stimulating, but heart rending as the difference between the needs of our patients and theirs is so vividly evident. It has given me a world view that is more in tune with reality.

Early in my career I strove to be the best doctor I could, sometimes to the neglect of my children. Their development did not seem to be basically affected, but a new relationship became necessary two years ago when both of them, within a year of each other, divorced and came home. I decided then that I would be the best human I could, and it was not health that was most important to them at that time. I accepted them without question, loved them as ever, and did what I could to motivate them to new lives. I recognized the talent that lay hidden in each of them.

My wife, Fran, and I have enjoyed a close relationship with our two children, Lynn and Steve. Just as we strove to influence their chances of success during their early years, we were still alert to the opportunities to enhance their present chances and to be of moral, spiritual, and financial help until they could gain their independence.

After much discussion we decided to develop a family business. We saw a family venture as a means to teach honesty, reliability, perseverence, and a my-word-is-my-bond reputation. After a period of searching for a suitable business we bought a country store in the mountains of North Carolina and developed a restaurant within it.[11]

I have noted with considerable pleasure the development of maturity, perseverance, initiative, and sound business practices during these two years. Our relationship is one of unity and love. If it were all lost at this point I would count it a gain. From a financial point of view, they are doing better this year than last and by next year should have a reasonable income as the reputation of the Country Store and restaurant grows.

I have tried to steer my family away from the narcissistic trends in our society, but I am concerned about society at large. Looking at the future we may ask: What hope is there? What may we expect? Are the doomsayers on target or are there helpful signs anywhere? On the hopeful side, some social scientists say that the age of moral ambiguity in the United States is on the decline. Yankelovitch and Lefkowitz, in the prestigious journal, *Public Opinion,*[12] recently analyzed existing data regarding the expectations of the American public for the next decade. They concluded that there is a growing acceptance of resource limitation, of the need and even desirability of sacrifice. Furthermore, there is increasing doubt that technology can solve our problems. Finally, they say: "Americans speak enthusiastically about the moral benefits of a simple, nonmaterialistic life. But they have yet to incorporate these benefits into either their day-to-day behavior or their practical planning for the future."[12]

Thus, there seems an opportunity for doctors to consider a policy leadership role. They can do this first by asserting their values and beliefs and seeking some greater consensus on fundamental societal values.

As I mentioned earlier, doctors work with a means until it becomes an end and then that end becomes a mean to another end. Is there an ultimate end that is not a means to another end? Blaise Pascal, 17th century French philosopher, when asked to state his position on the existence of God and the eternal life of the soul, indicated that if he expressed his belief in such eternal life and was right, he had everything to gain; whereas if he expressed disbelief and was wrong, he had everything to lose. Therefore, he would wager on God and eternal life.[12] Whatever the relative merits of the various other options before me I will place my money with Pascal, because, among other advantages, his view promises to keep my life alive with hope, not filled with the pessimism of the doomsayers. As Thomas Sydenham[13] wrote in 1666:

> Whoever applies himself to Medicine should seriously weigh the following considerations: first, that he will one day have to render an account to the Supreme Judge of the lives of sick persons committed to his care. Next, whatever skill or knowledge he may, by the divine

favour, become possessed of, should be devoted above all things to the glory of God, and the welfare of the human race. Moreover, let him remember that it is not any base or despicable creature of which he has undertaken the care. For the only-begotten Son of God, by becoming man, recognized the value of the human race, and ennobled by His own dignity the nature He assumed. Finally, the physician should bear in mind that he himself is not exempt from the common lot, but subject to the same laws of mortality and disease as others, and he will care for the sick with more diligence and tenderness if he remembers that he himself is their fellow sufferer.

## REFERENCES

1. Rosovsky H: Educated Person: Interview. New Yorker 1978, 54:40–43.
2. Bigelow C, Scott T: The Works of Robert Louis Stevenson. New York, Davos Press, 1906.
3. Kipling R: A Book of Words. New York, Doubleday, Doran and Company, 1928, pp 44–45.
4. Osler W: Aequanimitas with Other Addresses. New York, Blakiston and Company, 1932, p 7.
5. Holmes O: The Professor at the Breakfast Table. Boston, Houghton, Mifflin and Company, 1882, p 41.
6. Webber R: Time is Money. New York, The Free Press, 1981.
7. Coope R: The Quiet Art. Edinburgh, Edinburgh and Livingston, Ltd., 1958, p 8.
8. MacKenzie A: The Time Trap. New York, McGraw-Hill Book Company, 1975, p 161.
9. DaCosta J: Selections From the Papers and Speeches of John Chalmers DaCosta. Philadelphia, WB Saunders Company, 1931, p 50.
10. Werber R: Dress for Success. Physician's Management 1981, 21(9):124–133.
11. Chandler T: A Physician Starts a Family Business. Physician's Management 1981, 21:9, pp 144–152.
12. Yankelovitch D, Lefkowitz B: National Growth: The Question of the '80's. Public Opinion Dec. 1979—Jan. 1980, 2:44–57.
13. Payne J: Masters of Medicine: Thomas Sydenham. New York, Longman, Green and Company, 1900, p 118.

# The Competitive Physician

Though physicians may find it difficult to acknowledge, competition is as natural for them as it is for the most aggressive fighting cocks. From their earliest days in medicine, students vie with one another, and competition does not end with retirement. The medical school candidate knows the stiff odds when applying to a school; for every person accepted two others will be rejected. Obviously, the candidate hopes to compete successfully against the other applicants.

Throughout medical school competition is constant. There is competition for grades, for the most desirable clerkships, for the most favorable scheduling, for the most interesting cases, and for the most sought-after instructors. Competition does not end with graduation. Far from it—if anything, it intensifies. There is rivalry for the better residencies, for fellowships, for grants, and for professional recognition. In short, competition is ubiquitous in life and in medicine.

Whenever a physician takes a new position, and as many as 40,000 do so each year, the new physician is quickly appraised by the other doctors. They critically assess the newcomer's strengths and weaknesses and they wonder where he or she will stand in the medical hierarchy vis-à-vis the others. The evaluation process is mutual. To understand competitiveness among physicians, it is necessary to understand competition as it affects everyone in all areas of life.

In this chapter Dr. Harvey L. Ruben analyzes physician competition, noting that competition is the fiber from which interpersonal relationships are woven. It may bind one physician to another or it may be a reason for separation. The rivalry may not be recognized, but it spills over from social and personal relations into recreational activities, economic pursuits, and political life.

*J.P.C.*

# 5

# The Competitive Physician

*Harvey L. Ruben*

The sense of competition is innate: each of us is born with it, and it is generally considered to be healthy, a part of being human. It may be a channeling of natural tendencies which once were savage into constructive modes which benefit society and provide gratification for the individual. Its source, however, is our instinct for self-preservation. We find it at every stage in the human life cycle. Anthropologists and ethnologists have documented it for us in other cultures and other time periods. Ethnologists have studied it in numerous forms of animal life. It very well may be genetically determined that competitive parents tend to have competitive children.

Competition is present in the play of young children from the middle of their second year of life. By their third to fourth year, we teach our children competitive behavior as part of enculturation. School children are taught to compete for grades, in athletic activities, for a part in the play, for a place in the chorus. Since children have been competing with their siblings for their parents' attention from the time they can crawl, it is not difficult for them to expand such behavior to these new areas.

Our sense of self-esteem and self-worth is based to a large degree on how well we compete in our early life. If we compete well, we develop "normally" without great difficulty. If we do not compete successfully in required areas, we often develop problems which become evident later. To the extent that we develop areas in which to compete and excel, we are able to develop the self-esteem necessary for personality growth; and in this way, developmental and later emotional problems are avoided. The unfortunate individual who cannot accomplish this frequently becomes involved in what may be termed unhealthy or unfair forms of competition and develops other emotional problems.

Because competition is a vital part of our lives, both professional and personal, it is important to understand who competes and how, what is healthy competition, what is unhealthy competition, and how one can compete successfully. Each of us must learn how to analyze our own personal strengths and weaknesses. If we are frustrated because of inadequate and unhealthy methods of competition, we must begin to understand the basic causes of failure and learn what we can do about it.

In my experience, many physicians were attracted to medicine because they believed it to be far less competitive than the business world or some other professions. During training, although they found themselves competing with other medical students or residents, they still believed that once they were in practice, the amount of competitiveness would be diminished. This obviously is not the case, as most physicians find out.

As physicians, we live in a world of increasing competition compounded by sociological changes, economic pressures, and moral confusions. While our patients and families look to us for guidance, we may be overwhelmed by these pressures. It is critical that we learn how to compete soundly and effectively in order to be in better control of our professional and personal lives.

## STYLES OF COMPETITION

The psychological benefit of competition is that through success we enhance our self-esteem and self-worth. Some of us are born with feelings of inadequacy and insecurity. To the extent that we are successful in our competitive endeavors, we are able to overcome these feelings of inadequacy and prove to ourselves that we are better than we feared. We are all competing on a continual basis in every aspect of our lives. Some accept this readily, and others find it hard to believe. The competition, however, is not all similar: some of it is direct and some is indirect; Some is aggressive and some nonaggressive.

All competitors can be classified according to the degrees of directness and aggressiveness of their competitive behavior. In addition, depending on a person's particular style of competition, different behaviors—competitive tools—are used. Certain competitive behaviors are common to all successful competitors; one who does not use a number of these modes is less likely to be successful.

I have developed a four-quadrant matrix, which I call the *competi-*

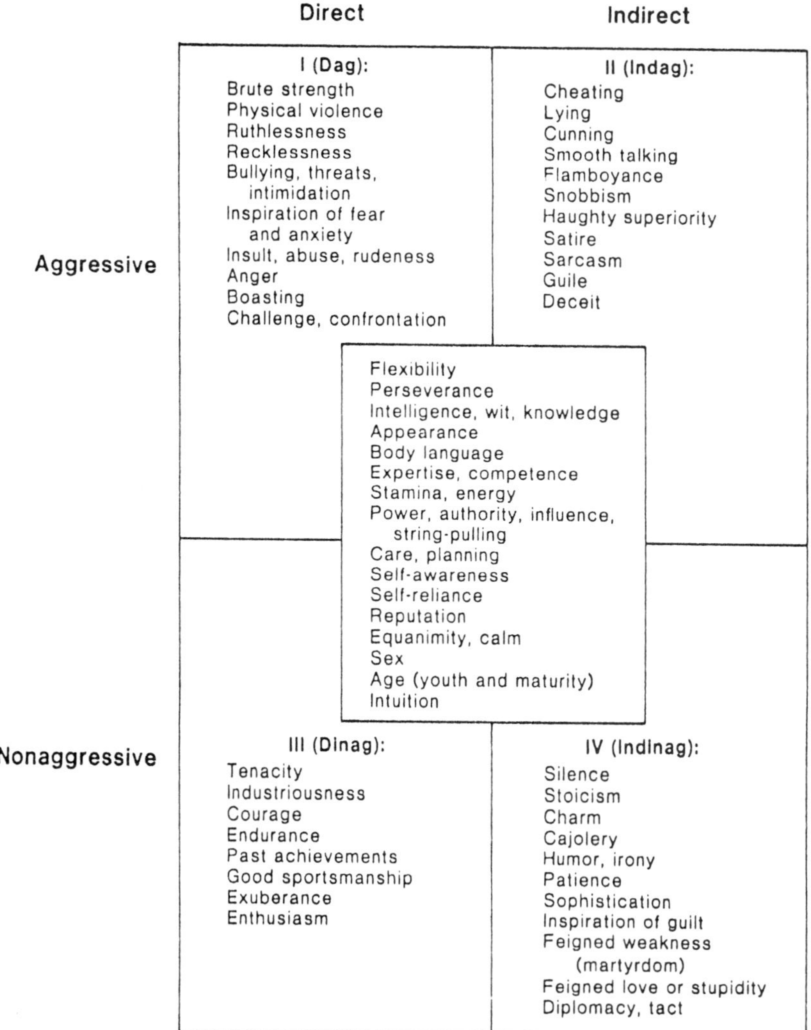


**Figure 1.** The competitor's toolbox.

*tor's Toolbox* (Figure 1). Those behaviors in quadrant I are characteristic of a **d**irect and **ag**gressive competitor (Dag); those in quadrant II, of the **ind**irect **ag**gressive competitor (Indag). The characteristics utilized by **di**rect **n**on**ag**gressive (Dinag) and **indi**rect **n**on**ag**gressive competitors (Indinag) are shown in quadrants III and IV, respectively. The tools described in the central area, which I call *Centerbox Tools,* are those common to all successful competitors. Each successful competitor usually utilizes a combination of quadrant and centerbox tools.

Through observing the particular kinds of quadrant tools physicians utilized I was able to determine which competitive style best characterized them. I also observed that if a person utilized only quadrant tools such as direct and aggressive tools or only indirect and nonaggressive tools without using a reasonable combination of the centerbox tools, he or she tended to be less successful in the long run. The physician who used only brute strength or violence, or ruthlessness, bullying, and intimidation, without using flexibility, perseverance, intelligence, stamina, care, or planning, was less likely to be successful in the long run.

It is true that you are unlikely to find too many physicians who fit into any one of the four quadrants precisely, since human beings are constantly shifting some aspects of their style—"borrowing competitive tools" other than their own. What makes a physician primarily one style of competitor rather than another is the fact that his competitive endeavors stress the importance of tools listed in a particular quadrant; most of his techniques will come from that quadrant rather than from the others. It is true that we all borrow tools from other quadrants at one time or another; however, we tend to use those tools with which we are most practiced, to increase the likelihood of success. When I assess what competitive style a physician uses, I find it useful to refer to the competitive toolbox and check off his predominant competitive tools or behaviors. Invariably I find that they tend to cluster in one of the four quadrants with a few perhaps coming from another quadrant and usually several coming from the centerbox.

Note that, although we might assume that those competitors who are direct and aggressive are frequently most successful and most difficult for us to handle, this is not necessarily true. Also, physicians who tend to be other than direct and aggressive (especially indirect and nonaggressive) frequently deny their own competitiveness. In my experience, you can be very competitive and very successful regardless of what style you utilize as long as you use your own tools effectively.

The intensity of competition, in terms of stress and anxiety levels, varies with the nature of the competitive situation. Figure 2 illustrates this principle and relates the intensity of competition to two factors: (1) whether the goal of the competition is fixed (there can be many winners), semifixed (the number of winners is limited), or unfixed (the best one wins) and (2) whether you know who the other competitors are or whether you are in a large anonymous field.

In cases where many people are trying to achieve the same fixed level of success—such as passing a licensing or board certification exam—there is a low level of interpersonal rivalry. It is not necessary to beat someone else in order to achieve the honor; anyone who meets

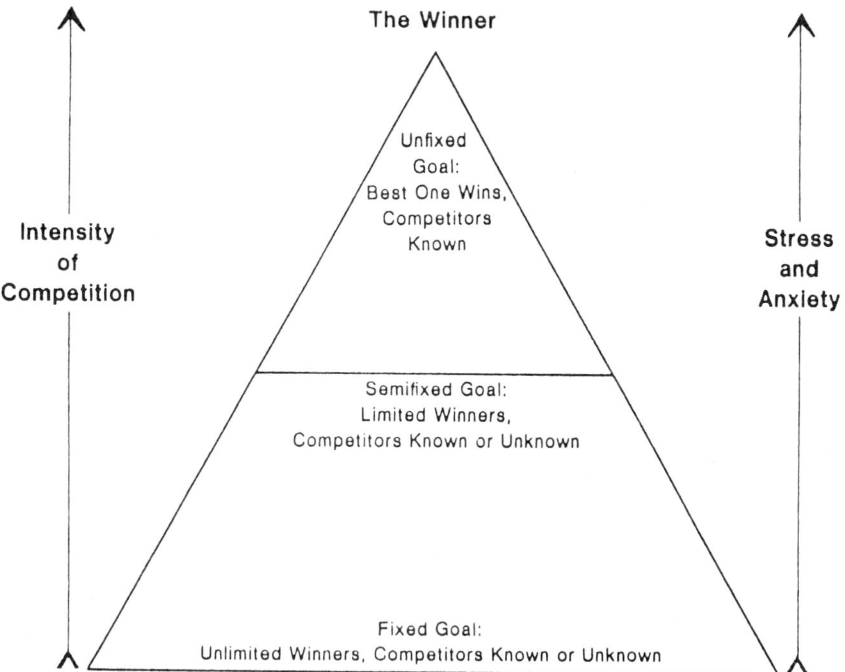


**Figure 2.** Situational variables.

the fixed standards can win. If you know many of the people with whom you are competing, it may even decrease the amount of tension, because you have a better sense of how you measure up against the others. Unknown competitors usually evoke greater anxiety and stress because we tend to magnify our opponents' strengths when we are in a poor position to assess their weaknesses realistically.

In cases where we are striving for the semifixed or limited-winner goal along with a number of other unknown rivals—such as being accepted into medical school or into a residency program—our sense of competitive anxiety may increase. This is unlikely to have an effect on the outcome, however, because whether or not you are anxious, there is still a possibility of being successful if you meet the desired standards. I refer to this as a semifixed goal because once you reach the acceptable standard you are still measured against other applicants in order to be the winner.

In situations where only the best contestant can win—such as receiving a particular grant or winning a particular research prize—the rivalry is bound to be more intense than it is when there can be many winners. In these instances even friends can become arch rivals. When the goal is quite simply to beat everyone else, interpersonal antagonism, stress, and anxiety are the most intense—no matter what kinds of competitors are in the running.

In these "best one wins" contests you are most likely to be successful if you are able to adjust your style to meet the demands of the situation. This may mean borrowing tools from other quadrants in order to meet certain exigencies. It certainly demands the use of an array of centerbox tools such as flexibility, competence, and perseverance. In these situations you almost always know your opponents, so you have an opportunity to adjust your own methods after making a realistic appraisal of your competition. If in spite of your best efforts you are still losing, you may wish to revise or adjust your style (including changing tools). You might also increase the intensity of your competitive efforts or perhaps consider ceasing competition in this arena and switching to a different one.

Another situational variable which should be considered is whether the competition takes place on a narrow individual scale or a wider group level. People compete differently when they are competing as part of a team. Therefore, it is useful to know, when analyzing competition, to what extent individual effort may be fused with (or confused with) a more general group or team effort. Individual competitive efforts can be considered microcompetition, which frequently merges into macrocompetition when we are involved in competition on a group or team level. Macrocompetition has an effect on our own individual competitive efforts. For instance, groups in which each member is dependent on the other members for the accomplishment of a designated task—such as freshman medical students dissecting a cadaver—constitute what behavioral scientists designate as a *positive interdependency group.* In such a group, each person's sense of well-being and self-esteem is enhanced while his or her interpersonal competitiveness with the other group members is decreased. Groups in which each member is directly competing with the other members, and can only get ahead at their expense—such as a pyramidal residency training program where only one person can become a chief resident—constitute *negative interdependency groups.* These tend to intensify microcompetition and diminish one's sense of self-worth and well-being. The specific type of group setting in which you find yourself necessitates adjustments in your competitive style if you are to be a success.

## COMPETING WITH YOURSELF

Thus far I have been discussing interpersonal competition. Some people believe that because they do not become involved in interpersonal competition they are not competitive; yet many reserve their most intense competitive efforts for themselves. Indeed, some find it all but impossible to compete with anyone but themselves. I have designated competition with one's self as an *autocomp*. Just as with interpersonal competition, an autocomper may employ almost any technique in order to achieve his or her goal, and may not even be aware of the competition.

Medicine is an intensely competitive area. The difference is that the competition is usually less direct than in other areas. In addition, in order to be successful in medical school and residency many physicians have become quite adept at auto-competition as well as inter-personal competition. Physicians also tend to be more nonaggressive in their competitive styles, whether they are direct or indirect.

An autocomp is a pattern of competition which substitutes an internal for an external standard of appraisal. A competitor pitted against him- or herself generally competes in a way which is not evident to others. Autocomps can serve three basic purposes: (1) enhancing ones sense of self-esteem without risking the loss of face associated with public failure; (2) avoiding direct interpersonal competition; and (3) practicing or training for interpersonal competition.

My basic premise is that our competitive urges and drives are tied to our primitive instincts for self-preservation and survival. These urges have evolved in modern humans to a point where personality development and psychological well-being are in part predicated on our ability to compete successfully. Successful development demands that each of us find an area in which we can excel. Traditionally, sports have provided a main arena for these competitive drives, but since not all are naturally athletic, it is obvious that only a few will ever be able to come out as winners in this area. The rest of us have to devise alternative areas of excellence if we are to maintain our early sense of self-esteem.

Autocomps are an excellent way for the unathletic person to overcome his or her feelings of worthlessness and inadequacy. When engaging in an autocomp you can set a goal without telling anybody about it, reach it or miss it, and receive no criticism except from yourself and your own conscience. You can change your goal every day and continue to feel better about yourself each time you reach your new goal. Even if on a certain day you choose not to work toward your goal, you are not accountable to anyone but yourself. Autocomps, therefore, are much less anxiety provoking and threatening than competition with others. They are a way of ensuring self-esteem without running the risk of invidious comparison.

I mentioned that some people may use an autocomp as a way of avoiding interpersonal competition; this especially may occur in people who fear success or failure. The success-fearing person may be afraid to compete and win, to evoke the wrath of the bested opponent, or to be exposed to the scrutiny that the winner often elicits. Unfortunately, just as such people tend to undermine themselves in interpersonal situations in order to cause themselves to fail, so may they also sabotage their own self-competitive efforts when they are forced to exceed a previous goal.

Similiarly, the failure-fearing person may also use the autocomp to prevent the fear of feeling like a loser. In an autocomp, if you fail to reach your goal, you have limitless opportunities to try again, without being censored by others. This, therefore, makes autocomps attractive to those who are competitively uncertain of themselves. However, if you are the type who has a need to punish yourself, you can surely use an autocomp to set yourself up to lose.

Not everyone who engages in an autocomp does so for negative or compensatory reasons. Many people who engage actively in interpersonal competition also utilize autocomps as practice, in order to prepare for the interpersonal competition. In addition, a person who is acknowledged as a successful competitor will often use the autocomp as a way of increasing skills and confidence to attain an even greater level. The marathon runner, for example, may autocomp on a daily basis in order to increase his or her performance level prior to running in public, interpersonal races.

Autocomps, like other forms of competition, have become so much a part of the fabric of our contemporary society that we frequently fail to recognize them. A number of the currently in-vogue autocomp activities used by physicians are running, skiing, and sailing. Physicians find that they need not compete with anyone but themselves, and these activities give them the opportunity to enhance their self-esteem greatly. As frequently occurs, once they become competent in a particular area, they may start to compete with one another and get drawn into interpersonal competition. It is the rare individual who can perfect a skill in private and not eventually feel obliged to compete publicly.

## GOAL-VAULTING

Most physicians who engage in autocomps in a productive manner have learned how to set reasonable goals for themselves and how to go about reaching them. Unfortunately, some use autocomps in a nonproductive and self-defeating manner. For these people, competing with themselves is an opportunity neither for practice nor avoidance, but merely for reiterating an already established feeling of worthlessness. Such physicians who are continually unsuccessful in their autocomps may have become what I have termed as *goal-vaulters*. The goal-vaulter is not content with achieving a reasonable goal, but must go on to achieve even greater, more outlandish ones, because he or she is unable to be satisfied with any achievement. In this sense, the goal-vaulter is fixated on the process of competition without paying true attention to the goal. This is an unhealthy form of competition because the goal-vaulter is compelled to move on to the next trial before being able to enjoy the psychological benefit of having achieved a goal.

"Climb every mountain" may be a laudable maxim, but when it is interpreted to mean that the last mountain you have just climbed was not worth the trip, then the climber is in a dangerous double-bind: obliged to climb the next mountain because it promises to give satisfaction, but knowing very well from past experience that, no matter how many goals are vaulted, they will all prove disappointing in the end.

Jill, a young energetic radiologist, was the envy of her colleagues and friends. At the age of 29, she had a doting husband, a healthy new baby, and a secure position in a group practice. To the casual observer, she was the Golden Girl, riding the crest of personal and professional success.

Inside, however, she was miserable.

When she came to me for help, Jill was an exceedingly troubled young woman. Fidgety and downcast, she confessed that the successes she had accumulated meant nothing to her; she was, in fact, considering both quitting her job and filing for divorce.

"I don't know what it is, Dr. Ruben," she complained. "Gary is a wonderful husband and father. We've been married for three years, with no problems. He's a hard worker and has been really helpful to me—especially since the baby came last year. But I don't love him anymore. I just can't stand what I'm doing at home or at work."

She laughed nervously. "You know," she continued, "it's almost as if I don't want to be happy. Every time I get what I want, I don't want it anymore."

I asked Jill to expand upon this revealing comment. It turned out that dissatisfaction with success had been a pattern in her life since she was a child. A direct, aggressive competitor, she found herself consistently dismissing compliments and poking fun at the laurels she had gained. Every step she had taken she saw as merely a prelude to the next step, in a perpetual cycle of overreaching. In high school she had been a straight-A student, but did not enjoy high school and she could not wait to get on to college. In college she made Phi Beta Kappa, but saw it only as a way to get into medical school. In medical school she yearned to be an intern, and during her internship she felt herself only biding time until her residency. When that too became boring, she decided it was because what she really wanted was to get married. Gary and she were married, therefore, while she was still a resident.

But neither marriage nor motherhood, which came two years later, solved her problem. Three years after the wedding, Jill had become impatient again. Her spouse had ceased to interest her, and she had come to the conclusion that what she needed now was a new husband. At this point, she ended up in my office—frustrated, bored, and unhappy.

Jill's type of discontent is not uncommon among Dag competitors—especially if they have come from a family background of similarly strong competitive urges—and is particularly prevalent among physicians and other professionals and executives.

I asked her to talk about her childhood, and what she revealed confirmed my suspicion that her obsession with achievements had started well before her whiz-kid high school days.

An only child, Jill was born late in the marriage of her successful, hard-driving parents, who always seemed to have more time for their careers than for her. Ever since she could remember, Jill admitted they had shown only a passing interest in her achievements. Her father, a banker, was detached and aloof; her mother, a publishing executive, acted like a meddling and hypercritical judge.

While neither parent had given Jill the approval she needed, it was her mother's negative responses that really hurt. "I never could please her," she recalled. As early as grammar school, she had worked hard to impress her parents, but had been rewarded with shrugs, silence, or outright criticism. No matter how well Jill competed, her mother remained unmoved. Neither her Phi Beta Kappa key nor her acceptance by a prestigious medical school had any affect on her mother; and, not surprisingly, it wasn't long before Jill herself ceased to consider her successes important.

She was caught in an agonizing dilemma: needing desperately to "come in first," but unable to believe that coming in first meant anything. So frequently had she been denied approval that, when she received it later in life, she could not believe it was deserved.

"I don't deserve to be content," she was really saying to herself. "Therefore, I am not content, and I have to move on to something else."

Probably her unmet need for approval was a principal reason for her initial attraction to Gary. Unlike her parents, he was extremely impressed with her, and as a husband very solicitous. For a while this seemed to be what she wanted; but then the childhood pattern reasserted itself, and she found herself, ironically, longing for the very denial she had so abhorred in her mother. So accustomed had she become to mistreatment, that she did not know what to make of applause. She expressed her confusion about Gary with the telling phrase, "He's just too good to me!"

In therapy I helped Jill see that by demanding that Gary be less solicitous, she was actually trying to elicit a response to which, however uncomfortable it made her feel, she had grown accustomed: the response of rejection. In conjoint sessions with Gary, I helped him understand what had been happening to his wife and how his ostensibly generous behavior had only aggravated her problems. He, I discovered, had been unwilling to compete with Jill at all, believing he was no match for his intelligent, successful spouse. Instead of giving her a realistic mixture of approval and disapproval, he had merely given in to her every whim, and this, predictably, had caused her to lose respect for him.

Since both Jill and Gary were committed to saving their marriage, we entered a phase of couples therapy in which Gary learned to make reasonable demands and offer the limited approval Jill needed rather than the adulation he thought she wanted. Jill responded well. As Gary became more of a friend and less of a cheering squad, he regained her respect; they reestablished the love and affection that had brought them together.

Thus while the goal-vaulter's obsession with achievement may stem from a childhood deficient in approval, such a competitive malaise cannot be cured by overcompensation. What the goal-vaulter needs is what any healthy competitor needs—realistic, balanced appraisal of how he or she is behaving. Jill ultimately learned to attend to both the process and the goals of competition rather than being overinvolved with one or the other. With this new attitude she was able to appreciate Gary's realistic input, and came to value the successes of her daily life without having to search about continually for new goals.

All of us move from one success or failure to another throughout our lives. To the extent that our successes have little meaning for us, in terms of our psychic economy and our sense of self-worth, we are compelled to leap on to new endeavors without pausing to savor the psychologically sweet taste of success. This is the goal-vaulter's tragedy.

The opposite end of the spectrum is occupied by the physician who pays no attention to the process but rather is fixated on the goals of the competition. Such a person would have the motto, "winning isn't everything, it's the only thing." Whether in an autocomp or an interpersonal competition, this person will go to any length to meet or achieve a goal. Unfortunately since none of us can win all the time, this person is frequently thwarted and ends up feeling like a loser in spite of a good performance—a "sore loser," in fact. We shall discuss this syndrome in more detail later.

## ARENAS OF COMPETITION

Competition occurs in all areas of our lives, throughout our life. There are basically five arenas of competition: (1) home and family, (2) school, (3) playing field, (4) work place and (5) community at large. A sixth arena of competiton which actually overlaps the other five is sexual competition, which we shall examine as a separate issue.

### Home and Family

The family is the training ground wherein we learn to compete. The way our parents and our siblings involve themselves in competition helps to set the tone for us in our competitive endeavors throughout the rest of our life. Competition within the family actually begins with the establishment of the marital couple. Whatever competitive patterns the couple brings to the relationship will influence their interaction throughout the marriage.

Once the wife is pregnant, the father may frequently become involved in what I have called "unintentional competition" with the developing fetus. To the extent that the father has to subjugate his wants and needs to those of the developing child, he may recognize the competitive aspect of this situation. When the expectant mother has to change her behavior because of physical demands placed on her by her pregnancy and is no longer able to relate to her husband in exactly the same manner—either because she is too tired, too sick, or too pregnant—this affects their relationship. Thus the new father finds himself having to make concessions and change his own life to meet the changes in his wife caused by the developing baby.

After the first child has taken his or her place in the family, the mother's second pregnancy serves to initiate sibling rivalry. Initially it is unintentional rivalry, but as soon as the baby is born it blossoms into full bloom. The core issue in sibling rivalry is the fear that with the advent of the new baby Mom and Dad will no longer be as loving as before. No matter how hard parents attempt to communicate to children that they have enough love in their hearts for all, older children continue to harbor the fear that they will be loved less.

As a result of sibling rivalry, older children "put down" younger children, telling them that they are dumb or stupid or inadequate in some way. On the face this seems ludicrous, for we know that for many years the younger child will rarely be as big or strong or smart as the older sibling. However, the older child who feels dethroned as King or Queen of the Mountain cannot help but continually attempt to prove that he or she is worthy of continued love. As the younger child grows older, the tension may shift, the younger child starting to compete with the older one, also to demonstrate worthiness.

In homes in which all the children feel frankly and equally loved, sibling rivalry, although it still exists, seldom becomes a major problem. In these situations the children can be confident that parental affection is not predicated on how acceptably they behave. Thus they can use sibling rivalry as a way of learning how to test themselves in competitive situations. If they are sure of their parents' love, siblings can use each other as practicing partners to spur each other on to a better realization of their individual characters without the fear that their failures will mean the loss of parental love. Children who grow up with this sense of security are far more likely to become successful adults. Physicians who have had this experience are most likely to be able to develop a true sense of altruism which is an essential ingredient of "the art" of medicine.

## Academic Competition

The next area in which future physicians involve themselves is academic competition. The various kinds of pressure encountered initially are those produced by the transition from the supportive family to kindergarten or nursery school. I call this transition the *early school crisis* because many young children have trouble accepting that the rules of the game have changed. Within the family the young child is usually able to get his or her own way; once in group learning with other children, the child is forced to learn that he or she can no longer always prevail.

Further along in school, the tension shifts from the initial pressure between convincing teacher and friends and conforming to their urgings, to a pressure and tension between performing (teacher/parents) and conforming, (peers). This is the *late school crisis,* which occurs usually in early adolescence, and the conforming tension usually pushes towards not doing so well in school. A child planning to go to medical school, of course, can not give in to such pressure, and the intensity of the competition increases. There can be no let up in performance during high school or college if one expects to go into medical school.

Once in medical school, performance pressures remain the same in order to graduate and obtain a reasonable residency. It is interesting to note that considering the various styles and tools of competition, a direct and nonaggressive approach is the most appropriate in school. Tenacity, reliance on learned facts, and burning midnight oil are helpful in academic competition.

When parents become overinvolved in their children's competitive endeavors, this may lead to problems. One young patient, Shirley, was brought to me by her parents when she was 16 because she was doing poorly in school. Both of her parents were physicians—bright, highly motivated, successful. They wanted the same for their daughter.

Shirley, who had inherited much of their intelligence, was having none of it. For some time she had simply refused to perform in school, and as a result, in spite of her intelligence, was barely passing most of her subjects.

Her parents' reaction was typical—and typically unsuccessful in motivating her to respond differently. With each new report card showing a lack of academic improvement, they chose to place severe restrictions on her as an "incentive" to do better. In the year before the family finally came for help. Shirley had lost car, TV, phone, and dating privileges; but none of these deprivations had had the desired effect. Resentful but unmoved, Shirley had simply failed to respond to her parents' competitive ambitions.

"If she weren't so intelligent," her mother confided, "I wouldn't care so much. But she's so smart, it kills me to see her doing poorly. That's why we've placed the restrictions on her, but it doesn't seem to help."

"What you're saying," I responded, "is that Shirley is being punished for being bright. If she were less intelligent and making the same grades, she wouldn't be on restriction."

But that was only part of the problem. The real issue was that, as Shirley herself recognized, her parents were trying to relive their own adolescent years through her. Her mother in particular felt that when she had been Shirley's age, she had never quite lived up to her own academic potential. She therefore wanted Shirley to make up for it, to become the whiz kid she had failed to become. As she pushed her daughter to excel, Shirley, in a not-uncommon pattern, rebelled against the parental attempt to direct her life. The placing of restrictions on her as punishment was, in effect, an acknowledgment that all other means had failed. All it did was to add a new difficulty to Shirley's performance—conformity tension. She now had to weigh her own needs and desires against those of her parents.

Parents who overidentify with their children's competitive efforts frequently elicit exactly the opposite kind of behavior from that they had hoped to receive. In this situation the best thing that the parents could have done was to retreat and allow Shirley to manage her own school tensions in her own way. Shirley perceived their demands as meddling; thus they actually had a counterproductive effect.

## Athletic Competition

Sometimes physicians use the athletic activities of their children to sublimate their own thwarted athletic ambitions in a very dysfunctional manner. One situation I handled concerned a neurosurgeon father who was an excellent surgeon, but a thwarted baseball player. He became overly involved in his son's little league activities—so involved that he attended every game, standing on the sidelines yelling directions to his son. Unfortunately, the more he yelled, the more likely his son was to make errors; the more errors his son made, the more exasperated and vociferous he became. He inevitably succeeded in "psyching out" the whole team, and they all had difficulty playing. It became so bad he eventually was asked by the parents of the other children not to attend the games, because he was actually disrupting the team's ability to play. The problem for this doctor was that he developed an overaccentuation on winning. As we saw earlier, winning is not everything; if it becomes everything, there will be problems for you and for your children.

**Economic Competition**

Competition in the work place or business world is something of which we are aware, but with which we may or may not be very familiar. Depending on the area of medicine and how far along you are in your career, you may still be more involved with academic rather than economic competition. As mentioned previously, many physicians are attracted to medicine because they perceive it to be relatively free from economic competition. This is obviously a naive view, but one that I have found to occur with some frequency in premedical and medical students. The belief is that by dedicating yourself to serving humankind, you can transcend economic competitive activities. At the same time you assure yourself a profession which provides rewards both in money and prestige. Thus, many young people who feature themselves as economically noncompetitive enter medicine.

However, as we have seen, it is virtually impossible to avoid competition. The young physician who remains in academia following training may avoid the business side of medicine, but for those who become involved in private practice, economic competition in medicine becomes a real and intense pressure. The physician/businessperson quickly learns the intricacies of the cash journal, accounts receivable and payable, and the balance sheet. There is also a great pressure to generate enough income to support the administrative side of the practice in addition to maintaining a reasonable lifestyle.

Physicians who become involved in group practice, partnerships, or professional corporations often become even more involved in the business side of medicine and economic competition. The complexities of managing different kinds of group practice can be just as great as those involved in running any small to medium-sized business, and the pressures to generate income are equally great. Thus, physicians experience the same kinds of job-related anxiety as occurs for other businesspeople. The corporate side of medicine, whether in the hospital or in one of the other areas of organized medicine, can create the exact same pressures as being in one of the Fortune 500 corporations. Thus physicians, like other corporate executives, are forced to make sacrifices in terms of family and recreational time to move up the corporate ladder, and are pressured to become more productive and generate more income in the group or corporate setting.

Physicians are not immune to what I have termed *executive vertigo,* which is common in the business world. Executive vertigo is the kind of pressure and tension that one experiences when moving up the executive ladder. There is a direct relationship between the level of responsibility that one achieves in corporate medicine and job-related pressures and anxiety. At a certain point the anxiety and psychological pressures may outweigh the positive benefits of the job; it is then appropriate to seek a new, less pressured situation in which to work.

In settings in which a physician is dependent on co-workers for the accomplishment of tasks, (a positive interdependency group), there is an enhancement of self-esteem when the group is successful. Conversely, in the negative interdependency group, each person is competing with other persons in the group to get ahead. A mixed interdependency group balances cooperation and rivalry among its members. For instance, you might find the members of a medical school department competing in a positive interdependent fashion to develop a grant in opposition to other medical facilities. At the same time each physician competes against the others to get ahead within the department, which creates a negative environment. How a particular organization deals with the competitiveness of its members ultimately affects the overall productivity of that organization.

Success in the corporate setting is not always to be equated with personal happiness. For many, achieving the pinnacle of success, whether chief of staff or chairman of the department, has placed such great demands on our psychic economy that even when we achieve these positions, we cannot truly be happy. The pressures and tensions of the positions and the sacrifices that must be made to handle them can be overwhelming. If you find as you rise up the ladder that your satisfaction decreases rather than increases, this is a sign that you should reexamine your goals and priorities. Sometimes it means switching positions; other times it may even mean considering a change of goals or even fields.

### Competition in the Community

Social competition is one of the main areas in which we are involved throughout life. Within the community we see a great deal of competition through status symbols. These, like all symbols, have little value in themselves; they are coveted mainly because of what they represent. When we buy an expensive car or house or boat, in addition to the psychological values of having the item itself, we are also making an outward statement. When our possession is seen and acknowledged as worthy of respect by our social peers, it enchances the value of that item.

This notion of status symbols as outward-directed gestures is very important to an understanding of social competition. Symbols tell us that we have met the standards of a group, that we have crossed some invisible finish line to earn our stripes as group members.

Group status symbols reinforce our feelings of belonging; they also make it clear who is not "one of us"—who is a member of a different opposing group. Most medical specialties have a few professionally elite groups which exclude the majority of the practitioners. We join these groups to be accepted by our peers, but also to be "one up" on those we consider outsiders or unworthy. Much of the subsequent interaction between this and other groups is a matter of macrocompetition, in which our personal competitive urges may be subsumed under the banner of a larger and more powerful grouping. Thus, group membership always looks outward; the proudly waved banner functions at the same time as a warning flag, telling all those who do not belong to keep away. The various Medical School Alumni receptions held at Major Medical Meetings or the various professional associations which select only a small number of specifically qualified physicians for memberships are examples of this kind of public statement. The meaning of this psychologically is that by belonging to a group we experience an enhanced sense of self-esteem and self-worth.

There is no doubt that, in some situations, status symbols such as fancy clothes and posh addresses can be a real asset competitively. The intern or resident who appears for a job interview at a conservative hospital in a T-shirt and sneakers is not going to stand anywhere near as good a competitive chance as one who comes in appropriate attire. There is a real difficulty that arises when something like appearance, which can be an effective competitive tool, is confused with overall competitive goals. Being driven to the hospital in a limousine may prove to be a good competitive gimmick; it may impress colleagues that one is far more successful than they are. However, if the whole point of one's efforts is merely to be seen, shadow has already been confused with substance, and priorities should be reassessed.

Much of what follows pertains not only to politicians and the political process in general, but also to physicians who become involved with politics within the community or, specifically, with the politics of medicine. Obviously, it need not apply to every physician who becomes involved in medical politics; but the fact that the American Psychiatric Association had to limit campaigning and expenditures for the organization's presidential candidates a few years ago suggests that medical politics can indeed get out of hand.

I consider medical politics to be a special kind of social competition. Political success in general or in medicine may be seen as the pinnacle of social success. The successful politician-doctor—that is, the one who gets elected—has achieved a kind of ultimate competitive victory in the social sphere by securing the fullest and, in our society, the most well-articulated expression of general approval and esteem. He or she has demonstrated "popularity." Getting elected, then, satisfies for the physician politician the very same inner needs that are satisfied for most of us by less grandiose social accomplishments, e.g., election to an honorary professional society or acceptance by a certain social set. It is no accident that many successful physician politicians serve their apprenticeship by being active on various committees or editorial boards of our professional societies. Becoming the leader of such a group fulfills on a nonpolitical level the same desires that getting elected to office fulfills on the political one; in both cases the competition for a sense of belonging has turned into a need for more particular, individual esteem. On a basic level, then, we can see political competition in medicine merely as an extension of competition between individuals and between groups, first for general approval and secondly for eminence.

However, politics has a psychological component which also makes it quite different from competition in the nonpolitical social sphere. For most politicians, the twin needs for approval and esteem are augmented by a third, and far more driving need: the need for influence and power. The motivation to get elected can clearly be related to a hunger for pushing through one's ideas, programs, and sense of self-worth at the expense of one's opponent. All of us have some interest in being carried aloft in the sedan chair; the politician (whether or not a physician) also wants to give orders while up there.

This need for power and influence may mask a deeper need for approval, which should lead us to look somewhat more sympathetically than is perhaps customary on those social lions and medical political giants who seem driven by a lust for power and control. Paradoxically, they may be the very people who are most in need of reassurance that they are worthwhile individuals; their yearning for the top may be seen as a transmutation of an older and constantly unsatisfied yearning for someone to say "You're all right."

The need for power, furthermore, seems to be a self-regenerating need. It is not only very seductive, but can also become, for the successful political climber, almost addictive. Many medical politicians, like entertainers, live on the sound of applause of approval; once they begin to hear that sound, it become extremely difficult for them to live without it. They may continue competing, then, not so much to further their society's programs as to keep hearing the voice of general approval. They are competing, in other words, for a symbol of success rather than for the chance to use that success intelligently. As peculiarly outer-directed people, they must be able to see themselves smiling in a thousand mirrors before they can believe in their own validity. Their consensual validation may have a much wider sphere than that of the members of most groups, but it has the same origin in psychological need.

Because political competition can be so addictive, it can become all-encompassing, forcing the physician to sacrifice practice, friends, and even health in a single-minded pursuit of the "position"—the desire for popular acclaim. Physician-politicians as well as others in political pursuits will attest to difficulties in their personal lives engendered by their competitive drive: we frequently hear of colleagues with domestic troubles that can be traced to this compulsion for power.

The pressures to which power seekers subject themselves can be overwhelming. Election campaigns frequently require that they work long hours with little sleep or little time to eat, and no time at all to relax. Since they are under scrutiny by their opponents and colleagues, they can never let down their guard, but must be continually alert. They have no certainty about success, and very little assurance that the campaign tactics that have worked last year will be equally effective this year. Since these tactics (or we might say styles) vary greatly, from the direct and aggressive to the indirect and nonaggressive, the campaigning physician is in the position of a competitor who is not quite sure of the rules of the game, but is aware that they may be changing every minute. As a result, there is a continual level of anxiety and doubt throughout the campaign. It is not surprising that drugs and alcohol may be abused in this period; such substances, whatever their later addictive effects, can at least alleviate the more severe pressures of the campaign for a while.

Once elected, the politician's worries do not cease, but take different forms: various pressure groups often converge to offer their own complicated, and frequently conflicting, programs; long hours must still be spent at work away from family: and then there are still the pressures of running the organization. The need to maintain an image of competence and reliability, while attending to manifold problems that promote self-doubt, leads many an ostensibly successful leader into a depression for which drugs and alcohol, again, often provide the only solace.

We are now touching on what is perhaps the most deep-seated problem of the would-be politician, and it is really only a variation of what we have identified as the central difficulty of social competition in general: I mean the confusion between image and reality, or the mistaken belief that what you are showing to gain external approval is identical with what you need to feel good about yourself. Numerous leaders fall into the trap of believing their own "press releases," their own campaign descriptions of themselves. They forget that competitive success in the social sphere requires a certain amount of lily-gilding, and they begin to believe that they are just as good, virtuous, hard-working, and resourceful as they must make their supporters believe they are. Frequently, they end up lying to themselves as much as to their constituents; they have allowed themselves to confuse mirror images with the real thing.

This is not to say that all organizational leaders are liars. Many of them surely believe their own campaign promises and would be shocked by the suggestion that they are dissembling. The point is that in order to win a popularity poll, you have to prove yourself not competent so much as deserving of popularity. In many cases this means remaking yourself in the image of what you think your supporters want. The problem is that many leaders start to fool themselves, and can continue to do so for long periods of time. They see themselves being successful competitively as they adopt new public images, eventually losing sight of the fact that those images were adopted in the first place to "win friends and influence people" and not because of any intimate connection they might bear to the competitor's real needs and desires.

The trouble with selling yourself on image rather than substance is that, like the person who uses status symbols as goals rather than tools, you may end up unable to tell your manufactured needs apart from those that are truly inherent. You may find yourself in the position of the person who, sporting a designer outfit and high-style haircut, looks in the mirror and asks, "Is that really me?"

Style is an extremely important tool in social competition, and an even more important one in political competition. However, the clothes one wears, the car one drives, and the smile one adopts for speeches not only "make the man" but become the man, in spite of oneself. In other words, there is a great danger in social competition of becoming engulfed by the many external symbols commonly employed to make climbing up the social or political ladder easier. When trapped by these symbols, a realistic distinction between goals and tools cannot be made. Though publicly acclaimed, one is privately without an anchor.

**Sexual Competition**

Several years ago a doctor and his wife, who had three teenaged daughters, came to me for consultation about the youngest of the three. Lisa was 14 at the time, and in the past year, they explained, she had become increasingly defiant and uncooperative, both at home and at school. Her attendance record was poor, and even when she did attend classes, the teachers could not manage to interest her in her work. At home she was sullen and nasty to her older sisters. The parents were at a loss.

I met with Lisa alone for the first time a couple of days later. It did not take long to discover that her parents' description had been fairly accurate. She confessed to me her hostility toward her sisters, and acknowledged readily that she was simply not interested in school. It was a fairly standard case of sibling rivalry, in which the younger sibling, overshadowed by the older and more "attractive" ones, felt herself rejected and unwanted by her parents. Her parents did little to correct this impression, since they were both quite busy—her father with his practice and her mother with community affairs. They could not seem to find the time to spend with any of their daughters, time the children obviously needed. Their lack of attention to Lisa aggravated her feelings of inferiority; it was not long before she began cutting classes and "acting out" to attract their attention.

The most interesting fact I discovered in talking with Lisa was that, in addition to rebelling against her parent's inattention by becoming disobedient, she was also extremely active sexually: within the past year, she told me, she had been to bed with over a dozen boys. She was, in fact, beginning to develop a "reputation" at school; the fact that her parents did not know this was an indication of their lack of awareness and sensitivity to her.

It was obvious that Lisa's promiscuity was provoked by her feelings of inferiority in relation to her sisters and by feeling unwanted by her parents. She had entered high school with grades that were not quite up to those of her siblings. She had just about begun to resign herself to being "second best" there, as she had been in grammar school, when she discovered a startling fact, if she went to bed with boys, they would like her. If only for a while, they would give her the attention that her family would not give her.

So, Lisa adopted sex as a prime competitive tool. It had a salutory double effect: first, it was a way of punishing her inattentive parents by flouting their own sexual standards; secondly, it got back at her sisters by making Lisa successful in a field in which they had not even begun to experiment. As soon as Lisa discovered that she could secure the image, if not the substance, of affection from her liaisons, she started using sex quite indiscriminately, gradually changing it from a mere tool into her entire field or arena of competitive behavior. Since she could not compete on the home front, she switched; in her new chosen field (sexuality), she perceived herself, for the first time in her life, as a success.

However, she was not genuinely happy about herself. For one

thing, she had changed arenas, so she was not really competing well with her sisters. Also, she was smart enough to know the difference between honest affection and attention paid to someone for the purposes of gaining sexual favors. The more boys she ended up with in bed, the more she began to see that, while this might have been better than no attention at all, it was really not what she wanted. Sexually, she was a good competitor, but she had chosen the wrong arena to fulfill herself. Inside she still felt like a failure; that, in fact, was one of the reasons she had to change boyfriends continually—she needed constant proof that she was desirable.

Fortunately, Lisa came into therapy while she was still young enough to reverse her dysfunctional behavior pattern. Through conjoint sessions with her parents, we were able to help the family become aware of how they were failing to meet Lisa's needs. They then began to interact with her more meaningfully. As she started to feel better about herself, she became more interested in school, learned to compete with her peers in less self-destructive ways, and ultimately settled down with one boyfriend.

Lisa's story illustrates only one of the many patterns in which that popular center-box tool, sex, can be used in a competitive manner and even transformed, unfortunately, into a person's major competitive arena. Promiscuity is a fairly common human response to the felt need for approval and affection; since our society has made it very easy to confuse sexual contact with affection, people like Lisa (both male and female) frequently adopt it as a way of getting the attention they need. Like the wide variety of games on the playing field, there are many sexual games or patterns which are no less common.

Lisa's use of sex falls into the category of behavior which I call *genital sexual competition:* the use of actual physical sexuality in a competitive manner. This type of behavior often arises in the early teenage years, when puberty naturally focuses a good deal of attention on sex as a new pleasure, forbidden fruit, and competitive tool. Before puberty, sex is already used competitively, but we do so in behavior patterns that fall into the category I call *gender sexual competition.*

Gender competition is competition between members of the opposite sex which is based on the simple physical differences between them. This pattern continues, with modifications, into adulthood, although by then it is frequently compounded by various types of genital competition. The "battle of the sexes" has its origin in gender competition.

Women in medicine and in the business world often tell me that when they get into a tense situation with a male colleague, the man frequently will turn to some type of genital sexual ploy as a way to defuse the situation or disarm the woman. This occurs in ways which would be totally inappropriate were two males interacting. A pinch on the cheek or a pat on the arm (or some other area of the anatomy) with the implication that the woman overreacted or is out of control and needs to calm down is actually a type of a genital competitive ploy. Telling stories that have sexual references or are vulgar or obscene is another way of attempting to disarm the woman by using genital sexual ploys.

An excellent example of this confusion of genital and gender sexual competition occurred to a woman surgical resident with whom I was working who had just received the position of chief surgical resident in a large municipal hospital. During the year preceding her appointment she had been competing for this position with a male resident with whom she had worked very closely for several years. They were intensely gender competitive (female vs male) as she attempted to prove that she was equally worthy to all the other male physicians in the program. When notified of her promotion to chief resident, she was overjoyed and could hardly believe it. When she shared her good news with her male colleague, she knew he would be disappointed because she had been competing with him, but she was unprepared for the response that she received. He looked at her and sneered, "The only reason that you got it was because you're a woman." The implication was that she had been given the appointment because she was attractive or perhaps had been supplying some sort of sexual favors to the chief of the department, not because she was exceedingly competent as a surgeon.

In this instance the male resident was attempting to turn the female resident's gender sexual victory (the woman besting the man based upon her own competence, skill, and expertise) into his genital sexual victory, implying that that was not the case, but rather that it was her genital sexuality that had gotten her the position. In fact, had the woman doctor thought even briefly that he was correct, she might have felt like a loser; she would have suffered a loss of self-esteem rather than the enhancement that goes along with successful competition. Fortunately, however, she was quite secure in her own sense of worth and merely looked at her male colleague and laughed. This only made him feel worse about himself and reconfirmed that he had been bested by a more able competitor.

Sexual competition overlaps all arenas of competition and spills into other areas of our lives. The case of the woman resident was an example of competition on the job, but it also illustrated how an unsuccessful person may attempt to shift the focus to the genital sexual area as a way to turn the tables. This happens not only consciously, but also unconsciously, especially in marriage. Often, when couple are having other kinds of problems, this will also affect their sex lives.

I recently consulted with a couple, Mary and Tom, who were residents at the same hospital and were having sexual difficulties. They had married during their internship and, although in different specialties, had experienced a great deal of gender competition in relation to their jobs. Mary was very bright, competent, and well liked; she was the shining star among all the residents in the hospital. Although Tom was also an excellent doctor, he felt lackluster in comparison to Mary. Whenever they were together socially, people paid more attention to Mary while Tom stood on the sidelines. Also, Tom received continual compliments about Mary which, unfortunately, only intensified his feelings of inferiority.

In reaction to this, Tom started spending more and more time attending to his work. He spent longer hours at the hospital and more time doing paper work and reading journal articles. Thus, they had even less time to spend together than would be expected, and eventually they did not even have time to make love. When Mary complained of Tom's lack of attention, he explained that he was just too tired after a strenuous day at work. When they did have intercourse, Tom suffered from premature ejaculation. Psychologically, he was getting sex over with in a hurry, so as not to give her too much pleasure.

Mary initially came to me complaining that she could no longer satisfy her husband. Tom had unconsciously managed to shift Mary's gender sexual success over him into his genital sexual "superiority." Mary actually interpreted Tom's sexual problem as her failure and identified herself as a "psychiatric case"; thus she sought help. I involved both of them in couples crisis intervention therapy, a form of brief treatment appropriate for their difficulties. In a relatively short period of time they were able to see how each of them had contributed to Tom's "tiredness" and "quick trigger." If his sexual interest and ability were to be restored, they would both have to make an effort to focus attention on each other as well as on their professional activities. This made them realize that time was not limited when it came to a sexual response; what they had been missing was not the time to deal with each other, but the will.

One of the most common difficulties associated with sexuality today is the failure of one partner to "perform" sexually to the satisfaction or expectation of the other. The new sexual freedom is placing increasing demands for performance on everyone; as a result, we are seeing a greater emphasis on competition in the sexual arena. As the media have intensified their emphasis on open and relaxed sexuality and sexual mores, each person experiences mounting internal pressures and tensions to start changing attitudes and actions in light of these new norms. I have heard many young people complaining of the pressures they have experienced to increase their sexual activity. They feel that in order to be accepted, to compete with their peers, they must do things that they might not do under other circumstances. These increased sexual pressures, which are experienced by young and old alike these days, can be quite severe, leading to a good deal of anxiety over "performance."

In addition to pressure generated by relaxed sexual mores, there has been a steadily increasing focus on performance as a goal of love-making. This can lead to a quantitative rather than qualitative appraisal of sex, with results that are both ludicrous and harmful for everyone involved. We have all heard amusing tales of all-night lovers who judge sexual performance on the basis of how many times they have achieved orgasm, or have helped their partners to achieve orgasm. Such an attitude can be psychologically damaging, because it detracts from the pleasure of the moment which is one of the real delights of sex. If your attention is all devoted to counting orgasms, you are unlikely to have a very good time on the way. In many cases I have seen concern for "getting there" at a specified time or speed lead to the common dysfunction of premature ejaculation for the man and resultant dissatisfaction for the woman.

In other words, a "winning is everything" attitude toward sexuality is no more effective in creating a real victory in the bedroom than it is on the playing field. In sex, far more than in almost any other endeavor, playing the game for the sheer fun of it is far more important in terms of final satisfaction than getting high scores.

## HEALTHY COMPETITION

The healthy competitor has a positive self-image, is not emotionally or physically constrained by competition, and enters into it in a hearty, unguilty manner, hoping and trying to win but realizing that failure is always a possibility and can be accepted. The healthy competitor may be quite aggressive and bold about getting ahead, but does not focus all of his or her identity on any particular competition. For the really healthy competitor, winning is the icing on the cake; the real name of the game is striving for personal excellence, win or lose.

At a marathon race some months ago, I happened to spot a rather overweight runner in the midst of a pack of much sleeker, obviously more expert runners. I watched him closely as he passed in front of the spectators, trying to get a glimpse of his face to see how being so obviously outclassed was making him react. He was being passed continually by better runners, and I thought this might be making him feel disgruntled: I expected to catch a frown, or at least an expression of physical pain.

As he approached, though, I saw that his face had an expression of utter delight. There he was, plodding along in his own markedly "unsuccessful" way, and he was radiant, exuding self-confident health. I realized that wherever he came in in the final "scoring," whether he ended up first or last, he would be a winner. That overweight runner (who I later learned was a urologist), intent on the process rather than the goal of his competition, was someone I would call not only healthy, but also successful—successful on his own terms.

By way of contrast, the unhealthy competitor, even if frequently successful, will experience various physical or psychological symptoms in the midst of the competition. Health problems like stomach troubles, alcohol or drug overuse, sexual difficulties, recurrent fatigue, insomnia or listlessness, all may be associated from time to time with unhealthy forms of competitive behavior. If you heed these physical symptoms you will realize that your body is trying to tell you something about the way you compete. The wise competitor, no matter what the present level of "success," pays attention to such warning signs. Beyond that, there are a host of vaguer psychological difficulties which frequently accompany unhealthy competitive behavior. These include anxiety, tension, frustration, anger, guilt, and shame experienced prior to, during, or after the competition. Again, if you are troubled by such emotions often, it may be time for you to reassess your competitive hopes, tactics, and style. All of these feelings are signals that your psyche is laboring under an undue amount of stress, and that it may be time to analyze how and why you compete.

Not all stress is harmful; in fact, a modest amount of anxiety may even provide a psychological boost in certain types of competition. Just as medical students or residents get keyed up before exams, so do athletes speak of getting "psyched up" before a game or meet, meaning they feel they have a better competitive edge when, just before the beginning of their event, they feel a little queasy, nervous, and impatient to begin. Actors and actresses about to go on stage speak of the same phenomenon. What is commonly identified as "butterflies in the stomach" may therefore be a special sign of readiness rather than true anxiety. As long as the student, athlete, or actor does not have to carry it around throughout the day, it may be a welcome spur to a stronger competitive effort.

Still, this kind of "beneficial stress" is a special case. For the most part, the presence of stress, whether chronic or acute, tells you that you are not competing in the best interest of your psychological or physical health. You may be competing compulsively, or opting out of competition because of a fear of failure, or of success. For whatever reason, if you are carrying a permanent butterfly jar inside of you, take a closer look at how you go about participating. Your own feelings about yourself, physical and emotional, are the first and truest guide as to whether or not you are competing in a healthy manner.

Beyond that, it is important that you balance your attention between the process and the goals of the competition. Many competitors fall into unhealthy behavior patterns precisely because they give so much more weight to one than to the other that they keep forgetting what the race is all about. It is like going to an AMA Annual Meeting and attending all the CME courses you can because you need the credits without paying attention to the relevance of the content for your practice. By keeping in mind both the process and the goals of a competitive situation, and attending to both relatively evenly, you are much more likely to accrue the beneficial aspects of healthy competition.

Knowing how to maintain such a healthy balance involves a good deal of self-knowledge and self-acceptance.

The healthy competitor realizes that there is a limit to the amount of revision you can do on your psyche and still call yourself "yourself." Also, avid as the healthy competitor may be to win, there is a final realization that not only can you not always be a winner, but that if you are constantly concerned exclusively with winning, you will never enjoy yourself while competing.

These qualities are perhaps the foremost characteristics of all healthy and successful competitors. Achieving them is no easy matter, but I think that learning how to visualize and accept yourself in any competitive situation may be facilitated by an attention to three important steps.

## Step One: Assessing Your Situation

The Socratic dictum "know thyself" is an especially useful guide for the competitive physician to keep in mind; without an adequate assessment of who we are, we can never hope to achieve any kind of competitive success. Knowing yourself in this sense means understanding both your particular strengths and weaknesses. While the former are, of course, generally much easier to identify than the latter, an awareness of both, and of the ways they work together, is essential to competing well.

Knowing your strengths and weaknesses helps you decide, first of all, what kinds of competition you want to (or should) enter, and which you would do well to avoid. If, for example, you have a quick mind but no patience with detail, it is unlikely you would make a very good researcher; knowing this before you attempt to compete with people who love to handle detailed protocols may save you a lot of unnecessary stress. Most of us at one time or another enter competitions which are simply out of our league; we could keep our losses to a minimum merely by becoming aware of what we do well and what gives us trouble.

In addition to knowing your own strengths and weaknesses, you must gather as much information as you possibly can about your opponents and about the competitive situation in which you are about to become involved. The more information you have, the more likely you will be able to perform adequately and not be caught off guard. Also, being able to predict how your opponents will perform based on a knowledge of their previous performance will enable you to have contingency plans or alternative modes of action set up for yourself depending upon how the situation is progressing.

### Step Two: Playing the Game According to Your Own Best Rules

Having assessed the situation adequately and come to terms with your own strengths and weaknesses, you can now utilize your strengths to your advantage, rather than being caught up in your own shortcomings. Many of us spend a great deal of time worrying about what we do not do well rather than attending to what we do do well. We spoke earlier in the chapter about competitive tools that are characteristics of our personalities. Although the best competitors may borrow competitive tools from quadrants other than their own, their style of approach tends to remain pretty consistent throughout all their competitive efforts; they usually rely on tools from their own quadrant, with which they are most comfortable. The physician who attempts to be aggressive when it is not part of his or her nature will not be very good at it. Utilize those tools characteristic of or consistent with your own style. If I am direct and aggressive and you are indirect and nonaggressive, I am far more comfortable using threats, challenge, confrontation, or boasting (some of my best tools) whereas you are best with such tools as charm, patience, and sophistication. I am far more likely to be successful if I force you to use unfamiliar tactics such as the direct and aggressive ones I use. Thus we have a much greater chance of being successful if we do what we do well, according to our own best rules.

When you observe that your opponent is beginning to use weapons rather than tools, you know he or she is in trouble. By a weapon I mean a competitive technique that is designed to harm another person—like using a hacksaw rather than a scalpel to do surgery. The distinction, I hope, is obvious. When you begin to use weapons rather than tools yourself, it is time to reassess your position.

### Step Three: Setting Reasonable Goals

Knowing yourself and playing according to your own rules will still not ensure your success in competition if you insist on setting goals so high that they are basically out of your reach. Nor will you come out ahead if you consistently set mixed or conflicting goals. Your best chance of succeeding rests on being able to predict the probable outcome of a particular competition based on a reasonable assessment of your own abilities and the apparent abilities of your rivals, and then going after a possibly attainable goal with all the energy and imagination you can muster. True, if you aim consistently low, you will only succeed in breaking even; but if you aim consistently too high, you will gain even less, and end up frustrated in the bargain. "Dreaming the impossible dream" may work on Broadway, but it seldom does in medicine.

Gauging an outcome, then, is a matter of weighing your own potential against the many situational variables of the particular competition in which you are interested. Your chances for success are enhanced the closer to reasonable expectations you set your goals, and diminished the closer they get to fantasy or mere wish-fulfillment. You may, for example, want desperately to become a famous surgeon, and you may say to yourself that you will become one, come what may, by the time you are 30. That is not likely to be a reasonable goal. There are so many variables associated with becoming a famous surgeon that no amount of "wishing it were so" will help you compete successfully if chance and circumstances are against you.

The reasonableness of a goal is something, however, that need not be left up to prediction or chance entirely. The most successful, healthiest physicians/competitors take frequent readings of their progress to see if they have overestimated or underestimated their capacities. Each new competitive situation affords you a new opportunity to do this. Therefore, competition itself can be a useful guide to further competition, for our success or failure in one event allows us to undergo a process of reality testing that is of value for our future endeavors. We can thus see if our perceptions of ourselves within a particular competitive situation are, in fact, accurate. The closer in line with your own actual capabilities your goals are, the less likely you will be to fall into the trap of chasing truly impossible dreams, and the more likely you will be, ultimately, to feel good about yourself.

## AVOIDING REPEATED FAILURE

Merely having your own style, of course, is no guarantee that you will be a successful competitor. Some personal competitive styles are actually self-defeating.

If you find yourself using a consistent set of competitive tools and a consistent competitive style, but are still failing to achieve the kinds of victories you want, it may be because you have learned to compete in an inherently unproductive way, and continue to do so not so much out of a sense of individual integrity as out of an obsessive need to go over the old familiar ground again and again. What you need in this kind of situation, obviously, is a reassessment of your qualities. You need to take a close look at yourself to see if you are "running the same loops" repetitively; you need to judge whether or not your consistency of style has turned into a detriment rather than an advantage.

Most unsuccessful competition can be traced to the competitor's failure to size him- or herself up accurately in a particular situation. Very often the unhealthy competitor is unsuccessful not only because of a current misunderstanding about his or her potentials, but because of much older patterns of unsuccessful behavior that were learned early in childhood.

Like all parents, physicians generally pass a legacy of competitive styles along to their children. If your ways of dealing with competition are unhealthy and unsuccessful, your children are likely to behave similarly. Extremely aggressive physicians, for instance, often elicit unsuccessful competitive behavior in their children; so do their opposite numbers, those who are afraid to compete at all. The children of compulsively aggressive competitors may become just as aggressive and single-minded about success as their parents, or react against their early role models and opt out of competition entirely. The children of passive competitors may grow up with the notion that there is something shameful about competing, and feel guilty whenever they win. In either case, the parents' own confusions about competition will have been passed on to the children, who will usually perpetuate their parents' errors.

There is a way to avoid this cycle of repeated failure, however; have the courage to evaluate your behavior on a regular basis. Such constant reassessment can help us to discern cases in which we are using competition, for example, as a way of replaying old family (e.g. sibling) rivalries. It can help us understand that our responses to competitive attacks are commonly grounded in the way we responded to similar attacks in childhood; this understanding, in turn, can help us escape the self-defeating cycle by making us realize the need for adopting new tools in a new situation.

This process is anything but simple: no matter how self-defeating the old ways of competing may be, most of us are still wary of changing tools or modifying our competitive styles, simply because the old ways are known and comfortable. When striving to increase your chances of competitive success, aim for a balance between the old tools and styles and new methods which, according to the particular competition in which you are involved, seem most appropriate.

Suppose you have followed all the steps for success I have outlined and still find yourself failing more often than not. What should you do?

Many people caught in this kind of situation go on bulldogging their way through defeat after defeat, always hoping that the next competition will prove to be the one in which the pattern changes and they see clearly the way to win. Actually, such perseverance is not always healthy—especially if you are involved in an old, repetitive pattern. Sometimes the best thing you can do is simply to withdraw from the game; take a breather and give yourself time to reconsider your options, to reassess what you are doing wrong, and why.

These steps for competing successfully can, I believe, save you from falling into the more blatant self-destructive traps which many competitors set for themselves. They cannot really guarantee, however, that you will be successful in all competitive situations. Chance and a host of situational variables can have a great deal to do with the outcome of any competition, and even the best prepared competitor is bound to fail sometimes. Accepting the outcome of your competitive efforts is one of the most difficult yet most important aspects of any competition. All of us are losers once in a while; learning to live with both victory and defeat is perhaps the single most important psychological lesson that we need to learn to become healthy and successful competitors. Learn to deal with both sides of the competitive coin: know how to be a graceful (that is, happy) loser as well as a guiltless, self-confident winner—a "sure" loser, not a sore one.

Now, we all feel lousy when we lose, at least as an immediate reaction; but the sore loser, having no realistic ways or workable contingency plans for dealing with failure, cannot accept defeat. All the energy of sore losers is geared to winning; when winning does not result from their performance, they are undone amd must resort to rationalization. The "sure" loser, on the other hand, is able to make an informed and intelligent appraisal of the possibilities of victory, and can therefore react realistically when defeat is the outcome. What one is sure of is oneself. The sore loser, on the other hand overvalues the importance of every individual competition; to him, every contest is a matter of life or death, and when he loses, he has no choice but to cry "Fault!" or shift the blame elsewhere: he is so unsure of himself that he interprets every failure as proof of his basic worthlessness.

Thus, for us physicians and our families, as for everyone, competition is a constant activity involved in every area of our lives, throughout our lives. To the extent that we understand our competitiveness and are able to accept and grow from our defeats as well as from our victories, we can be psychologically healthy, mature, productive individuals. To the extent that we do not understand this and continue to believe that we must come in first no matter what the cost, we are doomed to a life of dissatisfaction, frustration, and unhappiness. The choice is obvious, for those who are aware that the choice exists.

# part two

# The Troubled Physician

# The Physician and Peer Review

Physicians have commanded respect over the years and rightfully taken pride in their accomplishments. This is not to say that every physician has been a paragon of virtue. While there have been some charlatans who brought medicine into disrepute, it is safe to say that most physicians have made medical decisions conscientiously, performed admirably, and respected their own and the patient's privacy. This traditional situation may not continue indefinitely. Already the winds of change are buffeting the practice of medicine. Some of these forces are fair and friendly; others bode ill for anyone who gets caught in their stormy track.

Increasingly, the way medicine is practiced is being removed from the hands of physicians and becoming the bailiwick of bureaucrats, politicians, and health planners. Doctors who do not learn to tack with the shifting winds will find themselves foundering.

Physicians now not only have to answer to third party payers, hospital administrators, and the media but must also contend with an increasingly informed customer. It is not bad that consumers are better informed but if patients are to benefit optimally from the information they possess, physicians have to spend more time discussing and explaining rather than doing. This involves considerable change by action-oriented physicians.

A problem with increased lay medical sophistication is heightened expectations. Not infrequently consumers expect that there should be no such thing as a bad result and no one should die. Unfortunately that is not the state of medical art at present; good doctors get bad results sometimes and immortality is unattainable.

In the past decade doctors have had to become familiar with new jargon and acronyms. These include certificates of need, length of stay, peer review, and health systems agencies to name a few. The traditional right of a physician to make independent decisions about a patient is being replaced by multidisciplinary teams and consensus judgments, with concomitant increased scrutiny of what a physician does or does not do. A physician may have to answer to a review nurse who questions why a particular course of action was chosen.

No longer is privacy paramount; the patient's chart or data bank has become a reference source for almost anyone in the hospital. Students, social workers, secretaries, laboratory technicians, and many others all use it at will. A patient's most intimate revelations, if charted, are no longer for the doctor's eyes only. If they are entered in the patient's record they are open to scrutiny by others, from review persons to malpractice attorneys. With privacy lost, physicians have to bear in mind that what they write may appear one day on the front page of a newspaper.

What is the solution? Where are these changes going to end? In this chapter Dr. Harvey Mandell discusses transformations that are taking place and what the outcome is likely to be.

*J.P.C.*

# 6

# The Physician and Peer Review

*Harvey Mandell*

The practice of medicine is less private than it used to be, particularly in hospital. It was not so long ago that physicians of any or no specialty could bring their patients into a hospital and do whatever they wanted, confident that none of their work would be reviewed. For good doctors this seemed to work out fine, but bad doctors who might not know they were bad doctors had more license for mayhem than any good hospital would permit today.

It is hard to believe now but surgery was often done by physicians who had no more surgical training than that provided by a 1-year rotating internship. Until the 1950s, when the number of surgical residencies and fellowships increased rapidly, many community hospitals had predominantly untrained surgical staffs. The so-called G.P.-surgeon was often liked by his patients because he took care of the whole family, saw them at home, delivered their babies, and removed their diseased gallbladders when he thought necessary. When Dr. Paul R. Hawley, a former Director of the American College of Surgeons, fought to have surgery done only by trained and certified surgeons, he was vilified by some and accused of taking freedom from surgeons. That accusation was correct in part; for probably the first time, surgeons without formal training had to explain to hospital boards why they should continue to be allowed to operate in their hospitals. It is now taken for granted that a patient having an operation will have a physician trained in the appropriate specialty or subspecialty. Law courts hold executive commitees*

*Committees are called by different names in different hospitals. When I use the term "medical board" I mean a committee of physicians from the medical staff who make decisions and take actions. It is sometimes called the "medical executive committee."

of hospitals responsible for seeing that hospitals give surgical privileges only to qualified physicians.

Comparable movements have taken place in all specialties, although internal medicine and family practice sections of many hospitals have not effected such stringent requirements. Although most G.P.-surgeons no longer practice surgery, many internists, general practitioners, and family practitioners hold full privileges in their fields, including the right to admit and treat their patients in the Intensive Care and Coronary Care Units despite having had little or no formal training in critical care medicine.

Anyone concerned with maintaining high standards of medical care in hospitals would agree that it does not make sense to give every doctor who applies for privileges the right to do whatever he or she wants to in hospital. If the medical staff takes its mandate for self-governance seriously, privileges in hospitals are granted on the basis of proof of training and continued education in the specific field. Not every doctor likes this. It is easy to see how stressful it can be for a physician who has had general surgical privileges but who also liked to do an occasional genitourinary case or deliver a baby to be told not to do an orchiectomy for cancer because he or she has not mastered the new technique, or may have done only one such operation in 5 years. This may be hard to take for a proud surgeon; a confident and knowledgeable one should be glad to demonstrate his or her expertise.

This narrowing of privileges is but one indication of the increased tendency to scrutinize and review the work of physicians. Such review is performed by many people, including nonphysicians, physicians, and medical staff committees.

## THIRD PARTIES

Third-party payers have been prominent in examining the work of physicians in hospital. Doctors who practiced in the 1950s remember that Blue Cross paid the bills of patients only when they were admitted to hospital; thus it became common for the patients who needed diagnostic studies to request hospitalization because they had hospital insurance. Insurance companies, naturally, were not anxious to pay hospital bills for patients who did not have to be in hospital, so they examined patients' diagnoses and workups and eventually stopped paying for what they considered unnecessary hospital admissions. To

---

When I use the expression "executive committee" I mean the lay governing body of the hospital which has the ultimate responsibility for the work in the hospital. This committee usually includes one or two physicians from the medical staff.

do this, insurance companies had to hire personnel to review hospital records before making such determinations. Persons who knew neither patient nor attending physician could look at records and make judgments whether the physician or patient liked it, although there were always avenues of appeal and often the company sought medical advice. Then the patient might be notified directly or indirectly that someone had questioned the doctor's wisdom regarding the admission. The patient's insistence on admission or the doctor's suggestion of admission could cause the patient a great deal of worry unexpectedly and interpose a paying agency between patient and doctor—an agency that might indicate that the doctor's suggestion was not approved. If disapproved, it left the doctor owing an explanation to the patient who was, after all, the victim.

These early losses of privacy and freedom made most physicians uneasy. The worst physicians did not like it, of course, because their incompetence was in danger of discovery; but good doctors had problems too when, despite the best of intentions, their decisions for their patients might be questioned and disapproved by people who knew much less about the situation than the attending physician and who also might be blinded by rigid bureaucratic rules and regulations. Few physicians who admit patients to hospital have escaped the frustrations created by nameless and faceless auditors who have never had to make a decision based on clinical judgment. Review of a hospital chart after the patient's discharge is a lot different from making a lonely decision after midnight in an emergency room.

The paying agencies were only the first of many organizations or people who would open the doctor's hospital work to inspection. There followed a long parade of further intrusions into the doctor–patient–hospital relationship. Physicians who railed against Blue Cross a generation ago would welcome back these minor annoyances if they would only replace Utilization Review Committees, Professional Standards Review Organizations, malpractice attorneys, malpractice insurance carriers, Health Systems Agencies, and dozens of other daily interferences in their professional lives. We physicians sometimes let our frustration with such groups obscure the practical and potential usefulness of having doctors work more openly.

## LOSS OF PRIVACY

There are few aspects of in-hospital work today which maintain the privacy, or what some might call the secrecy, of a generation ago. The very nature of the patient's admission process starts the dispersal of information about doctor and patient. As soon as you call the admitting office, the admission officers and clerks know what you think is wrong with your patient. If you do not want anyone to know the diagnosis you may try a euphemism, at the possible risk of looking silly later. Within a very short time the paying agency, PSRO, and U&R will all know what you think is wrong with the patient; shortly thereafter your patient will be assigned an expected length of stay without any contribution from you except the admitting diagnosis. For the admitting physician this usually is only a working diagnosis: there may be very little firm conviction that this diagnosis is correct. For others, the admitting diagnosis takes on an air of permanence and shows up on all sorts of requisitions and reports sent elsewhere.

To be sure, the estimated length of stay assigned by others is a nuisance, but it does accomplish something; there are among us physicians who keep their patients in hospital longer than necessary. The reasons for this vary. Some of these physicians are honest but overcautious and if they have to explain why their patients are in hospital rather than at home or in a skilled nursing facility, they will have to think more clearly and perhaps use hospital beds more rationally. Keeping a patient in hospital too long invites complications, nosocomial infections, falls from bed, and a variety of horrors. There are also a select few among us who are dishonest and keep patients in hospital longer than necessary only to generate fees. These physicians may give all sorts of skilled explanations to rationalize their behavior but when their patients' average length of stay exceeds that of everyone else's patients, the explanations may ring hollow and peer pressure may alter their habits, especially if demand for hospital beds is increasing. We doctors are proud professionals and most of us value the esteem of our colleagues.

The admitting history and physical examination that we do and document is immediately shared with others who may know neither doctor nor patient. Very few of us write our workups in longhand any more so we immediately share information about our patients with a record room transcriptionist. The professionals who see this workup with the appended progress notes include not only colleagues in radiology, anaesthesiology, and possibly pathology, but also student nurses, ward secretaries, social workers, physiotherapists, data retrievers, record committee members, and conceivably anyone who strolls into the nurses' station with an authoritarian air, picks up a chart, and looks it over. If there is any question about professional liability, your words, dictated in what you thought was privacy, will be seen by both plaintiff's and defendant's attorneys and their staffs, investigators, and consultants. The administration officer of your hospital who is concerned with risk management will read it and get advice from a physician, and a whole host of people in the insurance company's offices, both centrally and locally, will get copies to peruse. They only need the patient's permission; your permission is not important. This means you are writing for a potentially large number of readers—some friendly, some unfriendly, and some disinterested. You are no longer writing for yourself, the doctors who consult with you, and the patient's nurse. Jargon useful to doctors and nurses is all too easily distorted by readers not familiar with in-family talk.

Once in hospital, the patient's care and your role in it are not top secret. There are some major advantages in this openness, despite the obvious nuisances. When I was first in practice, a colleague came in late one night and ordered two blood transfusions for a patient with barbiturate overdose. This patient was not in shock, there was no evidence of volume depletion, and her blood counts were normal. There was no suggestion of bleeding from any organ. Today in the same hospital the blood therapy committee would have picked this up and the physician who ordered such bizarre treatment would be expected to explain this departure from rational therapy to the quality assurance board and the medical board. The nurses might also call the chief of service and ask if they should carry out these orders. Continued peculiar clinical practice might easily be followed by semivoluntary leave of absence or suspension to give this doctor time to think things over. One response to this sort of case by some doctors is that physicians are being pushed into cookbook medicine, something none of us welcomes. It need not be the case, however, and keeping an eye on professionals who have no reasonable explanation for patient management which falls outside accepted standards should not confine physicians' practice so stringently that they cannot be innovative.

## COMMITTEES

There are a number of medical staff committees which may look over your work in the course of carrying out their assignments. The records committee tries to see that your patient's record is completed in time for it to be helpful to those who need it and to see that the quality of the record is such that it offers a good idea of what is going on with your patient and the reasons you are doing what you are doing. Completion of hospital records is a continuous source of frustration for the physician who just does not have the habits that get records completed quickly. I doubt there are many of us coming off a sleepless night, only to find a note or warning about incomplete records, who have not considered burning down the record room with the record committee inside. Perhaps there is such a thing as justifiable arson.

If your patient has an infection, the nurse epidemiologist will know about it soon enough and may make recommendations about isolation or remind you of certain hospital regulations for infected and infectious patients—regulations which you may be trying, at least subconsciously, to ignore. Many of us think that placing a patient in isolation is a sentence of solitary confinement, for personnel often avoid going into the isolated room because of the added nuisance of "gowning up."

If something goes wrong, your section chief may want to find out more about the case and you may even be asked to present the case to your colleagues for their discussion, helpful comments and, rarely, their amusement.

A review or an audit by the medical evaluation committee may lead to perusal of your patient's chart if it "falls through" on a survey. Forget to monitor the latest aminoglycoside as regularly as experts think you should and your chart will pop up for the physician advisor to the committee to review.

Other committees of the medical staff also look at the doctor's records. The infection control committee may want to take a peek if there is a postoperative infection or a group of nosocomial infections in the hospital. If you want to use an investigational drug you make your case before the human investigation committee. About the only committee that does not look into your records is the library committee.

There are physicians abroad in our land who have long cried, "Enough!" and hope the constant review of their hospital work will stop. If the evaluation studies are done well and the results are used for educational purposes—and if the clinicians have reasonably open minds—only good can come of all the auditing. If practicing doctors feel this is a threat to their well-being, or if those charged with the responsibility of maintaining standards of hospital care do not know how properly to use the information from the evaluations, it truly will be wasted time and effort and an affront to the physicians being surveyed. Still, if the audits and the evaluations are not used to embarrass anyone not deserving of the embarrassment, but to do what evaluations are intended to do—to search for weak spots, try to correct them, and do follow-up studies to see if the corrections hold—then no one should find fault with them. Reasonable physicians should be grateful.

This all requires good sense by everyone. In one hospital a study was done to see if the renal function of patients receiving aminoglycosides was monitored carefully enough to be sure the possibility of nephrotoxicity was reduced to as low a level as possible. Of the patients studied, 25% were found to be inadequately monitored using the most generous criteria. The information was made known to the medical staff without identifying any specific physicians. No more was said until a year later when a similar study was made. With mostly the same physicians ordering the drugs the percentage of inadequately monitored patients fell to 4%. Was the doctors' privacy invaded when the nurse data retriever looked through the charts? Yes, it was, but more important, it in no way injured the doctors and it helped direct educational activity. The improvement in performance was at least in part a gain from the loss of privacy and patient care was significantly improved.

The value of the prying eyes of others looking into your patient's charts is inversely proportional to the distance of the reviewers from the patient. Your own hospital reviewers, assuming they are intelligent, fair, honest, and disinterested, should have a lot to offer, even if only to confirm your feeling that you are doing the right thing. As the distance of the reviewer from the patient increases and the methods of diagnosis and care are compared to standards made by personnel further and further from direct care of patients, it is easy to see that one is verging into cookbook medicine. People who set lengths of stay by diagnosis but who do not recognize the many faces of diabetes mellitus or stroke are poorly equipped to give the practicing physician any helpful advice. It may be up to each physician to make the effort required to separate the sublime from the ridiculous, put up with certain nuisances, and then profit when possible from the constant intrusions when they provide useful information.

## HOSPITAL PRIVILEGES

Most physicians applying for privileges in modern hospitals do not know the scrutiny given their backgrounds by credentials committees. Any hospital which does not check every line of the application is not serving its patients well. Too many hospitals have been injured by extending rights and privileges to physicians applying for staff privileges only to find later, possibly after a disaster, that the accepted applicant was not as good as he or she looked on paper or, in some instances, that the applicant was not even a doctor. A careful reading of references, followed by prompt, discreet phone calls to the applicant's former chiefs and colleagues, can do wonders for the credentialling process. Our hospital like others nowadays takes this so seriously that we send members of our credentials committee to special training programs. These physicians return more appreciative of their responsibility. True, the credentials committee invades the applicant's privacy, but there is really no alternative if you want to work with a good medical staff in a good hospital. The physician who is rejected should have adequate means of appeal available if needed. Most of those rejected for good reasons usually drift away to apply elsewhere.

Surgeons have long had to put up with inspection of at least one aspect of their work. If the hospital tissue committee does its job it must review every tissue removed at operation. If the resected tissue is normal there must be an explanation satisfactory to peers, either in the patient's chart or in communications with the committee. If no tissue is removed, there must be an adequate explanation. Surely all physicians, but unfortunately not all lawyers and not all writers for the lay press, know that there are times when normal tissue will be removed from patients for honest reasons. An occasional normal appendix should not brand a surgeon a thief; but if all the others have 3% normal rates and he or she has a rate of 73%, the hospital has a problem and so do that surgeon's patients. That hospital is not serving its patients well and is obliged by conscience and the courts to solve the problem. Likewise, there may be operations at which no tissue is removed; e.g., abdominal laparotomy with lysis of adhesions. Again, the surgeon who does ten times more of these operations than his or her peers deserves an invasion of privacy. There may be good and honest reasons for each of these operations, and there should be every opportunity to present them; but if there is no good reason offered, there should be supervision or mandated consultations before surgery or a leave of absence for the errant surgeon to reconsider. Good surgeons should, and usually do, take this surveillance of their work in stride, although it can be annoying to be asked to write an explanation to the tissue committee for a procedure done after long and serious consideration. The tissue committee members, of course, must realize that they cannot deal trivially with the results of a physician who has made a lifelong study of his or her work.

The physicians who operate with the least review of their work are those who remove tissue which is not suitable for laboratory examination. Surgeons who remove cataracts without enjoying any other ophthalmologist's opinion do not share the same scrutiny as the appendix remover. The only reason the appendectomy doctor has to answer to the tissue committee and the ophthalmologist does not is the nature of the tissue delivered to the pathology department. It is not because the abdominal surgeon is thought in any way to be less honest or poorer in judgment. Why then the difference in review? Surely some way could be found to even this up—perhaps a version of the second opinion where cataract removal would be reviewed preoperatively. The same system could be routine in all types of surgery where tissue inappropriate for pathological examination is removed; in other instances where normal tissue is removed; or particularly, where no tissue is removed at all. No one wants to stay the surgeon's hand when he or she is looking for ruptured spleen, but most laparotomies are scheduled electively with plenty of time for consultation. Ultrasound, computerized axial tomography, and laparoscopy would seem to make exploratory laparotomy a rare event. If one surgeon's name is on the operating room schedule more frequently than all other surgeons for this procedure, why should he or she not be subject to a lessening of private decision? For that surgeon's colleagues on the medical staff, decisions to intervene depend on philosophies of the staff leaders. If the leaders believe hospital work is strictly a private business between patient and doctor, no matter how gullible the former and greedy the latter, then there should be no intervention. However, if the members of the staff have some pride in their institution and share my passion for our profession, then privacy must suffer a loss. For the hospital, the decision should require less than a millisecond of thought. A hospital offers its services to its patients with the implied consent that it will do all it can to provide a safe, modern environment where qualified and honest men and women will try to diagnose and treat sick patients. If the medical staff would prefer not to take care of this promise on the physician level, then the governing body of the hospital has that responsibility.

## GOVERNING BODY

Physicians presenting problems for patients, and thereby for the hospital, may be reviewed not only by their colleagues but by laypersons on the governing body. These lay governors usually have more knowledge of community affairs and finances than they do of medicine. Therefore, their review of a physician's work is a particularly difficult intrusion for a doctor to bear. At best it will be fair and disinterested; at worst, misguided and gossipy. The trend toward more lay governing body responsibility is not likely to slow and physicians are well advised to settle their problems with physicians rather than with businesspeople, bankers, and lawyers who cannot possibly understand the tensions and nuances of taking care of sick people.

Most physicians who limit their hospital work to the care of patients and avoid medical staff politics and committee work may not be aware of the increased mingling of medical staff and lay governors in the committees of staff and governing body. Doctors who have not been involved in hospital governance are often unaware of a whole world of joint efforts to make their hospitals work optimally.

The Joint Commission on Accreditation of Hospitals (JCAH) wants hospitals to have a hospitalwide board responsible for doing its best to see that the hospital functions well. The key to this is "hospitalwide," for many problems in hospitals cross the boundaries that separate doctors from nurses and from administration. If the doctor orders a serum calcium but the nurse does not carry out the order, or if the laboratory technician takes the blood from the wrong patient, no one is helped. It does not matter whether the doctor is expert or ignorant about calcium metabolism. If physician, nurse, and technician do not all function at their best, nothing is accomplished. The administration is responsible for making it all work; the governing body has the ultimate responsibility to see that the administration has the proper financing, management, consultation, and backing to make it go. Therefore, good quality assurance boards will have not only physicians but representatives from nursing, administration, and the governing body. This does not mean that an administrator sits in judgment of a physician who chooses to use ampicillin instead of penicillin V when he or she believes it to be the drug of choice. However, that administrator does have the duty to see that a physician problem which cannot be settled by the medical staff or the medical board is not dropped or ignored to the detriment of the patients in the hospital.

Doctors and nurses have so much to offer each other that it would seem needless to explain why they must have a site for reasoned discussion and exchange of knowledge, experience, and views.

## NURSE SPECIALISTS

Probably the phenomenon hardest for the inadequately trained physician to take is the rise of the independent-minded nurse no longer content to be the doctor's handmaiden. Nurses often know which doctors are better trained than others, which are more conscientious, and surely which are lazy. One difference between the "old time" nurses and most of today's college-trained nurses is that the former kept most of these opinions to themselves, at least in hospital, and the latter may sometimes express opinions to anyone who will listen. As you can imagine, it is not hard for a nurse to find listeners when discussing the perceived failures of doctors. Nurses also will not hesitate to question an order if it appears to be out of line, and not all doctors are prepared for this. If the doctors are of the Geheimrat Professor Excellency school and insist that, being doctors, they can order whatever they want without being questioned, they are likely to embarrass themselves.

The rise of the nurse specialist is particularly vexing to some doctors.[1] We now have nurses with specialization in narrow fields who often know more about that field than most physicians, unless the latter have had special training. Coronary care nurses become very good at cardiac arrhythmias and it is not unusual for them to make better electrocardiographic interpretations than almost all physicians except the cardiologists and some internists.

Why should the nurse specialist keep quiet and follow a senseless order when a physician orders a loop diuretic for an anephric patient who has no loops? This happened in one dialysis unit and the physician insisted that the nurse follow his orders. How much more sensible for that physician to change his order to something more appropriate and thank the nurse for the reminder.

Why should a nurse watch a patient slip into respiratory failure when she knows endotracheal intubation and mechanical assist will help while an out-of-date doctor assures her on the phone that there is nothing more that can be done? In one such instance which I witnessed, it was true there was nothing more that doctor knew of, but fortunately the nurse did and called higher authority. The patient was intubated and recovered so that he could leave the hospital and return home. An invasion of the doctor's private care of his patient? Yes, and the doctor did not like it. Fortunately he did not let this overshadow the satisfaction of seeing his patient recover. The doctor profited by the experience and now gets consultation in similar cases. He and his patients owe a lot to a nurse's failure to accept his serene words, "There's nothing more we can do."

Not every one of us is up to all this. We physicians take great pride in our accomplishments. Most of us have been the smartest kid in the class at one time or another and we have had more education and training than most other people. We have been examined and reexamined to satiety and have the certificates on our walls to prove it. It is hard for us to accept someone pointing out that despite passing all these examinations we are not omniscient and no longer have complete freedom to do whatever we want.

## AGING PHYSICIANS

Reactions to loss of in-hospital privacy varies. Often the types of response seem age-related; i.e., the level of tolerance of the physician is usually inversely related to his or her age. The reasons are easy to find. Doctors who practiced 30 years ago tend to think the hospital owes them something and, at the very least, should leave them alone. When doctors who are now middle-aged or older started practice, most hospitals had house or ward services and privately practicing doctors on the medical staff were responsible for lots of patients who did not pay them. Medicare and Medicaid changed this, and while we may not think Medicare and Medicaid fees are so great, it is true that almost all patients in hospital now generate some income for their attending physicians. Also, there were no full-time Emergency Room doctors then and staff physicians had to take their turn caring for patients who showed up for treatment. Those same physicians, 30 years later, are also faced with the insecurity caused by the arrival of younger colleagues more recently trained and often seeming to talk a different language. Whether this new language is superior to the old one is arguable but "preload," "afterload," "pulmonary wedge pressure," and "drug levels" may be a little unsettling for the physician nearing retirement. Couple this with the constant bombardment of universal scrutiny of the doctor's work and irritation is understandable. But still, surely he or she must bend to the new openness. Does not the hospital have an obligation to its patients to prevent an orthopedic surgeon with a tremor from doing hand surgery? Should an internist with loss of memory continue to write orders for patients with diabetic ketoacidosis? How long should a hospital put up with physicians who are not available when the nurses call them or who have a few drinks before they scrub?

## INFORMED PATIENTS

Another daily nudging of the doctor's privacy in making decisions comes from today's better informed patients. Any person who watches television or reads a newspaper cannot help but come across discussions of all manner of ailments and treatments. Suggested therapy is given and often the reporting, while improving all the time, fails to give much depth to the discussion. It seems the network news broadcasters and the *New York Times* get their copies of the *New England Journal of Medicine* a day before most physicians get theirs. If the information is good, it is not unreasonable for the patient to ask many questions. Most of us doctors are neither good educators of patients nor patient educators: we do not always have the time necessary to discuss all the ins and outs of every diagnosis and every treatment. Not that this is not a good idea; but most physicians who have to take care of sick people all day long often just lack the temperament required for explanation. Nonetheless, the decision the physician makes for complicated therapy often depends upon the approval of the patient and his or her family. It is no longer so easy to say to a patient, "You have a lump in your breast; if it's malignant I am going to do a modified radical mastectomy." The patient may well have heard that there are groups studying radiotherapy for certain types of breast lesions and her desire to know more about alternate therapy is reasonable. The very process of hospitalization for patients brings them into "the involuntary exposure to, and participation in, this social complex [the hospital] while undergoing treatment for diagnosed or discovered malfunctions."[2]

Gone are the circumlocutions of yesterday. One of my medical school professors was a master at discussing the most horrid complications with students at the bedside. His most elegant euphemism was "systolic retention" when describing death. Today's patient might well want to know if there are any hazards to systolic retention.

The loss of privacy affects patients as well as doctors, especially if the patient is admitted to a small, more personal hospital in a smaller community. The trade-off of less confidentiality for the possibility of better performance by doctor or hospital should be in the patient's favor. Ideally, those who look through patients' charts must be pledged to observe as much confidentiality as possible; doctors should maintain confidentiality instinctively. What the patient loses should be compensated by the knowledge that if management of the illness does not meet high standards, there is someone in the institution who cares about it and is responsible to take action. This is, of course, the best situation. In the worst case patients could find themselves objects of hospital and community gossip and poor medical management simultaneously. A hospital and medical staff which permits this to happen must look into its corporate soul and decide to make some changes, no matter how stressful to medical staff, administration, or executive committee. Lay membership on the executive committee of a hospital can no longer be a prestige post with never an unpleasant responsibility. If the lay board will not take such responsibilities voluntarily, the courts will see to it that they do: plaintiffs' attorneys are now naming members of boards in their suits. Even those doctors who still view hospitals as their workshops must be involved in working with lay boards who depend on physicians for explanations of medical affairs.

Some would have it that we are not our brother's or sister's keepers. This is a reasonable alternative opinion, but today's society with its judicial system, regulatory agencies, accrediting agencies, and (I think) higher moral accountability does not allow us the luxury of perfect freedom when other people's health and life may be compromised by that perfection.

Those who hold absolutely to maximum freedom and privacy for physicians working in hospital must answer the following questions. Should good-natured incompetence prevail among hospital physicians merely because the officers of the medical staff and the incompetent physicians are old friends? Should this cycle of tolerance for ineptitude leading to ever greater incompetence be permitted endlessly?

## REFERENCES

1. Mandell HN: The physician and the nurse specialist, or the tiger and the lady. Postgrad. Med. 1978, 64:24.
2. Shiloh A: Equalitarian and hierarchal patients and investigation among Hadassah Hospital patients. Med. Care 1965, 3:87–95.

# The Divorced Physician

Statistically, almost one out of every two marriages in the United States fails, but unions between physicians are considerably more durable. A study of 100 randomly selected physicians showed that their divorce rate was 8.8%, approximately one divorce per twelve marriages.[1] A survey of female physicians in Connecticut revealed a similarly low figure: only 10% were divorced.[2] In addition, the couples in the first survey rated their marriages better than an age-matched sample of the general population.

When medical marriages do break down, the sequelae can be devastating to a physician and the physician's career. The twin blessings of a competitive nature and a compulsive personality frequently ensure that a physician will succeed in medicine. These same traits can become anathemas in marriage. Many physicians are poorly equipped to accept defeat and tolerate it so poorly that they are shattered by the misfortune of a failed marriage.

Most data on medical marriages come from couples in which the physician is male and the non-physician spouse is female. As an increasing number of women become physicians the data may change and issues may become less sexually stereotyped. In the past, unhappy medical wives have complained that their husbands were "undemonstrative, stilted, cold, domineering, compulsive, perfectionistic and frequently absent."[3] In the future, it may be medical husbands who will complain that their physician wives are "irresponsible and poor parents."[3] A medical wife has lamented that, as she drove past the hospital, one of her children observed "That is where Daddy lives."[3] The same may be said of Mommy within a few years.

The best marriages, medical or otherwise, appear to be those where neither partner continuously dominates the other. Marriages seem to work best where both spouses are mutually supportive enabling each to find the time and the opportunity for self-fulfillment to realize their full potential. According to Dr. H. Waldo Bird, clinical professor of medicine at St. Louis

University, "Marriages resemble a teeter-totter. You cannot have a good ride unless someone is willing to sit on the other end of the board in the lower position some of the time. In time, he or she gets a turn on the top end."[4]

In this chapter on The Divorced Physician Dr. Hal Gillespie and his second wife, Sherry, give a detailed account of his previous medical marriage that failed. The marriage's strengths, weaknesses, dynamics, and the reasons for its ultimate demise are analyzed in painstaking detail. Failure may not have been inevitable and perhaps other participants could have written a different scenario. Other medical couples may be able to learn from the Gillespie experience as it is discussed here, in graphic detail.

*J.P.C.*

---

[1]Garvey M, Tuason VB. Physician Marriages. J Clin Psychiatry 40: 129–131, 1979.

[2]Callan CM, Klipstein E. Women Physicians in Connecticut: A Survey. Connecticut Medicine 45: 494–496, 1981.

[3]Evans JL. Psychiatric Illness in the Physicians Wife. J Amer Psych Assoc 122(2):159–163, 1965.

[4]Bird HW. Physician's Marriage. Joys and Sorrows Part 4: Spotting the Danger Signals. Facets 40: 18–20, 1979.

# 7

# The Divorced Physician: Autopsy of a Medical Marriage

*Hal G. Gillespie*
*Cheryl L. Gillespie*

***Case History.*** I watched the judge in his black robe disappear through the back entrance of the courtroom. His grim and firm pronouncement apparently was justified in his mind. I then saw my estranged wife and her lawyer exchanging gleeful and triumphant grins. I was numb with disbelief at what had happened. Seventeen years of complex interactions had been reduced to one fact. I had committed adultery, and as a result my estranged wife and children were entitled to continue living in the manner to which they had become accustomed. Two-thirds of my pretax income was to be the price of my separation. As a university-based physician, I had worked 65–70 hours weekly in order to reach that level. I felt I was being punished as a villain for events in which I was only one of the participants. There seemed to be no consideration of my pain.

Memories flashed through my mind. On August 3, 1974, I had packed my belongings in my car for the purpose of moving out. My 2½-year-old son had run up to me to say merrily, "Goodby, Daddy." There was agony in knowing that he felt Daddy was merely leaving for work: little did he realize, Daddy would never again leave that house in the morning. During the following months, my son was to develop a phobia and become terrified when anyone packed a suitcase for a trip. Never again would I be part of his daily life. I would relinquish my role as participant in his growth and development. A few weeks later, he drank some detergent and was taken to the emergency room. I, as a physician, was only to find out about this months later. I was never again to attend a piano recital by a son who was 10 years old at the time.

My heart had been heavy knowing that my 16-year-old son sobbed nearly all night after he was told of the impending separation. The boys had insisted on an elaborate birthday dinner for me on August 1st, two days before my departure. Never again were they to share actively in that event.

Another painful memory occurred one Sunday evening when I had gone back for some dialogue with my wife. Our conversation had rapidly deteriorated into a bitter quarrel, and she had demanded that I leave "her house." I walked out of the beautiful home in the country club section which had been the only house I had ever owned. In the prior years of training and military service, my children had always longed for a "home with a chimney." As I sped down the driveway in anger, I saw my wife standing at a window watching, and there was immense sorrow, recognizing the finality of the moment. Seventeen years of an intense relationship was ending, 17 years of tremendous change, immense joy, and intense struggle. Now I was compelled to search for a relationship with more joy, spontaneity, and relaxation.

For five or six years, I had felt extremely depressed and confined. I had seen myself as unappreciated and constantly criticized, resulting in a withdrawal and a smoldering anger that manifested itself even in my work. The years of depression, negativism, criticism, and conflict had become so burdensome I could bear them no longer. No matter how much I loved my children, I felt I was no model for them as a depressed and angry person who experienced home life as control and defeat. So it had all led to this courtroom and the humiliating revelation of partial truths. Not only was I experiencing a major failure for one of the first times in my life, but I was also being publicly condemned. This added to the sense of rejection I had experienced through vicious community gossip, criticism and embarrassment by respected colleagues, and rejection by my religious family which had never had a divorce in it. It seemed incredible that such defeat and failure should come to a bright young man who had always excelled, been a good boy, and, most of all, worked so diligently. That moment in court was the culmination of a growing sense of vulnerability, fallibility, and powerlessness in the area of my life that was important to me. I was perplexed in trying to understand how I had arrived at this point; and it is only after eight years that I can view it with some objectivity.

***Comments.*** Physicians are poorly prepared to participate in courtroom divorce proceedings. Having been trained in the scientific method where objectivity and the pursuit of truth are the ideals, they are surprised to find that courtroom drama involves only the letter of the law and how the "facts" can be portrayed by skillful attorneys. The oversimplification of complex issues leads to a disillusionment with the law, previously viewed idealistically. Physicians tend not to anticipate the intense bitterness and alienation brought about by the adversarial system in which lawyers profit from increased conflict. In many troubled marriages, problems escalate to a point of no return precisely when legal counsel is sought. Also, many states still require that one partner be found at fault in the dissolution of the marriage. This adds to the sense of public embarrassment, shame, and guilt to which doctors are unaccustomed. Few people are aware of the availability of trained divorce mediators in many areas of the country. Also, doctors tend to be somewhat compulsive people with great facilities for rationalization. Therefore, they tend to deny the pain involved in a separation, especially from the children, and paint an unrealistic mental picture of how things will work out after the separation. In the effort to get out of a painful relationship, doctors do not anticipate the depression and loneliness which result from a separation. Doctors in their success become accustomed to praise and respect and often are surprised at their reactions to the gossip and criticism. These social reactions are especially important in small towns where the doctor and his or her family are known and are seen as cultural heroes. Most of all, doctors, accustomed to success, are ill-prepared for the perceptions of failure and defeat which often accompany a separation and divorce.

> ***Case History.*** I identify my childhood with a lonely appearing little blond-haired boy in overalls pictured on a TAT card.* I was lonely and isolated, and there was constant family turmoil. I found refuge in the *Lincoln Library* and other reference books on the family bookshelf. I dreamed of places and things far away from my Appalachian home. This modest home was quite well-to-do in the world of poverty that existed around me. My mother was chronically psychotic with a fixed elaborate paranoid delusional system, producing constant family arguments. My father endured this crazy world through a deep religious faith and belief that "we'll understand it better by and by." The family hero was my oldest brother who had finished dental school when I was 6 years old. The next brother, who was eight years older than I was, supplied much of the protection, guidance, and nurturing that I desperately needed. He was in medical school when, as a high school student, I decided to become a doctor. In high school I met Peggy, an attractive young lady with "most dependable" as her class superlative. She was highly organ-

*Thematic apperception test

ized and gave structure to my chaotic world. In spite of being bright and quite popular in school, I felt terribly insecure and lacked confidence. I felt secure with Peggy's stability. Together we built the future dream of the 1950s of a successful doctor with a two-car garage and split-level house in the suburbs. Our plan was to marry after the first year of medical school. After a year and a half of college, Peggy became pregnant. A quick marriage was arranged, and Peggy soon assumed the role of working wife and mother, earning a "P.H.T." (Putting Hubby Through). Peggy herself had been denied a college education by her hard-working, lower-middle-class parents who saw no need for children, particularly girls, to go past high school. She had started to work and had been quite successful as an efficient secretary and bookkeeper. In her family of origin, interactions largely consisted of chronic complaints, grumpiness, and hostility, and she was glad to escape the confining negativism through marriage. With limited resources, we faced the prospect of two years of college and four years of medical school.

My mother had been an extremely bright and ambitious young woman who had been deprived as a child and was not allowed to finish high school by her cruel, tyranical, and abusive father. Longing for an education, she carefully taught her sons that homework must always take priority. This belief in the priority of academic excellence persisted into my marriage. True to my upbringing, my family life was centered around my school work, and Peggy took on the dutiful roles of family caretaker and breadwinner. She even took care of the automobile repairs. With a superior sense of organization, great endurance, and frugality, she orchestrated my way through six years of school. She obviously enjoyed and was quite good at her work although she chronically complained of lack of recognition and appreciation from her superiors, and of their unfair demands upon her. Mutual emotional constriction was tolerated by us and attributed to stress and fatigue. Although there were conflicts, we believed that they would disappear and all would be happy when the M.D. degree was achieved and Peggy could quit work and become the "doctor's wife." During these years, Peggy was seen by family and friends as having heroinelike qualities, sacrificing for the bright future which lay ahead. During these years my main task was to get my studies done, although I did help some with our child and I successfully sold cookware during my off-quarter. However, with both of us working and with some help from my family, we were able to finish medical school free of debt. I joined the army during my senior year in order to supplement the income and enable Peggy to quit work and have a second child just prior to graduation.

Following graduation, the dream was to begin. However, the move to a large city for internship was quite traumatic and disruptive. The rotating internship required that even more time and effort be spent in the hospital away from home. Peggy complained of loneliness, lack of support, and burdens of child rearing. She found that she missed the rewards of work outside the home. Then a completely disabling back strain became the first of a series of psychosomatic illnesses appearing throughout the remainder of our marriage. I reacted with resentment over the subsequent demands placed on me during these busy years. Then came the decision to enter psychiatric residency. Peggy had grave reservations about this and saw me as forsaking "real medicine" to enter a low-status speciality. The residency years of the late 1960s brought new interactions. Psychiatric jargon became a weapon. Even though the military setting did not require total devotion, I worked extremely long hours studying and seeing patients because it was "the opportunity of a lifetime" to train with such excellent teachers and interesting patients. Peggy became quite insecure and jealous concerning my obvious fascination with the subtleties of interaction with some long-term female psychotherapy patients. I was impatient, as no amount of reassurance or explanation could satisfy her that the therapy situation was only artificially intimate or that I understood transference phenomena. Peggy began to read the newly emerging feminist literature and voiced her severe dissatisfaction with the housewife's role. Peggy's unmet needs for attention, succor, and recognition were expressed through withholding and bitter criticism instead of being voiced directly. I was chagrined that she criticized me when I was working so hard and helping so many needy people. I withdrew further into my work and achieved further recognition and praise from my teachers, peers, and patients. I continued to believe that Peggy would be happy and everything would be alright once training was completed.

***Comments.*** In our experience with male physicians whose marriages get into trouble, we have frequently observed three major syndromes or characteristics. The first syndrome is that of a highly achieving but obsessive-compulsive and intellectualizing physician who has identified with the cultural stereotype of manliness in that he is problem-solving, analytical, self-sufficient, objective, and unemotional. Although he has a mechanical and rigid quality, he is seen as being strong and stable by others. He has often had a rather distant or absentee father who, although he may have been a high achiever, rarely gave direct approval to his son. The relationship with the mother was closer and more intense, although perhaps marked by greater ambivalence stimulated by the mother's control. In seeking a spouse, this physician is attracted to a woman who is more emotional and outgoing. She is more comfortable in a social setting and free with her emotional expression and approval. The physician perceives her as being far more fun-loving and flexible than his mother, and feels she will add more spark to his dull existence. The wife usually comes from a more chaotic and less stable family and perceives her husband as a strong man who will give her stability. The doctor's role as a caretaker emphasizes his ability to take care of someone. Though she may be quite seductive and dramatically sexual on the surface, the wife may be sexually inhibited underneath. Since the inexpressive husband has difficulty being physically aggressive, spontaneous, or demonstrative, sexual activity diminishes after courtship has lost its intensity. Also, the husband becomes critical of the wife's lack of organization and attention to detail, and she becomes upset with his tendency to isolate himself emotionally in his work or in journals, with his perfectionism, and with his lack of emotional expression. He complains about how she organizes her refrigerator or squeezes the toothpaste; she complains of the forgotten birthday or her experience that he is not any fun anymore. At midlife, the tradeoffs made early in the marriage may become unacceptable and an unarticulated standoff may result. This mechanical husband may start to get in touch with more emotional aspects of his life, such as spontaneity and tenderness, and may become critical of his wife who has by now learned some obsessive-compulsive habits in her efforts to please him. She is rightfully confused about these role expectations and is embittered that her efforts to please have not been successful. The husband may have difficulty recognizing the validity of his wife's complaints about his lack of emotional response. After all, his devotion to his work and his high standards are culturally approved. On the other hand, for the wife there is always the danger of involvement in an extramarital relationship in order to obtain romance and emotional involvement.

The second syndrome is the physician who suffers either emotional or physical deprivation as a child. Occasionally a physical defect, such as acne or adolescent gynecomastia, will contribute to the negative self-image. He has often experienced a deficit of nurturing in his home life. He is often basically shy, but is able to excel in his schoolwork. His prospective wife recognizes his intelligence and competence and assumes the maternal role in terms of nurturing and life organization. For the physician with a chaotic background, this structure is quite adaptive. However, he may reject the structure once he has finished his training and may decide that he no longer wants a mother in his spouse but rather a woman with whom he can play a more parental or adult role.

He may become dissatisfied with his own dependency feelings which, in his anger, may be projected onto his wife. Anger, which he has harbored toward his mother for excessive control or lack of nurturing, may become directed toward the wife. Also, the physician may have countered his negative self-image by achievement resulting in recognition and praise; however, at the end of training, he no longer has parental figures whom he is pleasing. His efforts have become routine to his wife by this time and he becomes resentful as he perceives her as being less supportive. Depression, along with alcohol and drug abuse, appear to be more frequent in this marital constellation.

A third syndrome we have observed is when both the physician and his family of origin are characterized by a high degree of social conformity. He describes a fine family and "perfect" parents with a high degree of stability. He has always been a "good boy" striving hard to please his parents and reflect positively upon them. Family interaction is seen as quite stable although it becomes very "routine." As the physician enters courtship, he chooses a woman who is socially, religiously, and personally compatible with him. They then reduplicate their families of origin in marriage and sense some reward in their conformity, although they may experience their relationship as monotonous. A crisis may arise in the marriage at midlife when one or both of the physician's parents die. Feeling a release from parental expectation, he may plunge into extramarital affairs or risk-taking activities, often of an adolescent nature. The wife may see her husband's behavior as a personal rejection and may be very upset about the social impact.

In all three types of relationship, there is a strong tendency for the physician to deny his dependency needs. In our case example, there were marked mutual dependency needs which were not recognized as such by either partner. This appears to be related to the physician's identification with the cultural stereotype of masculinity. In all three types of marriage, the lack of psychological intimacy and dialogue, the constricted roles and unrecognized dependency needs lead to great difficulties at times of loss or grief. The loss of a parent or a child by death, a severe disappointment or the failure of children to develop as expected, brings about an unshared grief with alienation and loneliness and a tendency to seek solace in extramarital relationships.

In his book, *The Seasons of A Man's Life,* Daniel Levinson[6] describes men as going through a life transition at about age 30 when there is a major reevaluation of their life goals and relationships. At this age, the physician is still often in specialty training or starting to set up his practice. The high cultural, family, and personal expectations involved in a medical career leave little chance for him to question or modify his life dream, vocational choices, or personal relationships. It is easy for him and his wife to deny basic conflicts and to attribute unhappiness or lack of fulfillment to stresses of training. It is easy for them to persuade themselves that the high investment in medical training will eventually pay off and everything will be straightened out once medical practice is actively established.

Once the marital deterioration has progressed, the spouse may be so emotionally distraught that her primary concern is to guard her "property rights", her investment of time, money, and emotion in the relationship. Rather than experiencing feelings of "I love you", she may feel "I own you".[13]

> ***Case History.*** At the end of residency, I was assigned to a rather isolated hospital in Germany. Again, the move was marked by Peggy's severe back strain which was totally disabling and required hospitalization. The assignment turned out to be very unrewarding from a professional standpoint. Peggy was extremely unhappy about the remote assignment, the social life, and the field grade quarters which were rather good by military standards. The accusations of affairs with patients became overt and began to sound to me like challenges or invitations. Even though I worked harder than most of the doctors, I was home more than ever. Yet our conflict escalated and Peggy began to predict divorce "when the children are big enough." She still despaired of not being able to go to school or to work outside the home. On transfer to the beautiful city of Nuremberg in northern Bavaria, there was no improvement. Peggy was still unhappy because of our quarters, our furniture, the commissary and post exchange deficiencies, and so on. We withdrew from one another, and our exchanges became more hostile. I continued to plunge into my work as an escape. I despaired that the tremendous opportunities of living in Europe were experienced as negative by Peggy. I recognized none of my withdrawal and lack of support and projected all the blame onto Peggy. I knew that the commissary or the living room rug were not the real problems, but I was unable to discern the true difficulties. Considering myself to be one of the best psychiatrists in the area, I was reluctant to seek help in a straightforward fashion. Peggy's negative evaluation of psychiatry appeared to rule out any kind of marital therapy. With so many positive external factors present, I began to lose my belief that one day things would get better. Then Peggy became severely ill with a Butazolidin-induced thrombocytopenia—a frightening event when you are in a foreign country. She was critical of my lack of support although I felt that I did well considering my work obligations and the care of our two children.
>
> Our marital relationship deteriorated into periods of smoldering

anger with increasingly frequent outbursts of hostility, along with a few interspersed episodes of joy and pleasantness. My resentment focused on Peggy's sexual withholding, her needs to control, and her incapacity to say "I love you" more than a couple of times a year. I was bitter because I desired more children, and Peggy, being determined to go to work or school, wanted no more. Feeling angry and deprived, I entered into an extramarital affair. My conflicts deepened as this relationship provided excitement, admiration, and approval which I seemed to need. Then two jolting developments occurred. My father suddenly died. Then Peggy became pregnant, a move she had consciously and secretly planned in an effort to save our obviously faltering marriage. Overwhelmed by grief for a father I admired, I determined that like him I would try to endure the marriage for the sake of my three children. In spite of its positive aspects, I began to withdraw from the affair with its implied dreams and commitments.

I returned to the United States determined to make the marriage work and hoping that at last the dream of the '50s would be fulfilled. I began to work in a university-owned private hospital, and our financial situation improved considerably. However, my income was still only one-fourth of that of my brother who was in a high-income surgical specialty, and Peggy felt her privileges were minor compared to the wives of "real doctors" who had considerably more leisure and abundant household help. I berated her for her refusal to decide on a course of returning to work or starting college. Her differing needs for achievement presented contrast in life goals. My much higher energy level and drive which prevented me from sleeping in on weekends became a sore point. My needs for orderliness appeared to decrease while hers seemed to increase. The shoes left on the bedroom floor or the coke bottle left on the kitchen counter became major battle grounds for control. I resented Peggy's continued back problems and peptic ulcer disease, blaming them on her inability to express emotions. I continued to ignore her unmet dependency needs and saw all of her demands as efforts to control. Peggy's unhappiness seemed to interfere with her social life, but this was blamed on my being a psychiatrist and my social nonconformities. My smoldering resentment extended into my work, where I gained the reputation of being angry and explosive. I continued to project and saw the difficulties as being related to Peggy's "neuroses." I mainly pictured myself as a victim in the situation. Then my former mistress moved to the small city where we lived. I saw this as intrusive and rejected her, remaining loyal to my marriage. Peggy's overt and covert anger over this event resulted in further depression and withdrawal on my part. With much denial and repression, Peggy chose to endure in the marriage. She saw herself as continuing to sacrifice for the sake of the relationship.

Because of my depression, I started seeing a psychoanalyst in therapy. Being traditional, he apparently never considered couples therapy. Month after month my relationships were examined, but always from my point of view. The therapist pointed out my excessive need for praise and recognition and introduced me to a taoistic philosophy of passivity and service to the needs of others. I attempted to carry this out, and my marriage deteriorated further. My depression continued, and my withdrawal became more pensive. I carefully kept a log of my marital interaction for weeks and saw no significant change occur. At this point, I decided that my endurance and passivity were pathological. I quit therapy, and my anger erupted. Then Peggy sought out a psychiatrist for psychotherapy. He called me to ask if I would participate in couple therapy after a few weeks of individual therapy, and I replied that I would gladly participate. Week after week went by without the anticipated phone call. Peggy became increasingly aggressive and blaming. After nine months, she announced that she was quitting therapy because she and her therapist were convinced that she had no problems and that I was psychotic.

I felt hopeless and despondent. Throughout our marriage, we had been able to enjoy some mutual interests, and we were certainly proud of our three sons and enjoyed watching them grow. In spite of these limited pleasures the elements of joy and spontaneity were lacking and the negativism was oppressive. I felt so depressed that I saw myself as a negative and dominated example for my sons. I was bound to Peggy with a remarkable intensity, but I realized that we were destroying each other in the process. Peggy articulated her sense of entrapment and a determination to get out of it. I grimly accepted that one day we would part. Because of my intense emotional binding and dependency I would hang on in the meantime in spite of my discomfort.

***Discussion.*** Several clinical studies have noted how a spouse's illness may serve to attract the attention and nurturing of the care-giving physician.[3] "I have to get sick and make an appointment in order to see him" is a frequently heard phrase that is more than good-natured humor. It has been noted that often by the time a spouse is identified as a psychiatric patient, the physician has been involved in giving medications, including intramuscular injections. When marital stress occurs, the physician often defends himself by identifying his wife as the patient, carefully outlining her "neurotic symptoms." The physician's marital partner is often presented to the psychiatrist with the expectation of a diagnosis, definition of pathology, and the outline of a "cure." The physician, in his authoritarian role, has difficulty identifying with a patient role and his well practiced defense of rationalization helps fortify his conviction that he is not part of the process. Again identifying with the culture's stereotypic male ideal, he sees himself as needing to be self-sufficient and thus has great difficulty accepting help from another physician. We have noted that doctors and their spouses are often more comfortable seeing a therapist who practices 50–150 miles away from their home. Another obstacle to therapy is the spouse's awareness of how doctors identify with each other and her subsequent distrust of the therapist, often fearing that the therapist and husband will gang up on her to make a joint diagnosis and treatment approach. In our opinion, probably the greatest difficulty in dealing with physicians' marriages is the tendency for the physician and spouse, as well as the therapist, to elect individual therapy where the problem is actually a marital conflict requiring marital therapy. Many times therapists appear eager to communicate respect and special status to the physician and also protect the narcissism of both partners. Unfortunately, this fits in with the physician's need to deny his involvement in the marital deterioration. Individual therapists often struggle along dealing with the distorted presentations of individual partners and frequently end up making recommendations which increase the marital conflict or else become used as weapons in marital battles. Whitaker and Miller[15] state:

> Where the marital tie is weak and divorce threatens, intervention with one of the pair seems routinely to be disruptive. We are impressed that moving unilaterally into a marriage relationship, taking one of the two as a patient and referring or ignoring the mate, is very often a tactical blunder.

***Case History.*** Then the shattering event occurred. I attended a two-week course at the Institute for Sex Research at Indiana University. I called home on one occasion but did not talk with Peggy, as she was not at home. I talked with my sons and gave them the number for their mother to call me back. Since she did not return my call, I assumed everything was alright at home. At the conference, I met a young professional woman, Sherry, who was obviously intelligent, beautiful, spontaneous, and energetic. Sherry was in an unhappy marriage, but she was still committed to it. We became involved in a romantic interlude but we both left the conference anticipating that we would not be likely to see one another again. I called home to announce that I was arriving a day earlier than anticipated and was greeted with flagrant hostility. After arriving home, I passively sat through a six-hour tirade on my negligence before I began returning the barrage. After fighting almost continuously for 48 hours, Peggy expressed her feelings of entrapment and her desire to get out of the relationship if she could only save face with family and friends. I immediately confessed my two extramarital involvements and, in anger, offered them for her purposes of face-saving. Then followed a month which seemed truly insane. We went to see her psychiatrist who seemed bewildered as I took the offensive in the couples session. He expressed surprise and astonishment as I reeled out irrefutable facts. At this point, Peggy angrily walked out of the session and slammed the door. She refused to attend any more couple sessions.

I contacted Sherry and again met with her briefly to reaffirm my first impressions. It seemed unlikely that I could create anything positive with her since she was determined to make her marriage work. However, I decided that there must be other women with whom I could have a similar positive relationship. The conflicts at home seemed unbearable with Peggy's demands that I leave the house immediately. I grimly and sorrowfully arranged for a place to live and, while waiting for the available date, went through the process of informing my children.

During the first few months following the separation, I experienced tremendous depression, loneliness and despair. I had suicidal fantasies and engaged in rather reckless behavior, such as careless driving and open courtship of women, much to my attorney's dismay. I saw Sherry for a few brief encounters which were joyous but still offered no hope of commitment. I dated several other women, but the encounters were unsatisfactory. Peggy and I attempted to start all over again by renewing a courtship. We often would have several hours of very positive exchange in which our dialogue seemed better and more mature than ever before in our relationship. However, this would often be disrupted by a sudden outbreak of heated and abusive arguments. On one occasion this proceeded to a physical exchange of pushing and wrestling. It seemed when one of us would move to come closer to the other, the response would be rejection. However, some of the exchanges were so positive, during the third month, I proposed moving back into the house. At this point, I was unaware that Peggy had contacted a lawyer who had assured her that she could obtain a very generous settlement and could indeed "take that goddamn doctor to the cleaners." Because of this lack of apparent progress in reconciliation, I decided to keep pursuing my relationship with Sherry. With her next visit, a detective was stationed outside my cottage documenting that she stayed there all night.

As the months dragged on, Peggy and I were still unable to settle on separation terms. I continued to support her generously, refusing to deprive my children in order to put pressure on her.

During the years in Germany, we attempted to divert our attention away from the marriage by travel and the purchase of European luxury items. During the separation, these items became objects of intense struggle. I also learned early in my marriage that any mention of Peggy in anything other than a positive vein to relatives would result in enormous disruption. Therefore, our relatives were unaware of the extent of our conflict. My closest brother was quite blaming and rejecting toward me, and our relationship remains distant to this day.

During the public phase of our conflict, my very conservative colleagues at the private psychiatric hospital were alarmed at the negative gossip and publicity and were concerned about the image of psychiatry at our hospital. At times this resulted in overt avoidance and hostility. Considerable time elapsed before my colleagues came to accept the changes that I had made, recognizing a basic change in my mood and disposition as a result. They also gradually began to accept and deeply respect my second wife over a period of time.

During the divorce proceedings, complex interactions of 17 years were deemed unimportant in the eyes of the law; the only factor to be considered was my adultery. North Carolina law is extremely punitive in such instances. The judge was a devoted family man and apparently felt judgmental toward this erring doctor. In the years that followed, with inflationary trends, the generous judgment did not truly prove satisfactory to maintain the previous level of living. This apparently added to Peggy's bitterness. She appeared to feel like a person who had been totally rejected and devalued. She appeared to feel deprived of the returns of a tremendous investment. She seemed to lambast me verbally and bitterly on every possible occasion to any possible listener. This bothered me less as time went by and indeed helped to resolve any remaining ambivalence about the breakup on my part. However, the attempts to control are continued in the form of restricting visitation privileges with the children, which resulted in further court appearances. There were also conflicts over the timeliness of support payments, since my major paycheck came ten days later than the appointed payment date. Peggy became friends with several other doctors' wives who were undergoing divorce and together they sung a chorus about the awful attributes of doctors and medicine.

Now, after eight years, Peggy's feelings have apparently begun

> to modulate. Although necessary exchanges continue to be unpleasant, her attitudes about my contact with the children appear to be more compromising. She has done well, attending college for four years and obtaining a bachelor's degree with good grades. She obtained a job which she apparently feels is quite satisfying. Her health, including her back problems, has improved immensely and dramatically. She has become more active socially. She also has remarried an apparently fine man whose needs and habits are compatible with hers. In spite of both of us becoming more satisfied in our second marriages, our necessary interactions are marked by continuing awkwardness and some bitterness.

*Comment.* As marital deterioration takes place, certain milestones seem to occur even though they are not always in the same sequence. The revelations of marital conflict and impending separation to children, families of origin, friends, colleagues, and community appear to constitute individual steps in the disintegration process. Another event that can be quite disturbing to the well controlled physician is the occurrence of near or actual physical conflict. The decision to contact an attorney is a marker event which often increases the fear, anger, and defensiveness of the marital partner. Each step of the court battle appears to increase the subsequent bitterness, as well as the self-depreciation. The bitterness and hostility do not stop when the divorce papers are signed, and this is often surprising to the participants. Since the marriages were formed to meet intense emotional needs, the couple often continues to have intensive emotional binding for years after a divorce. This can even result in repeated legal skirmishes over control of the children and property with the obvious payoff being the opportunities to see the other partner in the courtroom. We feel that the pain generated by these long standing conflicts is one of the tragic aspects of divorce. It often appears that the hostility generated in the divorce process is so strong that the partners have difficulties in admitting the value of the lost partner. In striving to protect their own self-concepts, they continue to blame the other partner. Thus, when the loss cannot be fully appreciated, the individual cannot go on to complete the brief process. This results in a dual tragedy; the partners cannot go on to develop their own lives without completing the grief process, and the bitterness becomes an issue with which the children have to deal.

## DISCUSSION

Whenever there is a cultural hero, mythology abounds. The doctor, as a cultural hero, is no exception. Indeed, Wilson and Larson[16] referred to the physician being seen by society as a "heroic God-like person—a super-intelligent, self-sacrificing, moral, trustworthy, perfect, reliable individual who has leadership abilities that are sacrificially presented to society for its use." Much has been written in professional, as well as the lay literature, regarding this God-like individual. Often these articles indicate that the physicians' marriages are more troubled than marriages in general. Some articles even go so far as to state, "Never marry a doctor."[9] The typical reasons cited for failing in medical marriages are the long hours, the medical practice being seen as a mistress, the physician's need to be omnipotent, role strain, and developmental differences between the physician and his spouse. Also, Dr. Mead states "Much of the estrangement between doctors and their wives comes down to her not knowing what his day is like."[10] However, little objective data is known about the intimacies of the physician's life and marriage, and what objective data is published is drawn from a very select population, usually a clinical one.[2] Rose and Rosow[12] reported in 1972 that "marital stability is the rule rather than the exception among physicians."

Though it could be argued that divorce is only one criterion of poor marriages, recent literature does indicate physicians having fewer divorces than individuals in the general population. An important question needs to be raised here: Do physicians and their spouses stay in poor marriages rather than divorce because of such factors as financial security for the spouse or concerns over social status in the community? Doctor Taubman was quoted recently as saying, "There are powerful social, cultural, and economic pressures on a doctor and his wife to stay together. One of the occupational hazards of physicians is marital misery, but it's hidden by the mask of marital conformity."[8]

Future areas of research need to be focused on obtaining objective data as well as examining both the physician and spouse's view of their marriage. A recent survey in *Medical Economics* did obtain physicians' opinions regarding their marriages. Doctors identified the following as marital problems: physician not home enough, conflicting ideas on how to spend leisure time, failure to communicate, unsatisfactory sexual relationship, financial problems, child rearing, religious differences, physician's extramarital romance, spouse not home enough, spouse's drinking habits, doctor's drinking habits, and spouse's extramarital romance. In responding to the open-ended question, "What is the most important factor that led you to rate your marriage as you did?", the happiest survey respondents used words as compatibility, companionship, common interests, good communication, and just plain love. In those marriages self-reported as happiest, the longer it lasted, the more likely that the doctor was to credit his spouse.[4] Nine out of ten physician's wives who remarry say second marriages are more successful than their first.[10]

These responses are typically found in marital satisfaction surveys. However, some authors have argued that medical marriages are unique not only in their problems but in their development and structure. This question can best be answered in part by examining the life cycle of the medical marriage with a critical look at its strengths as well as its stresses. Most of the objective data on the family backgrounds of physicians has been taken from a clinical population or, for instance, disabled physicians. These distressed physicians frequently describe a childhood dominated by overprotective parents with rejecting attitudes. The parents of disabled physicians may even have failed to acknowledge and support childhood successes. There seems to be excessive dependency on the mother continuing beyond childhood. The father seems to be emotionally detached, whereas mothers were often more demanding, controlling, and seductive. Interesting to note is that a physical illness during childhood may stimulate and support the mother's behavior.[11]

It is also thought that doctors come from families who value achievement. In the literature, physicians are often described as possessing personality characteristics such as obsessiveness, a need to control, and a tendency to intellectualize. These characteristics are often seen as making for a successful medical student, as well as for being a competent physician; however, they can interfere with communication in marriage.[5]

Not only do the characteristics as described of physicians lead to problems with marital communication, but also the physician's professional role may permit him an opportunity for avoiding an attempt to solve marital conflict. In interactions with patients, the physician may tend to be directive and even authoritarian. As one author puts it, "The physician listens, decides, and directs."[7] "To a woman, the doctor is a strong, wise, considerate, saintly man who listens patiently to her complaints. . . unless, of course, the doctor happens to be her husband."[3] The doctor, who at the hospital, is involved in miracles, at home is also seen as human. At the hospital, he may be seen as superefficient and decisive; at home he is the husband who keeps his journals and notes in chaos and cannot decide what he wants for dinner. Indeed, the place where a doctor is least likely to be treated as "doctor" is at home. Having a special status in society, the doctor may find it degrading to come home and be asked to take out the garbage.

This role discrepancy often creates role strain, which occurs when there are gaps between one's expectations and performances, between promise and delivery, and between one's values and norms.[14] Role strain also develops when the physician strives to meet most of the demands of his professional role, as well as the need for personal gratification. In this society physicians are not unlike other men who are accorded social status on the basis of their achievements in the work world. To be a real man in this culture requires a certain amount of occupational success and, in this regard, the physician has become the cultural hero. There are few other careers, however, which seem to create the degree of status anxiety as medicine. The doctor looks to other physicians for his concept of his own self-worth. His reference group becomes other physicians, not other men.[1] Indeed, when mortal men strive for heroic standards, the achievement of a caring and compassionate marriage is the miracle.

## REFERENCES

1. Coombs RH, Vincent CE eds. Psychosocial Aspects of Medical Training, Charles C. Thomas, Springfield, Ill., 1971.
2. Garvey M, Tuason V. Physicians' marriages. J Clin Psychiatry 40:129–131, 1979.
3. Himler LE. What's happening to the doctor's home life? Medical Economics 41:61–69, 1964.
4. Kirchner M. After hours—sharing your life with somebody else. Medical Economics Oct 1:11–49, 1979.
5. Krell R, Miles JE. Marital therapy of couples in which the husband is a physician. Am J Psychother 30(2):267–275, 1976.
6. Levinson DJ. The Seasons of a Man's Life. New York, Alfred A. Knopf, 1978.
7. Lewis JM. The doctor and his marriage. Texas State Journal of Medicine 61:615–619, August, 1965.
8. Manber MM. Being a doctor may be hazardous to your health. Medical World News August 20, 1979.
9. McCall's. Never marry a doctor. September, 1969.
10. Medical Economics. Medical marriage dilemma: Mend it or end it? 88–101, April 30, 1973.
11. Roeske NCA, Stress and the physician. Psychiatric Annals, July 1981. 11(7):10–32.
12. Rose KD, Rosow I. Marital Stability Among Physicians. Medical Aspects of Human Sexuality, June 1973, pp. 62–78.
13. Towsley AC. The doctor's wife: problems of a medical marriage. Medical World News 8:137, 1967.
14. Vincent MO. Doctor and Mrs.—their mental health. Can J Psychiatry 14(5):509–515.
15. Whitaker CA, Miller MH. A re-evaluation of 'psychiatric help' when divorce impends. Am J Psychiatry 136:6111, 1969.
16. Wilson WP, Larson DB. The physician and spouse: physician, know thyself—and they mate. North Carolina Medical Journal, February, 1981, pp. 106–109.

# Burnout

Life is an ever-changing ocean with constant movement and depth. There is the surface which can be smooth or stormy depending on external conditions. There are the shallows with their shoals; and there are the deepest depths no person has explored. Life is variable, with its calm and rough passages, its eddys and currents, its unsettled periods and its doldrums and it has its profound levels which remain uncharted.

Humans, in common with animals, exhibit goal-directed behavior. Achieving the goal brings reward and reinforces the person's behavior. If the goal remains unattainable constantly, frustration occurs and the person adapts by altering either the goal or the behavior. If neither the goal nor the behavior can be changed readily, as happens in medicine, the person is placed in a position where there is constant frustration. This continuous frustration makes one susceptable to decompensation or "burnout."

A physician is dedicated to ministering to the sick with the goal of having them recover. If the ill do not cooperate by recovering, the stage is set for frustration and eventual burnout. One or two setbacks where patients do not get better will be taken in stride by most physicians, but a series of therapeutic failures can make even a most dedicated physician vulnerable to burnout.

In this chapter, Dr. Austin McCawley describes some of the forces causing burnout, discusses who is likely to get it, outlines its sequelae and recommends what can be done to prevent it.

*J.P.C.*

# 8

# The Physician and Burnout

*Austin McCawley*

> Doctors are oxydable products, and the schools must keep furnishing new ones as the old ones turn into oxyds: some are first-rate quality that burn with a great light,—some of a lower grade of brilliancy, some honestly, unmistakably, by the grace of God, of moderate gifts, or in simpler phrase, dull.
>
> *Oliver Wendell Holmes*

The term *burnout* has been applied in many different ways, but in essence it describes the situation where a person's resources and ability to cope are exceeded by the demands of work. The term was originally applied to the kind of emotional exhaustion and disillusionment experienced by counselors in the human services field—social workers, psychiatrists, psychologists, or paraprofessionals whose resources were drained by too many frustrating and difficult patients, insufficient support from the organizational structure, and overwhelming demands on emotional responsivity. Since then, the term has become something of a fad, overused to describe almost every type of job dissatisfaction. Nonetheless, it does describe a very real experience, one that has been given other names; for example, role strain or the overwork syndrome.

Some years ago, I took part in a seminar for first-year medical students in which the lives of two physicians were examined. The seminar, which was part of the social sciences curriculum, studied social adjustment in various stages of the life cycle. However, the class was also very interested in obtaining a picture in depth of the kind of career they were entering. The presentation took the form of videotape interviews of about 45 minutes long and the interviewer's questions were quite comprehensive covering every aspect of the personal life.

The first physician was a full-time chief of service in a university affiliated hospital, a man who had left private practice for a full-time academic career. He had a rather flamboyant personality and was an individualist with a rather offbeat lifestyle. He had many interests outside of medicine and seemed to be fortunate enough to have adequate staffing to cover patient service responsibilities; he was able to combine a satisfying professional career with a full personal life. The class was intrigued but realized he was most unlike an average physician.

The second physician, a successful internist who practiced in a small town, was active in medical affairs and gave some time to teaching the occasional resident doing a rotation in the local community hospital. This man's day started at about 7:30 AM, when he arrived at the hospital to do rounds. At 9:30 AM, he was in his office where he saw patients until 5:30 PM, with a short break for lunch. He then returned to the hospital to see patients on evening rounds and would get home sometime after 8 PM. His evenings were occasionally interrupted by late calls; sometimes he had to return to the hospital to see a patient. He took Wednesday afternoons off but frequently spent these attending a course at a medical school in a neighboring town. He worked all day Saturday and made rounds on Sunday morning but generally had Sunday afternoons and evenings off for relaxation. He played an occasional game of golf and took few vacations. He was quite content with his lot, even proud of himself.

The students were appalled. Their vision of the good life which combined an appropriate amount of hard work with a full gratifying personal life did not jibe with this crushing commitment to patients and practice. To the students indeed, this physician represented the endpoint in a long downhill course of personal deterioration. This was not what they had signed up for; it was not the popular image of the quality living enjoyed by physicians. Up to this point, I believe, they had regarded themselves as a fortunate elite, lucky to be chosen for medical school and assured of a satisfying future. Although in theory they all realized that physicians work hard, they had never quite realized how hard some physicians work. They had never heard the kind of advice expressed by Sonderegger when he wrote,

> Medicine must be (and everything depends on this) your religion and your politics, your fortune and misfortune, therefore, do not advise anyone to become a physician. If he still wants to become one, warn him against it, repeatedly and earnestly; if nonetheless he persists, then give him your blessing; if it is worth anything, he will have need of it.[1]

Four years later, I observed some of the same medical students working 70 to over 100 hours a week as interns. Some of them presumably would have difficulty maintaining their equilibrium in the face of such a schedule and would run into trouble in the internship. In the practice of medicine all of them would work hard, some as hard as the physician in their seminar years before. Some would thrive on it, others begin to burn out, and still others become casualties.

## SIGNS OF BURNOUT

The burned-out person is unable to maintain work performance and shows a consequent decline in efficiency and initiative. He (or she) becomes increasingly cynical and disillusioned about his work. Sometimes, he conceals this by a rigid, inflexible attitude which in a more subtle way expresses a basic negativism. He experiences many upsets of health including loss of energy, irritability, disturbance of sleep and eating habits, difficulty in concentrating, dejection, depression, tension headaches, and other symptoms of stress. Not infrequently, he attempts to self-medicate with alcohol or drugs. Although work performance declines, the person may spend increasing amounts of time in the office in an attempt to compensate. Outside of the office, he is unable to relax and to enjoy recreational pursuits.

The burned-out physician may spend increasing amounts of time in the hospital or office while accomplishing less; in other cases, he changes his work schedules in significant ways, e.g., making hospital rounds at unusual hours on a schedule different from colleagues, or making rounds less frequently and avoiding medical staff or society meetings. Burnout can also manifest itself in more subtle but quite destructive ways; for example, a cold, unsympathetic, and brisk manner that conveys an essential disinterest while going through the usual routines of a medical interview. However, the influence of medical tradition is still strong and although the physician may become indifferent to patients, the essential philosophical values of medicine are still held positively on an intellectual level. This is in contrast to burnout in other disciplines and businesses where the values of career, whether business or therapeutic counseling, may be completely rejected by the individual. This may make it more difficult to detect medical burnout.

While some physicians stay at the stage of being burned out, others develop frank impairment; in this sense, burnout may be regarded as a prodromal stage. The tertiary problems that result are well described in other chapters of this book. The statistics are impressive: high rates of suicide, alcoholism, drug addiction, and depression, not to mention the casualties in spouses and children. A comparison with statistics for other disciplines and professions indicates that physicians are not alone in having a high casualty rate. Many other professions—for example, trial lawyers, politicians, senior executives, air traffic controllers, and others—experience high levels of stress. However, high statistics for stress-related illness in other professions does not reduce the figures for medicine. The fact that medical students undergo such a long period of training and are screened for staying power gives an additional significance to the statistics for impairment in physicians.

The occupations listed above are well known to be stressful and the reasons for stress are quite evident. People who enter these occupations know what they are getting into and presumably like it. Although medicine is recognized as an arduous profession (perhaps more so in some particular specialties), the degree, quality, and type of stress is not appreciated by the lay public. In fact, the students who took the seminar on lifestyles knew very little about medicine as a profession; this seems to be true of most students entering medical school. In one study, 13.2% of male and 6.7% female first-year medical students had never discussed a medical career with a doctor or worked in a health care job.

## RESPONSIBILITY FOR OTHERS

Some of the stresses of a medical career are well known but their full impact is poorly understood until experienced. The anxiety of major decisions and taking responsibility for others is an intrinsic part of medicine; nevertheless, the special anxiety of being responsible for another's life affects the young doctor in unexpected ways. It is a major learning experience and a major stress in the internship. Similarly, it is generally understood that doctors are on call a good deal of the time, must be available at unusual hours, and work at times when other people do not. However, the emotional drain from being on call almost continually to the public is not really appreciated until one has to live with it. One doctor expressed it this way: "It's not being called to the telephone; it's the state of just expecting the phone to ring at anytime." When responding to a call, the doctor is expected to perform at peak level; this expectation of the public that the doctor will always be functioning optimally, even under the most trying circumtances, is a hard demand to meet.

The lay person thinks of the stress of medical practice in connection with an individual patient. The problem, however, is not simply the type of stress but the frequency with which it is repeated. In other words, it is not the emergency call itself but rather the next two calls from the Emergency Room that arrive when the physician has just finished the last call and started to relax. The lay person would find it difficult to comprehend the number of patients that a busy internist or orthopedist, for example, might see in the course of an afternoon. A lawyer, accountant, or salesman might only deal with a few clients in the same period of time. In terms of the number of patients including difficult personalities seen in the course of the working day, dentistry is the only comparable profession. The statistics for impairment in dentists are on a comparable level.

## ROLE STRAIN

There are some paradoxes in the practice of medicine which create role strain for the physician. A doctor is required to be sympathetic, sensitive, understanding, and compassionate; at the same time, there are some very tough decisions to make while maintaining one's performance unaffected by suffering and tragedy. As one physician put it, "Medicine can sometimes be a dirty business." In fact, Osler has described a certain measure of insensibility required for the practice of medicine and used to counsel medical students to "acquire early the art of detachment."[2] The physician, moreover, has to be capable of moving from this attitude of detachment to one of compassion. This is not always easy.

Most paradoxical perhaps, is the overwhelming attraction that medicine seems to possess for its practitioners, in spite of all the stress: the fascination and challenge keep them returning for more. This maintains and escalates the pressure. Oliver Wendell Holmes advised Phinneas Barnes, "If you would wax thin and savage like a half-fed spider,—be a lawyer; if you would go off like an opium-eater in love with your starving delusion,—be a doctor."[3]

Rhoads has described the characteristics of physicians who overwork.[4] Some individuals attempt to overcome fear of failure and insecurity through work; in others, identification with a perfectionistic parent is the driving force. Compensation for other defects such as poor health or aging can also be a motivating factor. Almost all physicians who overwork have in common an excessive need for approval and a compulsive approach to work as a defense against problems of aggression. Rhoads comments that "in physicians, particularly, the need to be loved by everyone was a major component of the drive to overwork."[4] Not only does an exaggerated attention to the practice of medicine enhance self-esteem and gain social approval, it also helps the physician maintain a clear conscience by demonstrating to the world that he or she has even worked to the edge of total exhaustion and is therefore blameless.

The compulsive traits of physicians are well recognized. Perfectionistic attention to detail and the need for omnipotent control are reinforced by the demands of medical practice. The physician's accessibility to the general public encourages the tendency to take responsibility for everyone. Doctors are always subject to what has been described as the tyranny of "the should"—things they should be doing.

The observations of Rhoads on the problem of burnout indicate factors in the individual rather than the external realities of medical practice, implicating personality problems that go back long before the time of choice of a medical career. Similar conclusions can be drawn from the studies of George Vaillant and colleagues[5] involved in an intensive study of a population selected in college and followed throughout their lives over a period of 30 years. The subjects were selected on the basis of having no easily detectable health problems, mental or physical, and for easily meeting the academic demands of college. From this group, 47 attended medical school and 46 graduated. These 47 were compared to a control group of 79 men, not physicians, who were randomly selected from the larger sample.

The 47 physicians, especially those involved in direct patient care, were more likely than controls to have relatively poor marriages, use drugs and alcohol heavily, and obtain psychotherapeutic treatment. Dr. Vaillant's study indicated that the presence or absence of these difficulties appeared to be strongly associated with life adjustment before medical school. Only the physicians with the least stable childhoods and adolescent adjustments appeared vulnerable to these occupational hazards. These findings indicated that stress of a medical career seemed to be less important than is usually assumed. The study also raised questions about the motivation for the choice of medicine as a career. Dr. Vaillant suggested that some physicians may elect to assume direct care of patients to give others the care that they did not receive in their childhoods.

## MOST VULNERABLE

The reaction to stress is a product of the particular quality of stress and the individual personality. The stress of medical practice is undeniable, yet many people seem to handle it well. As might be expected, those who break down are those who are most vulnerable. Medicine becomes a strain only when the physician has to give more than he or she has been given. There are of course many rewards and gratifications in the practice of medicine that maintain the necessary psychological supplies to a physician. Foremost among these is the gratitude of patients and the general social approval for someone whose job is to help others. Also important is the boost to the ego and the enhanced sense of importance produced by that special authority which a physician exercises within the medical field. As this authority, indeed omnipotence, is not matched in the physician's other social contacts, it is not surprising that some more insecure individuals prefer to remain within the context of their professional role.

It is interesting that Vaillant's studies showed the highest number of symptoms in the group of nonsurgical practicing doctors; in contrast, doctors in administration, surgery, and research had significantly less emotional difficulties and also more stable childhoods. Statistics on suicide indicate that the highest rates within health care are for psychiatrists, ophthalmologists, otolaryngologists, and anesthetists.

Several explanations may be advanced for these figures. The factor of self-selection may indeed be important notably in regard to surgery where the more aggressive, assertive individuals would tend to select themselves and psychiatry where students with problems of their own might feel drawn to studying the problems of others. However, the statistics may also be explained on the basis of the balance between psychological demand and reward in different types of practice.

Contrasting the four vulnerable specialties with surgery as an example of a specialty with a low casualty rate, the following distinctions may be made. In surgery, the demands and pressure of practice are heavy but the rewards are considerable. The obvious tangible achievements of the surgeon in terms of operative results, technical skills, and the special status enjoyed in the community and with patients constitute rather substantial personal rewards from practice. The otolaryngologist and the ophthalmologist do not usually have the same quality of personal relationship with patients: their skill is more technical and their contact with patients is often brief or at best intermittent; hence, the personal approbation that they receive from grateful patients is limited in comparison to some other specialties. This would of course vary with the type of practice: an ophthalmologist doing a great deal of eye surgery or an otolaryngologist doing more than routine tonsils and septums, would have much the same relation to patients as the general surgeon. The anesthetist obviously has much less personal contact with patients. In all three specialties the professional demands are onerous.

The psychiatrist has intense personal contact with patients but the protracted nature of psychiatric work, the delay in achieving positive results, and the rather intangible quality of those favorable results which are achieved combine to reduce the personal rewards experienced in psychiatric work. Some studies show that a large number of psychiatrists are happy with their choice of specialty, but the suicide statistics indicate that a significant number feel rather differently.

In other words, in three of the specialties with high suicide rates there is less close patient contact than in general medicine; in the fourth, psychiatry, there is a lot of close personal contact but in a very frustrating way. In this balance between reward and punishment, the practice of medicine seems in some individuals to resemble neurosis: the individual needs the neurosis while suffering from it. Like other neuroses, there are characteristic defense mechanisms: among them, detachment, isolation, obsessive compulsive, perfectionistic control, and intellectualization. As occurs in neurosis, the individual encounters difficulties when the defense mechanisms cease to function effectively. They are least effective, of course, at home; the spouse and family are also traumatized, and often the first to suffer.

## PREVENTION

Medical societies have become more concerned about the impact of stress on the medical practitioner. In addition to the numerous programs to help deal with the impaired physician, many of the societies have been running stress workshops or other projects designed to help the individual practitioner with personal problems. These help, at least, to raise the level of awareness; but one has to question how valuable any one workshop can be in producing lasting results, however entertaining and interesting the program may be. The attempt to change deeply rooted patterns of behavior is never easy.

It would seem that a start might be made in early training. Teachers, clinical supervisors, and chiefs of service rarely advise medical students or house staffs on the value of being able to pace oneself. Rather the ethos is "We did it when we were residents, and you ought to be able to do the same." A pattern is set during the residency experience that persists for a lifetime.

Rhoads compared his patients suffering from the overwork syndrome with a group of executives who handled extremely demanding schedules successfully without damage to themselves or their families.[4] These individuals were accustomed to carrying responsibility and a work load well above the norm but seemed to thrive on it. Among other characteristics, two traits were very noticeable in this group. First, they were able to postpone thinking about problems until the time for action on the matter arrived. Secondly, they were able to recognize when they were under strain and take some appropriate action, either taking a vacation, delegating responsibility, postponing a project, or some other response to reduce stress. It has to be recognized that medical practice will not always allow a doctor to slacken off. Nevertheless, there are many times in every physician's life when there is an option between a further commitment to work and leaving it to a colleague; often, the choice of the practitioner is to commit. Recognition of the need to back off occasionally might be an important factor in preventing the development of unmanageable stress.

Doctors as a group receive very little training in administration and management. Skills that could be acquired in such courses are certainly of value in organizing a daily schedule, and efficient organization of work can reduce stress. Effective working relations with colleagues and adequate coverage are also important supports; it has been a common observation that the solo practitioner is at higher than average risk for impairment. Professional association in the societies of the medical community is of course a great resource to alleviate stress for physicians who gain support from relaxing and sharing experience with colleagues.

Many other aids to reducing stress have been advocated including relaxation techniques, jogging, transcendental meditation, hobbies, self-hypnosis, and such basic commonsense measures as taking reasonable vacation time. Although most people are aware of these possibilities, the problem is to encourage the individual to take some positive action; it is surprising how often intelligent hard-working physicians neglect the most obvious basic needs. It is not uncommon to hear the wife of such a physician complain that they have not taken a vacation in years.

## COPING

In certain sections of general hospitals where the level of stress is particularly high—for example, the critical care units, dialysis, and oncology services—staff support groups have been particularly effective in reducing stress in members of the staff, including nurses and physicians. In discussing the problem of morale in groups under a high level of stress, Patrick McKegney[6] has described some survival values which the individual staff member should acquire. He calls this a "survival kit." The values include a sense of self-respect, an appreciation of human limitations, an ability to set priorities and to set limits, including limits on personal responsibility, attention to self, the capacity to recognize and accept the natural course of events, and, perhaps most important for physicians, the recognition of personal vulnerability. He also lists as most valuable qualities in dealing with stress the gift of laughter and a sense that the world is mad.

At first glance, the sense that the world is mad may not seem helpful but it recognizes a fundamental reality. We are not in control of our destinies, however skillful, knowledgeable, and sophisticated we may be. The world is unpredictable and not always kind. Physicians who are asked to treat the ills of the world and have mastered a few of them often develop the conceit they can control the uncontrollable.

Many physicians do not admit their personal vulnerability.

The ability to recognize when one is under stress is the most important single prerequisite—the ability to recognize danger signals and change direction. A capacity for self-awareness and self-knowledge is essential; when a problem is recognized, then appropriate strategies for reduction of stress and personal change can be worked out. The actual techniques for dealing with it are perhaps less important than the fact that the person recognizes the need to do something and attempts to organize and develop an appropriate plan of action. If the physician cannot do it alone then psychotherapy with a therapist knowledgeable about physicians may be indicated. In a pressured existence one needs a sense of where one is vulnerable to anxiety. It has been said that, " 'tis not work that kills but worry."

## REFERENCES


1. Jakob Laurenz Sondregger 1826–1896, Letter. In: Strauss MB (ed), Familiar Medical Quotations. Boston, Massachusetts, Little, Brown, 1968, p 381.
2. Sir William Osler. Aequanimitas, with other Addresses, "Teacher and Student". Philadelphia, Blakiston, 1932, pp 5, 32.
3. Holmes OW: Letter to Phineas Barnes, March 1831.
4. Rhoads, JM: Overwork. J Am Med Assoc 1977, 237 (24): 2615–2618.
5. Vaillant GE, Sobowale NC, McArthur C: Some Psychological Vulnerabilities of Physicians. New Engl J Med 1972, 287: 372–375.
6. McKegney P: Personal communication. Adapted from Lipp M: The Respectful Treatment. Hagerstown, Maryland, Harper and Row, 1977, pp 214–215.

# Physician Suicide

This week and every week two male physicians in the United States on the average will kill themselves. In addition, every month of the year a female doctor will also take her life. These are somber statistics. The male physician suicide rate is similar to that of other professional men; the female rate is four times that of her nonphysician counterpart. It is paradoxical that physicians, a group that holds life so sacrosanct, should have such a significant rate of self-destruction.

Suicide is an intimate act yet a public statement. There are few private actions that have such a profound effect on others. It has been claimed that suicide is not about death but rather is about life. According to Wilfrid Sheed suicide is the sincerest form of criticism life gets.[1] That may be so but a majority of physicians do not view life so negatively. Whatever the tragic reasons for suicides in physicians, a group above average in influence and income, the causes of it are puzzling.

Suicide has been pondered through the ages by priests and poets, philosophers and physicians; attitudes toward it vary from culture to culture. Whatever the cultural differences it appears to be an act that is uniquely human. Animals do not share our propensity toward self-destruction even though they act in a manner at times that leads to their death. There is no compelling proof that lemmings or a dog that dies of starvation following his master's death actually mean to kill themselves.

In this chapter Dr. Patrick Friel analyzes physician suicide from different perspectives and describes how you can spot danger signals that a colleague is troubled and may be contemplating his or her own demise.

*J.P.C.*

---

[1]Sheed W: The Good Word: and Other Words. New York, EP Dutton, 1978, p 68.

# 9

# Physician Suicide

*Patrick Friel*

Suicide, the intentional taking of one's life, is difficult to document from the standpoint of statistical accuracy. Retrospectively proving intention can be troublesome and intricate unless there is a genuine suicide note, previous abortive attempts, or pronouncements regarding intent. The almost universal social and moral opprobrium surrounding suicide pressures families and those others charged with reporting the cause of death to smudge facts and to use the widest latitude in extending the victim the benefit of the doubt. Economic elements play a part since insurance companies may refuse death benefits in cases of suicide. Single car accidents, plane crashes, and drownings are often masked suicides, but the cause of death is listed as accidental. It is generally accepted that suicide is under—rather than overreported.

These statements apply to physician suicides generally as well as certain additional specific considerations. Arguments are marshaled on both sides of the issue of whether a physician's death, by virtue of his or her standing in the community, is subject to greater or lesser scrutiny. Traditionally the doctor and doctor's family enjoyed positions of prestige, social status, and esteem in the community. Any suggestion that such an honorable person would commit suicide, bringing shame to the family and disgrace to its name would be rejected. The principle of *de mortuis nihil nisi bonum* (speak no evil of the dead) would receive the fullest application. The doctor's relationship with the coronor and the medical examiner was also cited as a reason for invoking special consideration. The day when the doctor was deified in the community has passed, and society's current almost voyeuristic obsessive need to learn "the facts" dispel any such protective desires.

## INVESTIGATIVE STUDIES

Beginning in May 1965, the *Journal of the American Medical Association* began to list suicide as a cause of death in their obituary column. The editor of the *Journal,* in a communication to Blachly,[1] cautioned that the data would not be valid statistically because listing in the *Journal* is allowed only when a statement has appeared in the public press. If the deceased's family request that the cause of death be omitted in a suicide, and there has been no public statement, the request is usually respected.

Rich and Pitts[2] reviewed the material collected by the Deaths Editor for physician deaths reported by obituary in the *Journal of the American Medical Association* for a five-year period from May 22, 1967 to May 30, 1972. The crude annual death rate for male physicians was 1179 per 100,000. Out of a total of 17,979 male physician deaths, there were 544 suicides. This works out to a percentage rate of 3.03. Thus, the crude annual physician suicide rate was 35.7 per 100,000. The overall suicide rate for white men over 25 during that period was 34.6. The suicide rate of the male physician thus parallels closely the rate for white males generally in the over-25 group.

Pitts et al.[3] reviewed the *Journal of the American Medical Association* obituary material for a five-year period and found 49 suicides in 751 female physician deaths. This works out to a percentage rate of 6.52. The crude annual death rate was 40.7 per 100,000 female physicians. The death rate by suicide of white women over 25 for the same period was 11.4 per 100,000.

It is obvious from these figures that while the suicide rate for male physicians approximates that of their white male counterparts, the rate for female physicians is nearly four times that of their white female counterparts.

### Age

The age at which male physicians suicided ranged from 27 to 84 with a mean average of 51.3 ± 6.[2] The age at which female physicians suicided ranged from 25 to 79 with a mean average of 47.8 ± 2.[3]

DeSole et al.[4] reported that 26% of all deaths occurring in physicians in the 25–39 age group are the result of suicide. For white males in that same age group the suicide rate was 9%. The percentage of deaths due to suicide remains twice as great for physicians in the 40–59 age group as in comparable white males.

### Method

Physicians have a definite preference for drug ingestion (55%) and an aversion for firearms (12%) in their suicidal acts.[5] The physician's knowledge of chemistry and pharmacodynamics has been suggested as a major factor in this choice. However, chemists and dentists—professionals who are also familiar with drugs—do not show the same predeliction (35% and 40%, respectively).

### Specialty

DeSole et al.[4] computed the suicide rate for various specialties based on reported suicides in the *JAMA* obituaries for a three-year period (May 1965–May 1968). They found that psychiatrists ranked highest with 58 suicides per 100,000; anesthesiologists, 44 per 100,000; general practitioners and internists were in the intermediate range with 34 and 31 per 100,000, respectively; and surgeons, general and orthopedic, were at the lower end of the scale with a rate of 22 per 100,000.

Approximately 100 physicians suicide every year. This amounts to an average medical school graduation class. Rich and Pitts[2] found that the suicidal rate for male physicians has remained relatively constant over the past 35 years. They conclude that some stable process or processes must be involved in the genesis of suicide. This is a tragic waste of human resource, most often at the peak of a productive professional career, and has naturally attracted attention and investigation.

## CAUSES FOR SUICIDE

DeSole et al. have written about *role strain* as a significant contributor existing when there are gaps "between expectations and performances, between promise and delivery, between values and norms."[4] Role strain is to be distinguished from *role conflict* or *role contradiction*, which would be more akin to Erikson's *identity crisis*.[6] There is no doubt about the role one is expected to perform; the trouble lies more in the lack of social institutions and norms to support that role.

Waltzer,[7] reporting on physicians hospitalized for psychiatric illness, found that 50% were abusing alcohol and drugs. The role strain of long hours, demanding patients, overwork, and fatigue contributed to physician suicide. The emotional demands of patients so drained the physician that the usual sources of renewal and support through relationships with spouses and children, friends, and recreation were avoided because of lack of incentive. This type of strain probably contributes to the doctor's use of alcohol and drugs to help cope with strain rather than seek recreational pleasure or social escape, as do nonphysician users. In taking drugs, physicians tend to use the intramuscular rather than the intravenous route because of the more sustained effect.

Undoubtedly there is stress and strain associated with the practice of medicine; but if this were the sole cause, then the suicidal rate of physicians should exceed that of the general population. While the rate for male physicians equals that of white males generally, there is a definitely higher rate of suicide for physicians under age 49. As previously mentioned, female physicians commit suicide at a rate four times that of their white female counterparts. However, Steppacher et al.[8] suggest that the death by suicide for female psychologists and chemists is similar to that of female physicians.

It is an accepted axiom in psychiatry that a healthy personality can cope with virtually any stress. Perhaps it would be fruitful to investigate this aspect of the problem and look also at the psychopathology of the individual rather than focus solely on the external stress factor.

Over 100 years ago, Sir James Paget traced the careers of 1000 of 1226 former pupils. He found that nearly 13% of his entering medical students were dead within 15 years. He characterized this as "a melancholy list," and concluded: "Nothing appears more certain than that the personal character—the very nature, the will of each student—has a far greater force in determining his career than any helps or hinderances whatever."[9]

An editorial in the *JAMA* addressing the issues of reasons for physician suicide stated: "It is not remarkable, in considering these facts, that failures must occur, that many of our professional brethren have to drop out of the profession in one way or another, and that weaklings, those morbidly disposed, and those lacking high principles and moral inhibitions, might very easily adopt suicide as the most direct way to end their troubles. That more do not do this, we think speaks well for the profession."[10]

## CONTRIBUTIVE FACTORS

### Personality

Altruism is one of the leading conscious reasons for interest in a medical career. The basic personality structure reveals fairly well compensated obsessive-compulsive traits: an ability to suppress feeling, postpone gratification, submit to discipline in the traditional authoritarian medical school teacher model. Most of the hard data on physician personalities come from studies about those who are disabled and mostly involve men.[11] The above-mentioned obsessive-compulsive characteristics can be an asset but instead become a liability contributing to the physician's impairment. It amounts to being consumed by a drive that under normal circumstances nourishes and supports. Excessive basic insecurity, dependency, depressive tendencies, and increased vulnerability to stress are more apparent in these personalities. The "I can't say no" syndrome is often a manifestation of a highly ambivalent attitude toward medicine, loving it yet clearly resenting its demands, but getting caught up in longer working hours that fail to grant the desired narcissistic need.

### Family Background

Disturbed and disabled physicians often describe a childhood dominated by overprotective but rejecting parents who fail to acknowledge or support success. There is prolonged dependence on mothers and fathers who are detached and who hurt. They also seem to lack warmth and understanding. Physical illness during childhood stimulated and supported mother's behavior. A significant number of impaired physicians have come from families where there was a history of mental illness, especially depressive disorders, suicides, and alcoholism.[11]

## THE MEDICAL STUDENT

Medicine is recognized as a prestige profession virtually guaranteeing social and material security. Too much emphasis on security and independence may indicate a reaction formation against hidden excessive dependency. Selection of medicine as a career based on too great a desire to please parents rather than on personal inclination and suitability can lead to unfortunate consequences.

Epstein et al.[12] conducted an interesting investigation at Johns Hopkins to determine whether there are recognizable psychological characteristics of predictive value in identifying future suicides. A retrospective–prospective design was used. The 33 subjects were a subset of a cohort of 1198 medical students at the school who were participants in long-term studies on cardiovascular disease. The 33 selected for this study consisted of nine subjects who were known to have committed suicide after graduation from medical school, two matched controls for each suicide, and six distractors. All subjects had been given among various other measures a battery of psychological tests in connection with the longer-term cardiovascular studies. The reviewing psychiatrist, blind to the number of suicides and controls (informed only that the 33 records included at least one completed suicide plus suicide controls) was able to identify the nine suicides correctly. Those subjects who committed suicide rated themselves on various psychological tests significantly higher than nonsuicidal controls in areas of thoughtfulness, anger, hostility, depression, negativism, suspiciousness, verbal expansiveness, dependency, and impulsiveness. Self-destructive tendencies and guilty self-concepts were also significantly higher in the suicide group. This study certainly suggests that students with such self-destructive potential can be identified.

Thomas[13] performed a follow-up study on 1337 former Johns Hopkins medical students from the classes of 1948–1964 and found that 49 subjects died prematurely. Suicide accounted for 17 (34.7%) of these deaths.

## THE MEDICAL GRADUATE

The youthful enthusiasm and idealism of the medical student, imbued with the glamour of dramatic life-saving adventures, often conflicts with the realities of life as an intern, resident, or practitioner. The 100–120-hour work week may be initially rewarding as a training experience, but it does not always mean working with interesting diagnostic and exciting therapeutic challenges. Chronic, multiproblem, demanding patients who do not respond to conventional medical approaches, and who require a social rather than a medical miracle, challenge idealism. It takes time to develop the pragmatic coping techniques required to deal with such problems. Failure to make an adequate adjustment will take its toll, and the resulting strain is often translated into conflicts in significant interpersonal relationships both professional and social. Spouses and children will complain about the frequently absent, undependable, or exhausted husband or parent who is too tired to listen to their problems and to the adventures of home life. This can lead to the oft repeated reports of "needing to make an appointment" to get attention from the physician whose time is so taken up with that demanding mistress—medicine.

The type of practice or chosen specialty seems to have some bearing on suicide. Vaillant et al.[14] reviewed the childhood experiences of 47 physicians and compared them with a group of 79 socio-economically matched controls. There was a high index of instability and a history of relatively loveless and unhappy childhood in those physicians involved in primary care as opposed to those engaged in research and administration. They concluded that one important motivating factor which leads some physicians to assume direct patient care is that they can give to others the care and attention they did not receive themselves in childhood. In effect, they are vicariously ministering to themselves.

Waring,[15] in a literature review in the early 1970s, mentioned the common assumption that the stresses that provoke psychiatric illness in the medical profession are the length and difficulty of medical training, the demands of the profession, the responsibility for life-and-death situations, and the ready availability of drugs. He concluded however, that "these explanations seem somewhat artificial."

Pond[16] held that there is not enough evidence to support the view that the conditions of work for the physician are more than minor precipitating factors. He believes that mentally ill doctors come from families with a history of mental illness, unsatisfactory homes, and make unsatisfactory adult relationships in marriage to much the same extent that their nonmedical patients do.

The higher rate of suicide among woman physicians has attracted particular attention. Pitts et al.[3] suggested that affective disorders such as depression may be a preexisting factor in the personality and predisposing in an unexplained fashion to their choice of medicine as a career. They felt it was possible to calculate the approximate morbid risk for affective disorder for any group for which the percentage of deaths due to suicide is known. This is a rather syllogistic type of logic that does not always apply to human systems.

The female physician faces certain problems and difficulties related to career goals. If in the interest of pursuing a career she remains single, she may then find herself in her 30s unsatisfied with the acclaim of professional competence. Marriage and children are significant events in the life of a woman, and their absence can lead to feelings of loneliness, alienation, and a lack of fulfillment. The married female physician has to cope with a situation significantly different from her male counterpart. She usually has a working spouse and, despite the demands of her own professional life, is expected to assume much of the responsibility for running the house and caring for the children. As currently constituted, there is more opportunity for conflict of identity as well as role strain in the wife/mother/physician than in the husband/father/physician model. This is not peculiar to the female physician: similar conflicts and higher suicidal rates are also common in female chemists and psychologists. Although there are stresses intrinsic to the practice of medicine as a profession, the weight of evidence would seem to incline toward the psychopathology of the individual as the more significant contributing factor in the genesis of suicide.

Ross[17] draws a composite picture of the typical American physician at high risk of suicide.

> He is a 48 year old doctor graduated at or near the top of his high prestige medical school class, and now practices a peripheral specialty associated with chronic problems where satisfactions are difficult and laggard. Because he is active, aggressive, ambitious, competitive, compulsive, enthusiastic and individualistic, he is apt to be easily frustrated in his need for achievement and recognition, and in meeting his goals. Unable to tolerate delay in gratification, he may use large amounts of anaesthetics or psychoactive drugs in his practice.

## PREVENTION

Since psychopathology plays such a significant role in the etiology of suicide, it is only fitting that possible preventive steps should be considered.

The profession both individually and through its institutions should be more aware of the problem and more active in seeking out those in need of help. Some state and county medical societies have established committees to review and make recommendation for impaired physicians, which is a step in the right direction.

Beginning in medical school, those students who are chronic abusers of alcohol and drugs should not be viewed by their colleagues as mere swingers but as individuals obviously needing psychiatric help. Students and faculty equally share the responsibility and should cooperatively address the issue rather than avoiding it with the rationalization that it is an innocuous social phenomenon typical of our times. The loner, the misfit, and those with other obvious manifestations of personality maladjustment should be handled similarly.

The practicing physician needs the support of colleagues and institutions including hospitals and medical societies. This responsibility is as old as the Hippocratic oath but too often ignored in the impersonal ambience of present-day practice. There are danger signals that should trigger appropriate action, including but not limited to the following:

1. Increasing reliance on drugs and alcohol.
2. Presenting in hospital for rounds or surgery while under the influence of intoxicants.
3. Making rounds at irregular hours or too infrequently.
4. Loss of previously recognized confidence in handling difficult diagnostic and patient management problems.
5. Significant recent change in working, eating, or sleeping habits.
6. Avoidance of close contact with colleagues.

Add to this list evidence of depression, recent loss of a spouse either to divorce or death, and disappointment in a career opportunity (in an individual in the 40–60 age span), and the risk is significantly and dangerously increased. The single individual with a combination of the above elements is an even greater risk category.

It is not easy to suggest to a colleague that psychiatric treatment is necessary; nor is it easy for physicians to accept such recommendations. Jones[18] recommends using peer pressure even to the point of discontinuing admitting and operating privileges as a more compassionate mechanism than legally revoking a licence. If such leverage is used and hospitalization is recommended, then arrangements have to be made for maximum care and supervision of the particular individual until admission is completed.

Physicians as a group have an almost phobic attitude toward illness in themselves, and especially toward emotional illness. Simon and Lumry[19] found that suicidal M.D.s tend to deny personal or physiological discomfort and try to cover up their suicidal impulses; thus, they are extremely resistive in admitting to emotional problems and the need for psychiatric help. This denial mechanism complicates treatment. Also, there is an axiom in medicine that whatever can go wrong will go wrong when one is treating a colleague or his family. The traditional doctor–patient relationship suffers distortion because of the extra demands, and the higher level of expectation. The resultant increased level of anxiety in the therapist raises the probability of complications and poor therapeutic results.

The American Psychiatric and American Medical Associations have announced the development of a year-long study to determine why some physicians kill themselves. The American Medical Association Board of Trustees said that the study "should help determine the nature and relative importance of the precursors to suicide, and in so doing give meaningful direction to efforts aimed at prevention and treatment of the predisposing conditions."[20]

Much work remains to be done in helping to clarify the relative significance of the various factors involved in the genesis of this problem. One hundred physician suicides per year is a human tragedy but a relatively small number from a dynamic investigative standpoint. A cooperative nationwide study over a long enough period of time offers the best hope of gaining the in-depth dimension that is required.

## REFERENCES


1. Blackley PH, Disher W, Rounder G: Suicide by physicians Bull Suicide NIMH 1968, 1–18: 2.
2. Rich CL, Pitts FN: Suicide by male physicians during a five year period. Am J Psychiatry 1979, 136(8):1089.
3. Pitts FN, Schuller AB, Rich CL, Pitts AT: Suicide among U.S. women physicians, 1967–1972. Am J. Psychiatry 1979, 136(5):695.
4. DeSole DE, Singer P, Aronson S: Suicide and role strain among physicians. Int. J. Soc. Psychiatry 1969, 15(294):297.
5. Rose KD, Rosow I: Physicians who kill themselves. Arch. Gen. Psychiatry 1973, 29:804, 805.
6. Erickson EH: Childhood and Society. New York, Morton, 1950.
7. Waltzer H: Physicians. *In* Hankoff LD, Einsidler B (eds), Suicide: Theory and Clinical Aspects. Littleton, Massachusetts, PSG Publ. Co., 1979.

8. Steppacher RC, Mausner JS: Suicide in male and female physicians. *J Am Med Assoc* 1976, 228:323–328.
9. Paget J: What becomes of medical students? *In* Paget S (ed): Selected Essays and Addresses by Sir James Paget. London, Longmans, Green and Co., 1902, pp 27–32.
10. Editorial—Suicides by physicians and the reasons. J Am Med Assoc 1903, 40:263.
11. Roeske NCA: Stress and the physician. Psychiatr Ann 1981, 11(7):297.
12. Epstein LC, Thomas CB, Shaffer JW, Perkins S: Clinical prediction of physician suicide based on medical student data. J Nerv Ment Dis 1973, 156(1): 19–28.
13. Thomas CB: What becomes of medical students: the dark side. Johns Hopkins Med J 1976, 138:185–195.
14. Vaillant CF, Sobowale NC, McCarthur C: Some psychologic vulnerabilities of physicians. New Engl J Med 1972, 287:372–375.
15. Waring EM: Psychiatric illness in physicians: A review. Compr Psychiatry 1974, 15:519.
16. Pond DA: Doctors' mental health. New Zealand Med J 1969, 69:131.
17. Ross M: Suicide among physicians. Dis Nerv Syst 1973, 34 (3).
18. Jones RE: A study of 100 physician psychiatric inpatients. Am J Psychiatry 1977, 134(10):1122.
19. Simon W, Lumry GK: Suicide among physician patients. J Nerv Ment Dis 1968, 147:105–112.
20. AMA Board of Trustees: Report to House of Delegates, December 1979.

# The Physician Drug Addict

Human beings show remarkable variation in their ability to withstand trial and tribulation. The faint hearted offer little resistance and surrender at the first sign of adversity. Others, more sanguine, never concede defeat and plough on regardless of pain or personal privation. A majority of physicians, it would appear, are at the latter end of this spectrum. This is not surprising because physicians have been trained to delay gratification, work long hours, accumulate enormous amounts of knowledge, and deal with circumstances that others would find beyond their capacity to endure. In short, physicians have better than average ability for coping with adversity.

However, a significant number of doctors, estimated to be about 500 annually, fall short of the high standards of behavior that society and the medical profession both expect from physicians. These physicians for one reason or another become drug addicts.

Why should this happen? Are these physicians suffering from chemical deficiency? Are they genetically predisposed or are they simply weak? Why one physician in a given situation becomes drug dependent and another does not is not readily answered. One fact is clear: drug addicted physicians can be treated and successfully rehabilitated.

In this chapter Dr. Perry Ayres, a physician who has studied drug addiction in physicians, outlines the cause, course, and cure of physician drug addiction.

*J.P.C.*

# 10

# The Physician Drug Addict

*Perry R. Ayres*

*It is Tuesday night at the Country Club and Joe, the bartender, is preparing for the monthly dinner meeting of the County Medical Society. Joe is a registered pharmacist. His stock of bottles, vials, ampules, syringes, and tourniquets is neatly arranged as the doctors begin to arrive.*

*"Good evening, doctor, what's your pleasure?"*

*"Hi, Joe. Give me a little of that demerol."*

*"Tablets, or injectable?"*

*"Make it the usual. Draw up about a hundred milligrams and let me use a tourniquet. It's been a rough day!"*

*"Next—what's yours, doctor?"*

*"Let me have one of those dexedrine tablets, Joe, and I'll take along a nembutal for after the meeting. Thanks. Hey, Frank, come over here and name your poison. I'm buying."*

*"Wow, we never know when the old tightwad might loosen up, do we Joe? Give me a couple cc of your best Talwin in a small syringe."*

*And so it goes. The doctors mingle in the lounge popping their pills, shooting up, and socializing as they let down, easing the tensions accumulated during a busy day in the service of suffering humanity.*

A ridiculous scenario? Of course it is. Disregarding a few younger doctors who may party with marijuana[1] and cocaine now and then, we know physicians do not openly use drugs other than alcohol in social situations. Drug use by physicians is a private, not a social thing, and addiction is a hazard. Until very late in the course, the alcoholics believe that they are drinking the way everyone else does: they are using a socially acceptable drug. Dependence on other drugs develops

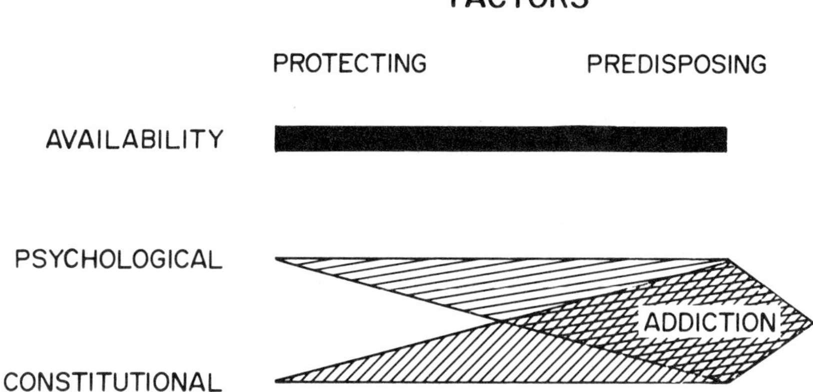


**Figure 1.** Factors predisposing to addiction.

insidiously, but self-prescribers are soon aware that their use of drugs is inappropriate and dangerous. They try to stop, but cannot. They are addicted.

## FACTORS FAVORING DRUG ADDICTION

Inscribed in spray paint on a freeway wall is this statement: "Drugs are bad but reality is worse!" The author was probably an adolescent, but could just as easily have been a physician, for some of our colleagues share this feeling and find themselves in the same dilemma. They use drugs to endure distress, whatever its source, and drug use then becomes the major source of distress.

The following three factors contribute to this vicious cycle (Figure 1).

***Availability.*** Recalling the days when pharmaceutical companies filled physicians' mailboxes with samples of amphetamines, sedatives, and even some "nonaddicting" anelgesics, a formerly addicted physician said, "While other doctors were reading their mail, I was eating mine!" Even in this time of stricter regulation and accountability, physicians have little or no difficulty obtaining drugs for their own use. Availability is a constant.

If drugs are so readily available to physicians, why are not more of them addicted?* Both psychological and constitutional factors explain this.

*There are no accurate figures regarding the incidence of drug addiction among physicians.

***Psychological Factors.*** Much has been written in this book and elsewhere[2–6] about stressful stimuli (stressors) peculiar to a physician's way of life and the psychological vulnerabilities of physicians. It is helpful to consider these in the general terms outlined in Figure 2, adapted from Selye.[6]

An extrinsic stressor impacting upon us produces stress that provokes an alarm reaction, followed by adaptation. This chain of events is modified by our external and internal conditioning. When the stress and the alarm reaction are disquieting or painful, we experience distress and adapt to it in healthy or unhealthy ways. Our vulnerability—here defined as the extent to which we experience distress and adapt in unhealthy ways—can be expressed as a spectrum widening from left to right (Figure 1). Maladaptation may be evidenced in many forms, one of which is the self-prescription of psychotropic drugs that may lead to addiction.

At some time in the past, many physicians have been given or have taken drugs for relief of distress. It may have been a narcotic to relieve physical pain, a sedative to help endure an emotional crisis, or a stimulant to defer sleep while cramming for an important examination. All certainly learned what drugs can do. Addiction is thus a maladaptive extension of their training.

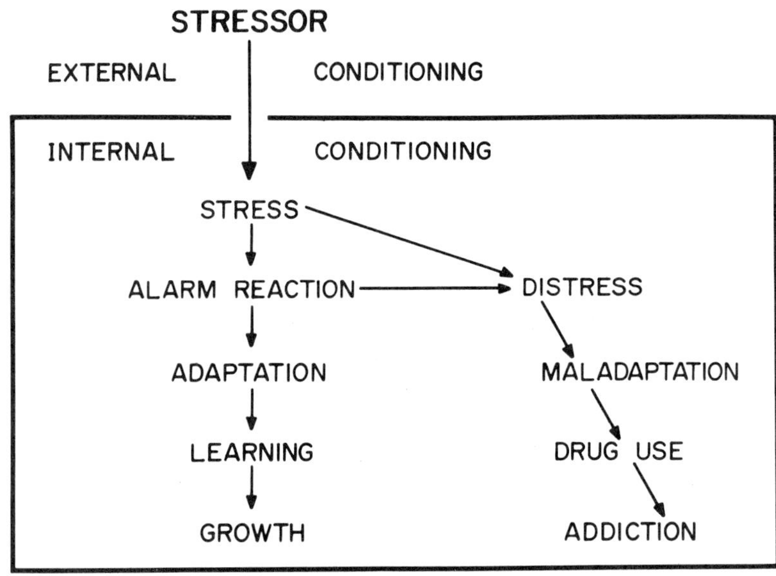


**Figure 2.** Pathway to addiction. (Adapted from Selye H: The Stress of Life. New York, McGraw Hill, 1976.)

*Constitutional Factors.* It seems likely that there are constitutional (neurochemical) factors determining susceptibility to addiction.[7,8] These may also be represented by a spectrum (Figure 1), widening from protection on the left to predisposition on the right. For a few at the left end of the spectrum, the effects of drugs taken in the past may have been so disagreeable that they will resist ever taking them again. They are protected from addiction to those drugs. Most were grateful for the relief the drugs provided, but were more or less impressed by other effects, so they are less or more protected from addiction. Some near the wide end of that spectrum experienced a salubrious effect far in excess of that anticipated. The memory of that experience is deeply imprinted. There may be no need or desire to recapture the effect for many years, but when the need for disinhibition, stimulation, or relief of pain arises for whatever reason, they know what agent to use. It is likely that these constitutional factors also determine which drug or class of drugs is selected.

Unfortunately, drugs produce a rebound effect that is always overlooked by the user, and often by his or her therapist. This rebound to alcohol and other sedative drugs has been described by Gitlow[9] as a large-amplitude, short-duration sedative effect, followed by a low-amplitude, long-duration agitating effect that is cumulative. Despite the fact that the sedative drug provides relief as anticipated, the user experiences a subtle increase in psychomotor activity or agitation for a time thereafter, which possibly justifies another dose. Clinical observations suggest that similar rebound effects accompany the use of narcotic and stimulant drugs.

The drug user trades off short-term relief for long-term distress. The stage is thus set for a self-perpetuating system. As the distressed physician moves from left to right on the psychological scale, the spectra merge, activating any constitutional predisposition.

## SOME QUESTIONS ABOUT ADDICTION

*Who Are the Addicts?* Estimates suggest that addiction is more common among physicians than among adult Americans of comparable age and socioeconomic status.[8] While statistics may show a greater likelihood in some groups than in others, neither age, race, religion, ethnicity, gender*, marital status, geographic location, academic stand-

*For convenience, the physician addict has been described as masculine throughout this chapter. This has been done with full awareness that women physicians may also become addicted and that they may encounter problems unique to their gender.[12]

ing, medical specialty, nor mode of practice precludes the possibility of addiction.

*What Do They Use?* Narcotic analgesics, sedative-hypnotics, and stimulants, alone or in combination, are the drugs of choice, but physicians may employ and become dependent on any psychoactive substance, with the likely exception of antipsychotic drugs. Some have used and abused nitrous oxide and other anesthetics. I have encountered two who were dependent on antihistamine-decongestant nose drops, and one who was at least psychologically addicted to amitriptylene. Cocaine, the drug used and praised by Sigmund Freud,[10] remains a favorite of some 20th-century doctors.

*How Much Do They Use?* Physician addicts are sometimes found to be functioning, with little or no evidence of intoxication, while using astounding quantities of drugs. For example, it is not rare for a physician to have been injecting 1000–2000 mg of meperidine or 300–600 mg of pentazocine daily for months while continuing to work. Among amphetamine addicts, daily doses of 60–90 mg, usually "balanced" with appropriate quantities of alcohol or other sedative drugs, are common. On the other hand, one occasionally encounters a doctor who has never taken more than the recommended daily dose of a minor tranquilizer, but who suffers severe physiological withdrawal symptoms when it is discontinued—the "low-dose sedative addict."

*How Do They Get It?* As addiction progresses, procurement may present problems. Physicians who have never before lied or cheated will begin to do so. They demonstrate resourcefulness and enterprise as they devise methods to ensure their supply. Each physician addict seems to think his methods are unique and innovative, but they are not. Procurement patterns are stereotyped, and pharmacists and narcotic agents are familiar with them.

First, having suddenly acquired a lot of patients tailored to his needs, the addict uses samples and office supplies. Sometimes, he writes prescriptions for himself based on self-diagnosed ailments: meperidine for migraine or back pain, amphetamines for narcolepsy, or barbiturates for sleeplessness. Next, prescriptions are written in the names of family members or office personnel. He then starts to fill prescriptions for patients, casually mentioning to the pharmacist that he will see that the drugs are delivered. Finally, he may pilfer drugs from colleagues or from hospital or clinic supplies. If his license to prescribe the addictive drug is suspended, substitutes are tried, often eventually leading to the legal drug—alcohol. That, at least, is always available.

*How Do They Use It?* Routes of administration are usually the recommended ones, but physicians injecting drugs tend to move rapidly from the subcutaneous or intramuscular to the intravenous route. Although they are generally more scrupulous about equipment and technique than are other "mainline" addicts, they, too, eventually destroy their superficial veins. Their knowledge of anatomy then serves them well; they may begin to use the femoral veins or even to inject into arteries.

## WHAT HAPPENS TO THEM?

Addiction eventually causes problems in one or more areas of the doctor's life: physical, psychological, family, social, or professional.

### Physical

Early in the course of addiction, physician addicts are generally cautious about dosage; but they develop remarkable tolerance and become less cautious as drug intake increases. They use "pure" drugs in predictable dosage, so accidental overdose seldom occurs. Physical toxicity from prolonged use of these drugs, in contrast to alcohol, is rare, and injuries while under the influence are also less common. However, if an intercurrent illness or injury interrupts drug supply, the ensuing withdrawal syndrome may not only confuse diagnosis and complicate therapy, but also add substantially to the risk of the complicating illness (e.g., withdrawal seizure after trauma).

Common problems include thrombophlebitis as well as ulcerations and subcutaneous edema, fibrosis, and abscesses at injection sites. Doctors usually treat these themselves, so they remain hidden unless they require examination for some intercurrent illness or injury. Serious, often life-threatening complications can occur.

Consider the following examples: a 55-year-old internist with an arteriovenous aneurysm at his wrist from repeated intravenous and intraarterial injections of pentazocine; a 28-year-old family doctor with bilateral femoral thrombophlebitis and embolic pneumonia after months of injecting meperidine into his femoral veins several times a day; a 40-year-old emergency physician (formerly a surgeon) with widespread obliteration of superficial veins and severe ischemic ulcerations of his legs and feet from intraarterial injections of various drugs, including amphetamines (he withdrew from a hospital and committed suicide when amputation was suggested); and a 48-year-old anesthesiologist who died of bacterial endocarditis from his addiction to intravenous Dilaudid.

**Psychological**

Although the bizarre, loose behavior so characteristic of alcohol intoxication is uncommon in sedative or narcotic addiction, anergy, apathy, cognitive impairment, and drowsiness ("the nods") are likely to be seen. With stimulants such as cocaine and amphetamines, impaired judgment, grandiosity, belligerence, paranoid behavior, and drug psychosis are common. In addition to these pharmacologic effects are the feelings resulting from preoccupation with drug use—guilt, displaced anger, grief (for real or perceived losses), and self-doubt. Such effects, impacting upon preaddiction character and personality structures, lead to major psychiatric disorders. The common result is depression. Depression is to addiction as the chicken is to the egg, each producing the other. It is universal among physician addicts and often leads to suicide.

**Family**

Addiction and its attendant depression and emotional isolation seriously disrupt communication within the family, even before the others are aware that the doctor is using drugs. Their assimilation of the reality of the addiction and their adaptation to it lead to sickness of the family and each of its members.* To the extent that they continue to adapt, their sickness progresses along with the physician's. Spouses and children often develop physical or psychological illnesses. Sometimes they seek relief in alcohol or other drugs and also become addicted. They may come to treatment before addiction of the physician is apparent to anyone else.

Many spouses of physician addicts demonstrate a remarkable capacity to endure this maladaptation of the family. Divorce, when it occurs, is usually sought only late in the course of addiction.

---

*"Recognition of the problem and its implications is slow. . . . However, once the reality of the problem becomes apparent, despair follows. . . . The only recourse for the physician's wife is to conceal the reluctantly perceived truth . . . and with each lie or half-truth, her guilt and shame grow. . . . The conviction is strong that no one would understand, and all would condemn. . . . Feelings of isolation give rise to resentment and a sense of outrage . . . which are repressed or sublimated. . . . and other family problems pale in importance. So, every member of the physician's family operates under a distorted perception of reality. It is tragic that most likely to suffer are the children, who fail to understand parental inconsistencies."[11]

### Social

Both the physician and his family isolate themselves socially in their continuing effort to conceal their problems, gradually relinquishing their usual social activities. Some even move to another community, vainly hoping to leave behind the addiction and associated problems—the "geographic cure."

In contrast to alcoholism, drug addiction seldom causes problems with civil authorities, unless the addict miscalculates his dose, has an accident, or suffers a drug psychosis. A surgeon who took a sedative drug before leaving his office was arrested because he fell asleep in his car while waiting for the traffic light to change at a busy intersection. A family doctor, addicted to amphetamines and barbiturates, was referred for psychiatric evaluation when the police apprehended him, with considerable difficulty, wandering about in a deserted shopping mall, carrying a loaded gun and wearing a ski mask. His wife had thought he was working late at the office. An internist was found dozing on a curbstone near his office after evening office hours due to barbiturates. In rare instances of advanced addiction, the doctor becomes a derelict with deteriorating health, abandoned by family and friends and moving from job to job and from state to state for as long as he still has a license to practice somewhere. Such people obviously have concurrent psychiatric illnesses.

### Professional

The physician addict lives in fear that his addiction will be discovered, and there may have been incidents to justify his concern. Perhaps a nurse complained of unusual difficulty in rousing him for the delivery he was awaiting in the doctors' lounge; perhaps, when making rounds in the morning, he did not remember orders he had given by telephone the night before. Perhaps he was observed nodding while doing his chart work, or worse, while monitoring an anesthetized patient. A pharmacist questioning a prescription could in itself be sufficient cause for alarm. But he is an addict, and problems continue to mount.

Early in his addiction, he is scrupulous and compulsive, not only in patient care but also in performing the chores of medical practice, such as office paper work and hospital records. Later on, his professional performance may deteriorate, especially with regard to chores not directly involving patient care.

Inevitably, the moment of truth arrives. He is confronted with the fact that someone else, who knows of his addiction, will tolerate it no longer. If this is family, a friend, or a colleague, the confrontation may lead to treatment. If it is an authority, confrontation leads to interruption of his professional activity through loss of (1) hospital privileges, (2) the license to prescribe controlled substances, and/or (3) the license to practice medicine.

## PROFILE OF PHYSICIAN ADDICTS

Although physician addicts may possess various character and personality traits that predispose to addiction, these are usually identified only in retrospect. Generally, he has a premorbid history of integrity, dedication, and professional competence that differs very little from that of most of his colleagues. However, there are some characteristics commonly encountered in physician addicts entering treatment that may help to identify the person at risk.

Impaired self-perception is his hallmark. The chaos of his life that is so obvious to others is only dimly evident to him. Long before he began to use drugs, the need was growing to bolster his physician identity while denying his vulnerability, his inadequacies, his anger, his grief, his guilt, and even his personal identity. As his addiction progresses, he develops denial and projection to a fine art. He becomes expert at identifying extrinsic stressors and assigning blame, for he cannot see and dare not examine his own role in the evolving disaster. His best defense is the shield of physicianhood, because he has long since lost contact with the person behind that shield.

Except in his role as a physician, he has difficulty relating to others, so no one really knows him. Often, his family background is characterized by the work ethic and denial of feelings, and his years of education and training reinforce this. He spends his emotional resources nurturing his patients, but he is unable to recognize his own needs and those of his family. Indeed, his spouse and children exhaust themselves attempting to nurture him. But in his isolation, he is unable to benefit from their support, except as it may fortify his physicianhood. He sees himself having value in only one dimension—as a physician. He is a giver, he cannot receive.

Most people maturing through late adolescence and early adult life are exposed to the problems of the real world and learn to cope with them as they prepare for their life's work. Physicians have spent these years in an institutional cocoon, in single-minded pursuit of education and training. He emerges as an educated and skilled professional, but he is emotionally stunted and ill-prepared to deal with life's crises. Like Sisyphus, he struggles to accomplish an impossible task. Since life and death depend upon what he knows, he must try to be all things to all people, must know everything, must keep up with medical progress at all costs. Although aware that such goals are not attainable, he is not capable of setting limits for himself. The resulting frustration and guilt drive him harder to prove himself as a physician, so work compulsion is his style. His status as a physician and the rewards for his "doctor" work, both material and personal, buffer him against life's stresses. It is to be expected, then, that his work and the pursuit of education and status will continue to be used as coping devices. Healthier coping skills have atrophied.

His family is caught up in this compulsive dedication to his work. They must not intrude, because he and his work are so important. They, and he, believe this implicitly. His family is sick too; other physicians and their families feel these same pressures and bend a little now and then, but they find healthy ways to adapt.

Eventually, problems arise that work cannot solve: indeed, work compulsion is generating some of these problems. He cannot reach out for help, for he cannot recognize that it is he who needs help. He begins to feel the pain of his lonely life and comes to believe that his selfless service to others is not appreciated. It is then that he starts giving to himself. He may indulge himself with compulsive spending, gambling, women, or drugs. If he possesses a constitutional predisposition to addiction, it is now activated. But, he denies this, rationalizing that he has special immunity.

Given this interplay of psychological and constitutional factors (Figure 1) addiction results—an acquired drive as powerful as the drives for food, shelter, or sex.[12] Sensitivity to stressors, whether extrinsic or intrinsic, increases in direct proportion to the time elapsed since the last dose of drug. Whether actual or anticipated, physical or psychological, distress demands more drug, and relief must be immediate. Drug use has become his prime defense, dominating his life.

The effects of his drug and preoccupation with its use lead to psychological and social dysfunction manifested by obnoxious and deceitful behavior as he struggles to ensure his supply, conceal his addiction, and preserve his physicianhood. Such behavior is more likely to be symptomatic of this new illness than of some underlying disorder of character or personality. No matter what sort of person he was before, he has become, in essence, a different person—a distortion of the original.

Colleagues and others find it difficult to look past such behavior and perceive addiction as an illness rather than a primary moral defect—to accept the physician addict as a sick person rather than a bad person. But, he is sick, and he can be treated. This sick person can be restored to a happy, productive life. If he is not treated, his patients, his family, his career, and his life are in jeopardy.

## STRATEGY OF MANAGEMENT

### Four Roles

Management of the physician addict entails sharply delineating four roles: patient, authority, colleague, and therapist (PACT). Those assuming any one of these roles must understand and respect the integrity of each other participant.

***Patient.*** Physicians adapt to the role of patient with difficulty. This is especially true of the physician impaired by drug addiction. By the time he reaches treatment, he has already tried more than once to usurp the other roles. He has lectured to himself as an authority, he has pitied himself as he believes only a sympathetic colleague could, and he has tried to treat himself. Now, he must be induced to accept the patient role. To the extent that he is able to do so, he has a chance for recovery. He must abandon his physician shield and enter treatment as a sick person, acknowledging that he is an impaired physician because he is an impaired person.

***Authority.*** This may be the courts, the licensing board, hospital administration, partners, or others—any person or body having the power to affect his life in a major way, especially his professional life. Such authorities may be helpful in identifying the sick doctor and motivating him to accept and complete treatment, and they usually must be dealt with in the process of reentry into professional activity. When the addict agrees to enter treatment, or his addiction is discovered after he has entered treatment, authorities sometimes defer action on privileges and licensure pending evaluation of outcome. In any event, they monitor the recovering addict, thus adding to his motivation for sustained abstinence.

***Colleague.*** Some branches of organized medicine recognized long ago that many physicians impaired by psychiatric disorders, alcoholism, and other drug addiction can be identified, effectively treated, and returned to professional activity. This notion gained impetus when the American Medical Association held its first National Conference on the Impaired Physician in 1975. Since then, most state medical associations, many county societies, some specialty groups, and some hospital staffs have developed programs for this purpose.[8]

These are programs of identification and intervention by concerned colleagues, who lead the sick physician to treatment and give him a chance for recovery. They are designed to provide help rather than punishment, and they employ persuasion before coercion. Some monitor the progress of the sick doctor and assist both in rehabilitation and in decisions regarding reentry.

The work of these committees is done by dedicated volunteers, many of whom have experienced and overcome similar problems.* These concerned colleagues approach the physician addict with firmness, but they convey a message of hope and understanding. They provide support during treatment and aftercare and are often helpful in the reentry process. Love, indeed, "has a place in professional practice and professional relations."[13]

*Therapist.* If he is able to reach out for help, the physician addict is prone to consult the wrong person for the wrong reason. Most often, it is a physician friend, who is ill-prepared to treat him and whom he manipulates disastrously. Doctors consulted in this manner must realize that the greatest kindness they can offer their sick colleague is to insist firmly that he accept help from a skilled and otherwise disinterested therapist. They should help him make arrangements for this and see that he follows through.

Selection of the proper therapist or therapeutic facility is crucial. Not all physicians, including psychiatrists, possess training, experience, attitude, and temperament suited for this difficult task. However, some psychiatric and general hospitals have special units or programs for treatment of alcoholism and drug addiction, and there are many excellent, free-standing rehabilitation centers especially structured for this purpose. Some have programs specifically designed for the treatment and rehabilitation of doctors.

## Four Steps

Management of the physician addict also entails four steps, identification, intervention, treatment and rehabilitation, and reentry. It is helpful to consider them separately and in sequence, since each step presents special problems and challenges.

*Identification.* Recognition that a physician is impaired is easy when addiction is so advanced that professional competence has been affected. Of course, this is already too late. Lawrence Durrell[14] has written, "Illness invites contempt. A sick man knows it." Certainly, drug addiction invites contempt. The addicted doctor knows this and hides his problem to the extent that he can. Remember, he perceives himself as having identity and value only as a physician. Preserving this becomes a matter of survival. This proud, compulsive person must main-

---

*Commenting on the principles of rehabilitation in general, Dr. Howard Rusk has said, "Those who . . . survive their illness or overcome their handicap and take their places back in the world have a depth of spirit you and I can hardly measure. They have not wasted their pain."

tain professional competence, and he does so at the cost of everything else in his life. As his illness progresses, the scope of his life begins to shrink, and all activities and concerns not directly related to patient care gradually diminish. Such changes can be identified as evidence of impairment.

In contrast to the alcoholic whose facies, breath, and drunken behavior often bring his problem to the attention of police, hospital personnel, and even his patients, a physician's addiction usually remains hidden from public view. Soon after addiction begins, however, someone close to the physician knows he is using drugs. This may be his family, office personnel, colleagues, or other friends. Not being aware of the inevitable and relentless progression of his illness, fearing disgrace and financial disaster that might result from disclosure, and just simply hoping it will all work out, these concerned people often keep silent. They may discuss the problem among themselves, but they are reluctant to confront the doctor. If they do so, they may be intimidated by his anger, or reassured by his rationalizations and promises. They thus find themselves in a conspiracy of silence, and their own illness progressing in parallel.

Often, they believe they are somehow responsible for his drug use and for the bizarre behavior associated with it. They are frequently angry, frustrated, fearful, and depressed. Sometimes, the physician's spouse resorts to alcohol or other drugs supplied by the doctor and also becomes addicted, or the spouse or the children develop physical or psychological symptoms. Physicians' spouses and children seeking medical or psychiatric care may provide early clues, helping to identify the sick doctor.

It is to be hoped that family, office personnel, colleagues, and other associates can be helped to see the inevitability of disaster if a sick doctor is not treated. They may then look past the stigma, overcome their own denial, and ensure proper care just as they would if some other illness were involved. It is better to proceed with intervention than to risk progression of the illness.

***Intervention.*** This consists of precipitating a crisis for the physician and limiting his options so that he will accept treatment.

The purpose of intervention is to make the addict aware that others know of his addiction and will not tolerate it, that treatment is available, and that disaster is inevitable without it. Not infrequently, physician addicts comply promptly and with a sense of relief once they know their addiction is no longer hidden. Often, more detailed confrontation is required.

Confrontation is most effective when it is arranged by someone skilled and experienced in this art. It is unwise for relatives and personal friends to attempt it alone, for they are likely to have difficulty avoiding emotional involvement and resisting the doctor's manipulation. Here is where the concerned colleague can be most helpful.

For those contemplating intervention, the following suggestions are offered:

- Do not try to solo; seek trained help.
- Include a few family members and close associates selected for their personal knowledge of the doctor's problem and for their ability to maintain composure.
- Plan ahead and school all participants.
- Introduce reality.
- Present evidence, not accusations.
- Be prepared to act promptly; make an advance reservation for admission to a treatment facility.
- Let the sick doctor know you care.
- Be prepared to get tough if necessary by reasserting your moral and legal obligation to inform authorities of his impairment if he does not comply.

***Treatment and Rehabilitation.*** Initial detoxification and treatment are best accomplished in an institutional setting by people experienced in such work (see preceding section on the role of the therapist), preferably in a milieu of other addicts. The goal of therapy during this period should be to achieve abstinence. Psychotherapy should be limited to supportive measures aimed at motivating the addict to abstain. In the early months, anything that heightens anxiety may lead to relapse and sabotage recovery. Later, more definitive therapy can be undertaken, and the physician will likely be more receptive and treatable than in the early phase.

Specific measures for treatment and rehabilitation must be individualized by the doctor's therapist, but the following principles are generally applicable. The doctor must:

1. Stop using all self-prescribed psychoactive drugs, including alcohol; the therapist should prescribe them with extreme caution (e.g., some antidepressants, notably amitriptylene, have potential for abuse).
2. Stop work while undertaking treatment.
3. Learn to play, being self-rewarding in healthy ways.
4. Learn that he is a worthwhile person, even if he never attends another patient.
5. Recognize the need to change.

6. Have family involved in treatment.
7. Be introduced to a healthy support system, and learn to use it.*
8. Accept and continue a relationship as a patient with a personal physician.
9. Assimilate the reality of his past into his new life, accepting responsibility for any obnoxious and deceitful behavior displayed during the illness.

***Reentry.*** To regain self-respect as much as to make a living, the physician addict should finally return to work; if possible, he should be encouraged and enabled to resume his accustomed professional activities. Unfortunately this often presents major problems with regard to assessing the doctor's competence, providing advocacy in such matters as professional privileges and licensure, and devising programs of surveillance.[15]

Now is when those functioning in the four roles of the PACT can work together to restore a skilled physician to a position of optimum service with optimum safety. The physician-*patient* is ultimately responsible for his own recovery and for negotiating reentry. Various *authorities* are obliged to safeguard the interests of the people and institutions they represent by seeking assurance that the doctor is complying with therapy and that his progress is being monitored (e.g., periodic drug screens). Concerned *colleagues* can not only provide understanding and support, but also serve as advocates in the reentry process. The *therapist* should insist upon a firm contract for aftercare and an agreement permitting him to report to authorities if the physician abandons treatment or relapses. While recognizing that such reporting may be abhorrent to many therapists, I believe it is their moral obligation in the case of a physician-patient.

## PREVENTION

Of the factors predisposing to addiction (Figure 1), only the psychological are amenable to change. Risk factors for addiction have been implied in the profile given earlier: an interplay of character and personality structures with a lifestyle that favors denial of feelings and emotional immaturity, but provides rewards sufficient to compensate for life's stresses until the tenuous balance is disrupted.

*International Doctors in Alcoholics Anonymous (IDAA), which welcomes addicts as well as alcoholics, maintains a central office (1950 Volney Rd., Youngstown OH 44511) through which physicians can be assisted to contact others having similar histories of substance abuse. Its annual convention is attended by several hundred doctors from all areas of North America. Similar support groups, meeting every week or so throughout the year, have been organized in many urban areas.

Regarding the factors determining psychological vulnerability (Figure 2), individual physicians can do little to modify external conditioning and stressors; but they can modify internal conditioning and adaptation to stress by attending to their physical, psychological, and spiritual health.[16] Also they can help each other.

The following suggestions are therefore offered to all physicians, but especially to those just entering the profession.

- Remember, you were a person before you became a doctor.
- Recognize your personal needs and attend to them.
- Pace yourself.
- Learn to give to yourself in healthy ways.
- Reach out to one another, and learn to receive.
- Be alert to problems among your peers in the brotherhood of medicine.
- Be prepared to help each other.
- Be your brother's keeper.

## REFERENCES


1. Lipp MR, Benson SG: Physicians' use of marijuana, alcohol, and tobacco. Am J Psychiatr 1972, 129:124–128.
2. Hall RCW, Stickney SK, Popkin MK: Physician drug abusers. J Nerv Ment Dis 1978, 166:787–793.
3. Johnson RP, Connelly JC: Addicted physicians. A closer look. J Am Med Assoc 1981, 245:253–257.
4. Lipp MR: Respectful Treatment. The Human Side of Medical Care. New York, Harper & Row, 1977, pp 200–216.
5. Roeske NCA: Stress and the physician. Psychiatr Ann 1981, 11:245–258.
6. Selye H: The Stress of Life. New York, McGraw Hill, 1976.
7. Bunney WE Jr (moderator): Basic and clinical studies of endorphins. Ann Int Med 1979, 91:239.
8. Wilford BB: Drug Abuse. A Guide for The Primary Care Physician. Chicago, AMA, 1981.
9. Gitlow SE: Alcoholism: A disease. *In* Bourne PG, Fox R (eds): Alcoholism. Progress in Research and Treatment. New York, Academic Press, 1973, pp 1–22.
10. Musto DF: A study in cocaine: Sherlock Holmes and Sigmund Freud. J Am Med Assoc 1968, 204:125–130.
11. Ayres HP: A rationale for therapy for the physician's family. Proceedings of ALC 80, International Conference on Alcoholism, Bath, England, September 20–24, 1980.
12. Bejerot N: A theory of addiction as an artificially induced drive. Am J Psychiatry 1972, 128:842–846.

13. Dorr D, Bonner JW III, Ayres PR: Love and the addicted physician. J Religion and Health. Fall 1983 (in press).
14. Durrell L: Mountolive. New York, EP Dutton & Co, 1961, p 22.
15. Robertson JJ (ed): The Impaired Physician: Building Well-Being. Proceedings of the Fourth AMA Conference On the Impaired Physician, Baltimore, Maryland, October 30–November 1, 1980. City, Publ., pp 103–107.
16. Schiedermayer DL: The heart man. J Am Med Assoc 1981, 246:2852.

# The Alcoholic Physician

Alcohol is both the nectar of the Gods and the curse of demons. In moderation, it brings good cheer, lifts flagging spirits, and encourages conviviality. In excess, it is the ruination of reputations, destroyer of homes, and an enslaving tyrant. Almost every physician drinks alcohol at one time or another and most never develop problems; but a few are unable to stay in control. For them, a thin line can separate their "social" drinking from "problem" drinking. Out of every fifteen physicians who start drinking alcohol socially, three on average will develop serious problems; one of these will become alcoholic. This means that there are approximately 15,000–25,000 alcoholic doctors in the United States.

Physicians see what alcohol does to their patients. They are familiar with cirrhosis, pancreatitis, esophageal varices, Monday morning "flu," and the myriad other complaints of chronic drinkers. Often they advise their patients that excessive alcohol is dangerous and recommend that the patient "do something about your drinking." The physician's frustration rises when warnings fall on deaf ears; they shake their heads wondering how the alcoholic can be so stupidly self-destructive as to ignore their advice.

However, this shortcoming is not unique to their patients. Many physicians have scotomas for their own failings, particularly that of alcohol. Doctors are as apt as anyone else not to see what alcohol may be doing to themselves, no matter how obvious it is. While they admonish others to cut back or abstain, they deny that their own inability to steady a syringe or their recurrent "indigestion" is due to daily imbibing.

Anyone can spot a terminal alcoholic; you do not have to be a doctor for that. But it takes sophistication to detect alcoholism in its early stages. In this chapter Dr. Thomas Kearney describes the early and late signs of physician alcoholism. He points out the subtle personality changes and other behavioral fluctuations that let you know a physician has a problem. These changes occur long before gross complications of alcoholism make such a conclusion obvious. Dr. Kearney also discusses what can be done to break a dysfunctional physician's mental and physical dependence on alcohol.

*J.P.C.*

# 11

# The Alcoholic Physician

*Thomas Kearney*

While the bibulous poet or artist may be seen as an amusing rogue, the thought of your surgeon being drunk while wielding the scalpel inside your bodily cavities is rather disagreeable. Since we have to surrender ourselves to our doctors and dentists, we have a not unreasonable desire to see them as persons of decency, competence, and trust. We want to look up to them, which is what we generally do when they have us in their grip. Their image of gravity and Oslerian *aequanimitas* is ill served when we see a physician fall into the cake at her daughter's wedding, or a surgeon punch his spouse at the hospital's annual ball.

Alcoholism is a disease, however, that like diabetes, arthritis, and high blood pressure, is no respecter of persons. Not only can it attack anyone from the most skilled surgeon to the humblest orderly; it is a condition for which there is no cure. The illness is progressive, whether the sufferer is drinking or not, so that a period of abstinence for six or 12 months seems to make no difference to the inability of the drinker to control consumption. If anything, it is possible to get drunk faster on less liquor when resuming drinking following a layoff. With treatment, large numbers of alcoholics are able to lead productive and happy lives, but these few successful people refer to themselves always as "recovering," and never as "cured"; in fact, clinical experience suggests that a physician who talks of being cured is almost certainly on the way to, or from, a gin mill.

The most important thing to establish about a physician who is alcoholic is that he or she is no different from any other alcoholic, with a few essentially favorable exceptions.

Peter, a doctor who has been sober for 30 years, told me that one seemingly trivial incident finally cut through the stout system of denial that he had developed to keep him drinking. He was seriously alcoholic because, as a result of drinking, he lost his practice in his small southern town, lost his wife and family, and almost lost his life while still quite a young man. He had made a few half-hearted approaches to AA, where he met a man roughly the same age as himself, who had been sober for about a year. This man became the doctor's sponsor and called him each day; he encouraged him and brought him to the nightly meetings of Alcoholics Anonymous. After a few weeks of this, Peter felt that his flesh and blood could stand no more sobriety and bought a bottle of gin and proceeded to get outside it. John, the sponsor, arrived that night and was dismayed to find his protégé in his cups. He didn't become angry but looked at Peter and said evenly, "You know, Pete, the only difference between us is that I'm a sober housepainter and you're a drunk doctor." That was in 1950 and Peter has been sober, happy, and reunited with his family since.

## THE EXTENT OF THE PROBLEM

It is very difficult to be sure how many people in North America suffer from alcoholism. Measurements are indirect, often derived from individual pieces of research in a particular district or ethnic group. Figures are available for the rate of hospitalization for alcoholism in public psychiatric facilities, but these tend to be very high for men of the poorer classes, and probably too low for women. Population surveys involving questionnaires indicate that as many as 2% of a district in New York City suffer from clearly defined symptoms of alcoholism.[1] If this figure can be projected across the United States, we find at least four and a half million alcoholics in the country.

Studies of general hospitals show that even in community hospitals, with little or no psychiatric service, 10–20% of the patients are admitted because of alcohol abuse.[2] Although the precise conditions for which they are being treated may be pneumonia, convulsions, broken bones, burns, frost bite, cirrhosis of the liver, or intestinal bleeding, their underlying disease is alcoholism.

Dr. John Norris, a physician who is a nonalcoholic member of The Board of Alcoholics Anonymous, has taken series of samples of persons attending meetings of that organization. His results suggest that there are probably a half-million people attending AA meetings in North America and that these constitute about 10% of the total number of alcoholics who are still drinking.[3]

One may summarize the available information by saying that alcoholism is a major public health problem, quite possibly *the* major health problem of our times; in addition it is linked to diseases of the heart and blood vessels, and the gastrointestinal system.[4] These are responsible for much premature, preventable death. Alcohol also causes death from accidents, suicide, and violence.[4]

In 1979, Dr. Anne Geller, the Medical Director of the Smithers Center, Roosevelt Hospital, New York, and Dr. LeClair Bissell, President of Edgehill at Newport, Rhode Island—each treatment and rehabilitation centers—expressed the opinion that one in ten doctors are affected at some point in their careers by an illness that impairs their judgment.[5] The largest group of impaired physicians, they find, are those suffering from chemical dependency, which is another way of saying the abuse of drink or drugs. (The further one goes in this field, the more one becomes aware of the euphemisms for this disease which lie about like leg-hold traps, and are found strewn around all the way to doctors' graves.) Geller and Bissell point out clearly that it is difficult for doctors to accept a diagnosis of drug-dependency, including alcohol, in a patient and almost impossible in a colleague.

Although younger doctors, who are still in residency training, seem more sophisticated about drinking problems, it is still very difficult for physicians to confront a colleague whose performance is deteriorating and say, "I think I can help you with your problem, and I think you have an illness called alcoholism."

Since it seems reasonable to believe, as Drs. Bissell and Geller do, that there are probably 23,000 alcoholic physicians in North America, one might tend to view the situation as needing rather urgent attention. A comparable number of drunk pilots or bus drivers would surely cause alarm.

In the past, the use of sedatives, narcotics, and stimulants among doctors had been thought to be largely caused by physicians' ease of access to them. However, in 1964 a study by Drs. Modlin and Montes[6] disclosed that 25 physicians studied, all of whom were in treatment for addiction to narcotics, had serious psychological problems, altogether apart from drug use. These would probably best be described as disorders of personality, or character, and are very difficult to treat. In 1970, Dr. George Vaillant and colleagues at Harvard Medical School concluded from a 20-year study of 45 doctors,[7] who were chosen, ironically, because of their ostensibly good mental health, that the doctors used far more mind-altering drugs, including tranquilizers, alcohol, and stimulants than a matched group of nonmedical people. In this case, the ease of acquisition and physician's grandiosity may well have been significant. Another work, a study by Drs. Richard Johnson and John Connelly of 50 alcohol-addicted doctors,[8] focused more closely on psychodynamics. This study had the advantage of using an inpatient unit at the Menniger Clinic, Topeka, Kansas, where nearly all the doctor/patients stayed six weeks.

Johnson and Connelly found that doctors under 40 years old tended to do less well in treatment and had more visible emotional problems. Most of their emotional scarring seemed to stem from parental deprivation or loss and was manifested by serious personality disorders. The doctors over 40 had more frequent neurotic problems (e.g., depression and anxiety) than personality disorders, and responded much better.

In general, while there has been discussion about the personality characteristics of alcoholic and drug-abusing physicians for more than 30 years, the picture which emerges of the alcoholic doctor is a person who may use some kind of solid drug as well. About a third of alcoholic physicians misuse drugs and they appear much the same as that of the nonphysician alcoholic American or Canadian. Such persons may be young or old; black, white or brown; probably from any kind of medical practice, although psychiatrists have a higher rate for alcoholism than others and are suspected of being more unstable. However, the kind of practice a physician has seems to bear no relation to the rate of development of chemical dependency. Actively alcoholic doctors tend to gravitate to salaried positions in institutions, like prisons, state hospitals, and the military, but this is secondary to their disease. Women are as yet underrepresented in medicine and there are therefore relatively few females in the ranks of impaired physicians; this will probably change as more female doctors graduate from medical school.

## PRESENTATION OF THE DISORDER

As with all alcoholics, the symptoms of the illness become more apparent, even if not correctly diagnosed, to the physician's family at an earlier stage in their melancholy progress than they do to outside observers. The spouse may become worried and sad, suffer from headaches, back pain, and vague bodily distress, and not infrequently is treated for depression by the family doctor, who knows nothing of the situation. The children become distressed in other ways, tending to do poorly or exceptionally well at school, showing deviations from average behavior and accomplishments; some are almost Rhodes scholars, others are expelled from school. Many of the children of alcoholics drink illegally, use drugs, and get in trouble. They may complain to their mother (usually) that "Daddy doesn't go to the Pony Club any more, take us to the ball-game or the movies, go fishing (camping, skiing) with me. Why is he so tired all the time, and cross? Is it something I've done?" The first leak in the security system may be a suicide attempt by an adolescent child.

As the illness progresses (1–11 years, average ~ 3), from the time the family realizes that the physician has changed for the worse, colleagues, nurses, and patients begin to talk to one another about their worry.

The doctor's work habits begin to change. Previously he (or she) may have been reliable and conscientious, now he becomes variable in his hours and unpredictable in his moods. He cannot be reached on the phone. Conversations with him after 8 P.M. are sometimes slightly incoherent and he forgets that he talked to you on the telephone last night. His appearance may change, as he becomes red-faced and heavy, or thin and pale. His nails and collar become grubby and razor scratches, along with a slightly shaky hand and hoarse voice, attest to the battle of the bottle. He may treat his hangovers with drugs, which will calm him down in the morning but play hell with his memory.

He starts to do rounds in the hospital at odd hours, like midnight, and his judgment becomes erratic. He discharges patients in the middle of the night, after telling them the day before that they should stay in the hospital for a couple of weeks for tests or treatment. At this time, he may be approached by a friendly colleague who says, somewhat embarrassedly, "Are you OK, Charlie? You don't look too great these last few months. Maybe you ought to cut down a bit, huh?" This is usually said with a sympathetic wink or grimace, although the colleague would not be embarrassed if suspecting syphilis, but would insist on treatment before the disease attacked the heart or brain. Charlie always responds, "Sure I will, Jack" usually adding for reinforcement, "Don't worry about it, I can take care of it." Again, if Charlie had tuberculosis we would not let him go like that. We would follow up and get him to a hospital where Charlie could get the treatment he needs, so he can get back to being a productive person again.

## APPROACHES TO TREATMENT

At present, it seems that at least a dozen states have well established programs for treating the physician who is disabled by alcoholism. Perhaps the best known, and certainly the pioneer, in the field is the Disabled Doctors' Program of Georgia,[9] whose prime architect is Dr. Douglas Talbott.

The essential features of the Georgian program consist of identifying the sick doctor—whose behavior by now has drawn attention—and having him or her confronted by two colleagues from a distant part of the state. In this way there can be no imputation of self-interest. If the doctor, as sometimes happens, turns a mastiff upon these visitors, they retreat and a fresh pair arrive the next day. This continues with a new couple arriving daily until the patient is willing to accept help.

The treatment consists of a period in a hospital which specializes in disorders of addiction, followed by further outpatient treatment, including time on special duties when the recovering doctor, under supervision, treats alcoholic patients. As long as the doctor cooperates, the illness is kept confidential. It must be borne in mind that a drunk doctor in a small town is likely to become the topic of local conversation. It is only if the doctor/patient refuses totally to admit to the sickness and accept treatment that licensing authorities are notified and become involved. By this time, the threat of loss of the license to practice medicine will almost invariably impel the patient into treatment.

Similar programs exist on a state-wide level in New York, Missouri, Pennsylvania, Maryland, Ohio, Michigan, Oregon, and California. Others have begun programs which are taking effect at the city or county level. For example, there is a recent law in Connecticut which empowers each county medical society to receive, in complete confidence, complaints about doctors who seem to be having problems with drink or drugs. The Connecticut Impaired Physician Committee, some of whose members are recovering alcoholics, sends a pair of physicians on a house visit after a complaint is judged to have substance. Of the visiting pair, one doctor is a nonalcoholic and one is recovering from the disease. The suffering doctor is interviewed and treatment possibilities are explored. If the doctor refuses to accept what the full committee would regard as adequate care, the matter is then turned over to the licensing authorities and becomes public. Although the program is new, it is expected that this final sanction will be sufficient to get the patient into treatment.

Many Americans believe uncritically in the efficacy of psychiatry, which often is seen as a modern cure-all, possibly because of how it is treated by the press, popular magazines, and television shows. If they have the capacity, psychiatrists can acquire a great deal of humility from their therapy of alcoholic patients, including doctors, who seem to evade the thrust of their ministrations as coolly and skillfully as the matador parries the horns of the bull. It is particularly to be deplored, in this context, when the drunk doctor is let off, after peer confrontation, with an undertaking to visit a psychotherapist once or twice a week. Although this approach may have cured some alcoholics (there *are* white blackbirds, after all), it is generally ineffective. The physician simply becomes more adept at the concealment of drinking, possibly abstaining for months at a time, until boarding the plane for three sunny weeks in Curaçao. There the doctor may drink in a bathroom which has a sunlamp, and return home with second-degree burns and delirium tremens. If unlucky, he or she may fall off the chartered sailboat and drown.

Another pitfall in the psychiatric encounter arises directly from the aversion to calling a sick person an alcoholic. The psychiatrist relieves everybody's feelings by saying that Jack is *not* an alcoholic—perish the thought. Rather, Jack is suffering from depression or possibly manic-depressive illness, which is more impressive still, and needs complex care and treatment. Jack is then sent to an expensive private psychiatric hospital, where the staff has difficulty recognizing a real live alcoholic. There he is encouraged to talk about his parents, his hated elder brother, and his mother-in-law, with all of whom he had previously seen himself as being on fairly good terms. In psychiatric hospital, the alcoholic physician begins to believe that the problem with alcohol is situational and secondary to depression arising from unresolved childhood anxieties.

A physician, who is now sober and has been attending AA meetings with scrupulous regularity for about five years, described his growing awareness, despite the formidable unconscious mental and societal resistance, to his terrible problem with drink. He had completely lost control of his drinking and drank daily, at times around the clock. He could never bear to look at television programs or even advertisements about alcoholism, and began to have frightening dreams of drinking himself to death—which were close to the mark, as it turned out. In the space of four years he was hospitalized four times to be detoxified from alcohol. He consulted four decent, highly competent, conscientious psychiatrists. The first, whom he promptly shunned like the Black Death, told him to go to Alcoholics Anonymous. The other three, who were personal friends, told him he had manic-depressive illness, should take lithium, and should cut down his drinking to three glasses of wine a day. This he did, buying a 20-ounce glass. On this regimen he really did become depressed, waking at three every morning with suicidal thoughts. He was then placed by the three wise men on anti-depressive medicine, which altered his electrocardiagram for the worse.

Two interventions now took place and proved to be life-saving. He was thrown out of a lower-class bar close to his hospital and he was arrested for drunken driving. These two events seemed to puncture the armor of his resistance and caused him to go for treatment to a hospital in a nearby city. There he was cared for by a psychiatrist who was himself a recovered alcoholic. This psychiatrist sent him for four weeks to a special unit for alcoholics at St. Vincent's Hospital and Medical Center, a general hospital in New York City, where he was able to accept his illness for what it was—alcoholism.

While there is a great deal of denial in alcoholism, it is not the only sickness marked by this primitive defense mechanism. Doctors have been known to show clear signs of heart disease (angina, for example) and dismiss them as indigestion.[4]

If attending physicians were sufficiently well trained in the early, prodromal (literally "running-before") signs of this disease, they might be able to take a better history with better results. This is what is done when suspecting a disease of other etiology; for example, a diagnosis may often be made in neurology by a detailed, careful, painstaking history, before the examination is even begun. Alcoholism is no different. Jellinek's 1952 paper entitled "Phases in Alcohol Addiction" has not been improved upon in 30 years and gives details of these signs very well. He describes what is really a growing obsession with alcohol, but one of which the sufferer is unaware.[10]

Classically, the alcoholic is a social drinker and does something like the following:

- always meets people for lunch in a place where alcohol is served, never in a coffee shop;
- sometimes arrives early for a meeting at the pub to have a drink or two before the friend arrives;
- serves guests drinks in the living room but has a second glass alone in the kitchen;
- becomes annoyed if drinks are not served at a meeting, or on a Sunday;
- drinks one or two before going to a cocktail party three doors away;
- becomes pervasively concerned about having enough alcohol at hand in the home and, possibly later, in the workplace; and
- drinks faster than others and begins to gravitate to the crowd who are recognized as heavy imbibers.

As time passes, this preoccupation with having alcohol available in sufficient quantity becomes troubling: a physician who is now a recovering AA member said that he reached the point where he could not look at a fish in a food shop without thinking of white wine. At about this point losses of memory begin, slight at first and then more bothersome. These may be as innocuous as forgetting that, at the end of a party, he or she had asked the neighbors over for lunch the next day. Lapses may be more of a nuisance if they have to do with patients, such as "Why did I admit that person to St. James' Infirmary last night?" or "What do I tell this dumb nurse who is calling me on the phone at 5 A.M. for orders on this jerk I never heard of?" An eye surgeon found it necessary to put triangular patches on the cornea of newly admitted persons so he would recognize his emergency patients next morning.

Some physicians go to their graves (usually early ones) without ever being confronted about their disease by their colleagues. This seems a pity, when we find a 1976 study[11] indicating that being admonished by a colleague was probably effective in getting the patient into correct treatment in 60% of the cases. This study involved a group of 98 recovering doctors, all of whom had been sober at least a year, and found that the confrontation by other physicians was much more effective than psychotherapy. More than a third of these doctors found that their therapists refused to accept a diagnosis of alcoholism, but rather saw the drinking as symptomatic of some deep underlying disturbance. This resulted in dangerous delays in obtaining proper care.

With all this in mind one may well wonder how does the alcoholic physician ever get better? In 1948 a small group of men met in a summer cottage and formed a club with the convoluted title of "International Doctors in Alcoholics Anonymous". The group now includes women and has more than 800 adherents in the United States and Canada, and a splash of overseas members in Britain, Ireland, Australia, and elsewhere. It meets annually like any other medical convention, and has regional and local bodies which meet often. For example, in Connecticut there are two meetings a week for doctors.

The cornerstone of recovery is the program of Alcoholics Anonymous, which emphasizes staying away from a drink one day at a time. Participants keep in close contact with at least one other member of the group, who functions as a guide and a counsellor and is called a "sponsor." They go to meetings of AA often and regularly, either to hear other members tell their stories and share experiences, or simply to sit around a table chatting over coffee and cake with a small group of friends. This mutual support program has a number of steps which members are encouraged to take as a part of growth in a human and spiritual sense. Much emphasis is given to the abandonment of resentments and the increase in tolerance of others. The program induces change, the key word in any form of psychological therapy, in the members' attitudes toward themselves, to those around them, and to life itself. Spiritual growth rather than spiritual perfection is sought and the recovery is sustained by living one day at a time.

Many of the principles of the AA program are drawn from the Oxford Movement, a type of Christian spiritual renaissance in England at the turn of the century. The patient progressing in sobriety begins to see there is much more to AA than not drinking; it is a way of life. Dr. Robinson's book *Talking Out of Alcoholism*[12] is the first study of AA from inside the organization and was carried out in England. It gives a great deal of support to the previously unsubstantiated claim that AA helps probably 50% of those who seek its assistance the first time around, and half the remainder on a second or third try. Getting three out of four drunks sober—regardless of class, race, sex, or religion—is a remarkable achievement, unequaled by any other form of ambulatory (i.e., outside an institution) treatment.

The most effective treatment for alcoholics, as opposed to simple detoxification ("drying out"), usually begins with a stay of three or four weeks in a special hospital, or hospital unit. There the doctor/patient is taught that this disease is progressive and fatal, but can be arrested if discussed with other people who suffer from the same thing; thus, it is much better than having cancer of the lung. The treatment center is directed by people who are themselves recovering alcoholics, or who are very familiar with the AA program. There is much emphasis on the nature of alcoholism as a disease (not bad behavior) that can be stopped by a simple program for complicated people, the essence of which is not picking up a drink today.

The members of the patient's group are told that whereas they had previously seen themselves in control of their drinking, their need for "control" itself implies a problem. Denial is dealt with extensively, and the mechanism begins to break down in this process of indoctrination.

One man, who had been drinking for almost 30 years, had completely forgotten being reprimanded 24 years before, as an intern, for his drunken behavior at the hospital's annual dance. He recalled being advised to go "on the wagon" for six months by the director of the hospital. Another described how he had naively determined to show his family he could control his drinking by having two margaritas every night for 18 months, at which stage he had made a dangerous attempt at suicide.

The educational and therapeutic process must involve the physician's family; the more successful centers insist on the spouse's participation in therapy. Some centers find that one-third (or more) of the spouses are themselves alcoholic. Spouses are encouraged very strongly to go to meetings of Alanon, the counterpart of AA, which exists to help those living with, or linked by love to, an alcoholic. Here they can be taught to "detach" with affection from the drinker and not feel guilty for the problem themselves. They are also taught not to become co-conspirators, not to cover up for the drinker, not to put him or her to bed, and so on.

Once a little steadier, patients go out of the center to AA meetings in the community. Members from the area come in to the hospital and talk about their lives and what happened to them as a result of alcohol. Patients begin to realize that there may be much worth learning from people with less intelligence or education than they. At this point they may be offered Disulfram, a medicine that makes one sick if alcohol is drunk. This is very helpful in some cases, especially for impulsive drinkers who know they have to wait five days for the Disulfram to leave their system. Thus, when upset, they can cool off, call their sponsor, and get to a meeting instead of picking up a drink.

*Finally,* a note of caution, lest the criticism of psychiatry's ineptitude in the disease of alcoholism seem too intemperate, one must never forget the possibility of (bi-polar) manic depressive illness in someone with a drinking disorder.

Dr. David Dunner and colleagues at Presbyterian Hospital in New York City have shown that almost 10% of a group of patients being treated for mania and depression were alcoholic as well, and needed therapy for their alcoholism in addition.[13]

Work done at St. Patrick's Hospital in Dublin, Ireland, (founded by Dean Swift "for fools and mad") has shown that almost 30% of male alcoholics admitted to a treatment service in a private hospital in Ireland (almost all of them natives of that country) have manic-depressive illness which requires independent therapy if they are to benefit from treatment for alcoholism.[14]

In summary: there are effective treatments for alcoholic physicians. It is therefore important to recognize cases and commence treatment as soon as possible. This means getting the alcoholics aware enough to submit. (Techniques of confrontation are described in Chapter 10.)

## REFERENCES

1. Bailey M, Haberman P: The Washington Heights Survey, Q.J. Studies of Alcohol, 1962, 23:610–623.
2. Kearney T, Bonime H, Cassimatis G: Impact of Alcoholism on a Community General Hospital, J Community Mental Health 1967, 3:373–376.
3. Publications of AA General Services Board, Box 439, Grand Central Station, NY, 1976.
4. Gitlow S, Peyser H: Alcoholism, New York, Grune & Stratton, 1980.
5. Geller A, Bissell L: The Impaired Physician: Advances in Primary Care, Baltimore, Wilmore & Wilkins, 1979.
6. Modlin H, Montes A: Narcotics Addiction in Physicians, Am J Psychiatry 1963, 121:358–363.
7. Vaillant G, Brighton J, McArthur C: Physicians' Use of Mood-Altering Drugs, N Eng J Med, 1970, 282:365–372.
8. Johnson R, Connolly J: Addicted Physicians—A Closer Look, JAMA: 1981, 245 (3):253–257.
9. Talbott D: The Disabled Doctors' Program of Georgia, Alcoholism, Clinical and Experimental Research, 1977, 1:143–146.
10. Jellinek E: Phases in Alcohol Addiction, Q.J. of Studies on Alcohol, New Haven, 1952, 13:673–684.
11. Bissell L, Jones R: The Alcoholic Physician—A Survey, Am J Psychiatry, 1976, 133:1142–1146.

12. Robinson D: Talking Out of Alcoholism, Baltimore, University Park Press, 1980.
13. Dunner D, Hensel B, Fieve R: Bipolar Illness, Factors in Drinking Behavior, Am J Psychiatry, 1979, 136:583–585.
14. Cooney J, (personal communication).

# The Dually Addicted Physician

The afflictions of alcoholism and drug abuse are common bedfellows. It has been demonstrated that 25% of all drug addicts would be classified as alcoholics even if they never took a drug, because of their excessive drinking. It is probable that figure is too conservative for physicians because physicians run a 50 to 100% greater risk than the general population of abusing drugs.[1] Authorities have estimated that up to one half of all physician alcoholics in the country are mixing drugs with alcohol and abusing both.[2] Thus, it appears that nationwide there are more than 10,000 dually addicted physicians taking both drugs and alcohol.[3]

The drugs consumed by physicians run the gamut from sedative-hypnotics through psychostimulants to synthetic and natural narcotics. However, physicians' drug abuse differs from the general public's pattern of abuse in two important respects. First, doctors seldom abuse heroin, so they are less likely to get arrested in a "drug bust" and undergo criminal prosecution. And second, they abuse more synthetic compounds such as Demerol, Talwin or the volatile anesthetics. Most develop a preference for a single drug of abuse but a few become multiple drug abusers. The reasons for particular drug abuse patterns are simple. Like manufacturing industries that developed from of the confluence of raw material and labor, physicians use the substances they do, because of the drugs' proximity, easy availability and personal preference. Licit drugs are as close as a hospital ward or a spurious prescription. Consequently, doctors who succumb to the dual temptation of alcohol and drugs are assured of consistent quality and a steady supply of "ethical" products to satisfy their cravings. Physicians who combine "street" substances with alcohol abuse generally have a greater degree of psychopathology than those who use a single chemical or "ethical" product.

Dually addicted physicians are difficult to understand and frustrating to treat. Most of them present with complicated psychodynamics which can be unraveled only with patience and consummate skill. However, they must be treated if they are to be steered away from their self destructive course and returned to medicine.

Dr Harvey Ruben author of this chapter is a physician with wide experience in the field of dual addiction. For four years, he was medical director of Blue Hills Hospital, Hartford, CT, one of the few hospitals exclusively devoted to the treatment of combined alcohol and drug addiction. His perceptive contribution to this book reflects his experience, knowledge and insight into the problem of dual addiction.

*J.P.C.*

---

1. Bissell L, Jones R: The alcoholic physician: a survey, Am J Psychiatry 1976 133(10):1142–1146.
2. Murray R: Characteristics and prognosis of alcoholic doctors, Brit Med J 1976, 2:1537–1539.
3. Steindler EM: The Impaired Physician. AMA Dept of Mental Health. An Interpretive Summary of the AMA Conference on the Disabled Doctor: Challenge to the Profession, April 11–12, 1975.

# 12

# Substance Abuse and the Professional: How It Effects You, Your Family, and Your Colleagues

*Harvey L. Ruben*

## NATURE OF THE PROBLEM

It is always easier to think about problems of drug dependence as someone else's problems; the truth is, the physician and family are far from immune from suffering these maladies.

With the general trend in the 1960s toward more liberal alcohol control laws, as more women and young people started to drink, there was a measurable effect on the lives of health professionals and their families. Current estimates are that 80% of the population of this country drink alcohol at some time during their lives. During the past decade there has been a 15–20% increase in heavier drinking by males and a significant increase in moderate drinking among middle-aged women. For both sexes drinking has become heavier during the younger years with a tendancy to decline in late middle age. Approximately 12 million people in our adult population, or 7% of those over the age of 18, can currently be classified as alcoholics or problem drinkers. Of all those adults who drink, over one-third can be classified as either current or potential problem drinkers. Estimates vary, but women are thought to constitute a fourth to a third of the nation's problem drinkers. It is also estimated that there are 3.3 million problem drinkers between the ages of 14 and 17 years. Alcohol-related deaths in the United States, including those from accidents, homicides, suicides, and various life-threatening diseases, are estimated to be over 200,000 per year. Deaths from cirrhosis have remained high during the past decade, and in 1975 cirrhosis ranked sixth among the most common causes of death in this country. Any evidence of alcohol problems in males increases their mortality rate 2–6 times over that of the general population. Internationally, the higher the level of alcohol consumption per person, the higher the death rate from cirrhosis. In 1975, alcohol abuse and alcoholism was estimated to have cost this country nearly $43 billion, as follows[1]:

| | |
|---|---|
| lost production | $19.6 billion |
| health and medical costs | $12.74 billion |
| motor vehicle accidents | $ 5.14 billion |
| violent crimes | $ 2.86 billion |
| social response programs | $ 1.94 billion |
| fire losses | $ 0.43 billion. |

These figures have increased since then. Considering these statistics, it is inconceivable that alcohol and drug problems would not effect physicians and their families. During the past 20 years, several studies have been published with remarkably consistent results. Asuming that physicians have drinking practices similar to others in our population, then about 384,000 of our 483,701 physicians are drinkers and between 20,000 and 25,000 are or will become alcoholics. Four times as many men as women are alcoholics and college graduates have a higher proportion of drinkers than those with lesser educational achievements—thus the high rate of alcoholism in this group. One English study reported a higher mortality rate from cirrhosis for English physicians.[2]

Although physicians seem generally to be reluctant to diagnose alcoholism in themselves or their colleagues, a recent AMA study indicated that 400 doctors are lost to the medical profession each year due to problem drinking. Small noted that the incidence of alcoholism among nonhospitalized physician/patients he treated was 17%.[3] Lee found alcoholism or heavy drinking to be a factor in 39% of physician's suicides he studied, with 19% being intoxicated at the time of death.[4] Other studies have shown that drug dependency in physicians is usually proceeded by alcoholism with the rate of narcotic addictions among physicians anywhere from 30 to 100 times that of the general population.[5] Modlin and Montes studied 25 physician addicts at the Menninger Hospital in Topeka and found that all used varying amounts of alcohol, sedatives, analgesics or ataractics in combination with narcotics.[6] Combined statistics from the United States, England, Germany, Holland, and France indicate that of known drug addicts about 15% are physicians and an additional 15% are members of the pharmacy and nursing professions.[7] In a study of 68 physician addicts at the U.S. Public Health Service Hospital in Lexington, Kentucky, alcoholism, chronic fatigue, and physical disease were all related to the practice of self-medication.[2]

Vaillant and his group at Harvard studied 45 physicians prospectively over a 20–year period and found that self-medication with drugs or alcohol was the cause of one-third of the total time this group spent in the hospital.[8] In addition 36% of these physicians compared with 22% of his control group were catagorized as being in the high drug use groups, which included heavy drinking or trouble with control of alcohol. Vaillant found that physicians, especially those who treat patients, were more likely than nonphysicians to be involved in heavy drug and alcohol use and to have relatively unsuccessful marriages. He stated that the presence of these occupational hazards, however, appear strongly associated with life adjustments before medical school: those physicians who had the least stable childhoods and adolescent adjustment seemed to be especially vulnerable to these hazards.[8]

## Risks

Bissell and Jones studied 98 recovered alcoholic physicians all of whom had been entirely abstinent for one year.[2] They found that psychiatry was the only specialty overrepresented in the sample. In addition, a disproportionate number of these physicians reported high standing in their medical school classes. Approximately half of the sample had also abused drugs other than alcohol. Although legal sanctions and admission to treatment facilities and correctional institutions were common among these doctors, relatively little in the way of formal response of a disciplinary nature from colleagues or medical organizations was noted.[2] These physicians reported that they abused sedative-hypnotics, tranquilizers, amphetamines, and volatile anesthetics. Codeine and terpenhydrate with codeine were frequently included in the narcotics. Many complained that a professional colleague refused to identify or deal with the problems of their drug and alcohol abuse, choosing to regard this problem as a symptom of another underlying condition.

The American Medical Association Council on Mental Health obtained figures from the boards of medical examiners of Arizona, Connecticut, and Oregon which showed the number of practicing physicians in each state subject to discipline action for alcoholism, drug dependence, and mental disorders. In an 11-year period, nearly 2% of Arizona's physicians came before the board for disciplinary action; in 10 years, 2% of Oregon's physicians were called; and in a 6-year period, approximately 1% of Connecticut's physicians were so censured. Thus in approximately a decade, 118 drug-dependent physicians were brought before their disciplinary bodies in three of the smaller states, with an equal number of physicians appearing for alcoholism and a smaller but significant number appearing for other mental illnesses.[7] The California Board of Medical Examiners estimated that at some point in their careers 1–2% of the physicians in that state had used narcotics; that board handles approximately 125 disciplinary cases a year involving alcohol and drug abuse.[7]

Jones reviewed the case records of 100 physician inpatients in a private psychiatric hospital in Philadelphia. He found that these physicians were more likely to have diagnoses of affective disorder (depression) for drug abuse than a general psychiatric hospital population. Their peak susceptibility seemed to occur during their late 40s. The percentage of substance abuse diagnoses in these physicians was about three times that of the general total hospital population during this period of time.[9]

Welner and associates in St. Louis studied 111 female physicians and 103 female Ph.D.s selected from the general population to see if they evidenced the signs of psychiatric illness. Among them, 51% of the M.D.s and 32% of the Ph.D.s were diagnosed as having primary affective disorders. Other psychiatric disorders were found in less than 10% of each group. Depression among the psychiatrists was significantly more common than among the other physicians (73% compared to 45%). Over 50% of the women reported prejudice against them in training or employment and the depressed subjects reported prejudice more often than the others. Presence of depression and children were shown to disrupt the women's professional careers. Welner found the high prevalence of affective disorder among female physicians was consistent with reported excessive suicide risk for this group.[10]

It should be recognized that substance abuse affects other members of the health treatment team. Levine and co-workers at Lexington studied the history of 12 nurses who abused drugs. These histories disclosed an early and extensive involvement in medical treatment—a"medical dependence"—manifested by a somatic orientation, chronic medical difficulties, dependence on alcohol, and finally, dependence on other drugs. He noted an irregular attitude in this group of women towards addictive substances: it was alright to take *medicine,* but alcohol and cigarettes were less acceptable and "drugs" (substances such as marijuana and heroin) were least acceptable. "Drugs" were rarely used. Alcoholism was found to be frequent and usually preceded the use of other addictive substances.[11]

## Reasons for Resistance

In a study of (male) physician attitudes in the Navy, Pursch[12] concluded that 75% of physicians are unable to deal effectively with alcohol-dependent patients for the following reasons:

1. The physician lacks useful training or education in alcoholism or drug addiction.

2. The physician has unresolved alcoholism or alcohol problems in his own family.
3. The physician himself is alcoholic, has a drinking problem, or is treating himself with psychoactive medication.
4. The physician is continually occupied with significant negative experiences with alcoholic patients in his own background.
5. The physician has a rigid personality structure with almost total inability to deal with any of his patients on an emotional level.
6. The physician fears that if he were outspoken about alcoholism he would lose some of his friends and colleagues who frowned on his forthrightness, and career advancement might be impaired.

Pursch found that in medical school, the physicians learned that alcoholism is not an important subject (2 hours or less is devoted to it in a 4-year period) and that it was a manifestation of underlying psychological conflict until cirrhosis, pancreatitis, or other medical illness was evident. In clinical experience the physician saw the alcoholic coming from skid row to the emergency room, ICU, and the morgue. Alcoholics were observed during limited stays on the medical-surgical ward where they were an interesting problem in electrolyte management and useful subjects in learning how to do a liver biopsy or a sternal puncture. These physicians seldom saw the alcoholic in a rehabilitative setting. The subtotal of all attitude-shaping experiences was that alcoholism appeared to be a behavioral problem which can lead to hopeless and eventually fatal organ damage. He concluded that the physicians he had studied had touched many alcoholic livers, but almost no alcoholic lives; thus they could not deal with alcoholism effectively. Only a few had ever known a recovered alcoholic.[12]

## CAUSES OF THE PROBLEM

Any number of factors may contribute to the development of substance abuse problems in professionals and their families. These include the constant pressures to perform at maximum level, continuous demands on time and knowledge, the requirement to maintain professional confidence, and the susceptibility to depressive symptoms that results from the gap between expectation and performance. Although physicians are supposedly at the top of the health care team, both in terms of knowledge and awareness, they are still at high risk for both alcohol and drug abuse in a country where substance abuse in general is at an epidemic level. When we consider that other care givers, such as nurses and pharmacists who appear to have at least as high an incidence of substance abuse as do physicians, the implications are serious both for our profession and for society as well.[5]

Modlin and Montes found that drug addiction in physicians ordinarily depended on three conditions: (1) a predisposing personality, (2) the availability of drugs and (3) a set of circumstances that brought the first two together. They further noted that the majority of the 30 physicians that they studied consistently denied serious addictive difficulties and shared the illusion that they could stop using drugs at any time they wished.[6] In addition to these factors, Bissell has pointed out several reasons why physicians are more prone to develop substance abuse problems and why they are more difficult for us to reach therapeutically. Very frequently the physician practices alone and does not have close interaction with professional colleagues. In addition the physician holds a prestigious position in the community; thus few people have any influence on his (or her) personal and professional actions. This leaves the physician in control, (and more than likely) to prescribe for himself when he feels the need.[13] This easy availability of drugs for physicians is an important contributing cause of substance abuse in the profession. Because they can prescribe for themselves at will with no professional or legal requirement for consultation with colleagues, they are quite likely to experiment with drugs, especially those they prescribe for their patients. The availability of samples at the office enhances the temptation to seek relief from discomfort or fatigue even though the choice of pharmacologic agent is often unrelated to the symptoms.[14]

The concept of drug abuse implies either self-medication or the use of a drug for a purpose other than its specific therapeutic potential. Any drug used for purposes other than its specific therapeutic potential has the capacity to produce drug dependence. Were it necessary for physicians to justify their needs for medication, many might ultimately not become involved in substance abuse. Instead, physicians, confident of their ability to prescribe properly and accurately for their patients, often believe that they can do the same for themselves. In fact, physicians frequently state that they would feel embarrassed to ask a colleague to prescribe for them when they are certain they are as knowledgeable. However, no matter how capable physicians may be in treating others, they may well be incompetent to treat themselves. Consider the fact that for the most effective therapy, dispensing physicians must carefully evaluate their patients' responses to the drug by consultation with the patients and by utilizing various laboratory studies which will reflect changes induced by the medication. It is exceedingly rare that any physicians involved in self-medication follow such procedures. Obviously, in self-medication physicians eliminate one of the basic needs for the successful practice of medicine: the physician–patient relationship. Although it is difficult to believe that people who have studied pharmacology in medical school would practice flagrant drug abuse, it is not uncommon for physicians to take analgesics to relieve fatigue and other symptoms when they occur.[14]

To understand better the causes of substance abuse in the physicians and their families it is useful to refer to the bio-psycho-social model of disease.

## Biological Causes

We know that there are no specific biological disease processes that precede the onset of alcoholism. Bissell and Jones found that many physicians reported a tendency to use various drugs in addition to alcohol to deal with both insomnia and agitation. As the use of various sedatives increased, frequently in the face of increasing alcohol use, the physicians often became confused as to how much they were taking; 23 men reported serious sedative overdoses which were not believed to be suicide attempts.[2] The study by Goby and associates at Lutheran General Hospital of 51 alcoholic physicians revealed that 28% identified a past or present medical problem, ranging from depression to coronary disease and carcinoma of the lung, as antecedents of their substance abuse. Five percent identified themselves as being in poor health and under treatment for one or more medical conditions.[15]

Although no physical antecedents of alcoholism and drug abuse have yet been found, a number of studies have shown a higher rate of alcoholism among the relatives of alcoholics than in the general population. Studies of adopted children suggest that male children of alcoholic parents are more likely to have a drinking problem whether or not any contact with the alcoholic parent occurred. One Swedish study of 2000 adoptees showed a significant correlation between identified alcohol abuse among biological parents and their adopted out sons. If alcoholism could be associated with other characteristics known to be inherited, such as blood type, salivary secretions, and color blindness, the case for the genetic cause of alcoholism would be much greater. However, studies to identify such genetic markers have yet to be proven conclusive.[1]

## Psychological Causes

The evidence of psychological factors which relate to substance abuse in the professional is far more substantial. The amount of denial by substance abusing professionals is great. Denial is an unconscious mental mechanism that enables one to resist recognizing some aspect of reality. Physicians dependent on alcohol and drugs frequently exhibit this primitive psychological mechanism as a conviction that "it can't happen to me." Many physicians seem convinced that they are immune to the organisms causing their patients infective diseases; in fact, some act as though they have aquired a general immunity to physical illness of all sorts. They also tend to avoid annual physical examinations, which they emphatically recommend to their patients. It seems especially true that physicians feel immune to the problems that they treat within their specialities. One of the malignant aspects of this denial is that it may interfere with the early diagnosis of the illness at a time when treatment would be most effective. Lack of early diagnosis is most evident in emotional disorders and is related to the most universally denied of illnesses among physicians—substance abuse. Physicians rarely if ever seem to consider the possibility that their practices of self-medication may lead to substance dependence. Even when physicians have treated patients for drug abuse or alcoholism or have known colleagues dependent on these substances through self-administration, many still maintain the "it can't happen to me" attitude. Thus many physicians continue to deny their substance abuse even when confronted with unequivocal evidence of the persistence of this state. The inner realization that the physician is addicted, a premise too painful to be dealt with consciously, provides a powerful motivation for denial.[14]

Rationalization is also another powerful psychological defense used by physicians in these instances. Most patients dependent on substances make excuses for their dependency. Physicians who are dependent on substances tend to justify their actions by stating that they take the drugs only to permit them to perform their responsibilities—not for "kicks" or personal need. Overwork and fatigue facilitate the physician addicts' ability to rationalize their pathologic dependency. Some even come to feel that "a little personal drug abuse" is necessary and permissible to fulfill the demands of medical practice. Often these physicians state that without their drug dependency they could not practice; they are convinced that their responsibility to their patients overrides any personal consideration stemming from the "required drug dependency."[14]

The existence of this massive denial and rationalization in the emotional life of substance-dependent physicians makes them impervious to receiving help. It is important to understand that this process is not mere lying. It is a genuine self-deception in which substance-dependent physicians are unable to appreciate the significance of drug use even though it may be obvious to colleagues and family. Because of physicians' free access to numerous mood-changing drugs, their use of these drugs and alcohol may not be characteristic of other substance abusers. The abusing physicians are able to present convincing and accurate arguments that they are not drinking or using drugs at all excessively. Therefore the use of mood-changing drugs, particularly when self-prescribed in order to function in everyday life, lends supportive evidence to the diagnosis of substance abuse.[13]

The individual personality of a physician is obviously also a determinant in the development of destructive alcohol and drug use practices. At times it is difficult to determine whether certain personality features cause or are a result of substance abuse. Diminished personality controls, impulsiveness, and antisocial trends are considered predisposing personality factors. This may be true, but drug intoxication also releases such behavior.[17] Regardless of the encouragement provided to the physician by the availability of drugs and the tendency to self-medication, the majority of physicians do not become victims of drug dependency; those who do have underlying personality problems. The genesis of drug dependency is therefore principally related to the patient and the manner in which he or she takes to a pharmacologic agent rather then the drug's intrinsic chemical or physiologic activity; it is the physiologic properties of the drug that determine to a great extent its continued use.[14]

The addiction of the physician can truly only be understood by understanding the personality of the addict. The physician addict has a unique relationship with the chosen addicting substance: it is required in order to deal with the stressful factors in life. Even though the self-treatment is rarely successful, it still must be recognized as an attempt to help oneself, however ill advised.[18] It is possible to become dependent on a drug even after taking a single dose. Rado's concept of this process is helpful in understanding this fact. He points out that prior to acquiring drug dependency, a precondition or "ripeness" must exist: the physician experiences certain psychological states that encourage susceptibility.[16] Preparedness for drug dependency includes psychological frustrations which, if unrelieved, produce mental anguish and feelings of helplessness. Self-deprecation and depression may then develop. Inability to solve these problems produces tension, which contributes to a further lowering of self-esteem. At this point—a condition characterized by the term "tense depression" develops—the physician is "ripe." The intensity of such a state and how effectively a substance relieves the painful condition essentially determine the rapidity with which drug dependency develops. When the individual is provided with a drug that changes pain to pleasure, and when depression is replaced with increased self-esteem, the first phase of substance dependency has occurred. The mind experiences an event it will never forget. It may be likened to a return to a blissful state of childhood when the mother attempted to keep her infant's frustration minimal by anticipating and gratifying every wish. To be taken care of and mothered seems to be a constant universal wish of every human being—a wish exemplified by some patients who when under the influence of drugs say, "Now I'm not afraid of anything or anyone; I can do anything I wish."[14]

Perhaps the most important psychological aspect of addiction for the physician is the need to distort reality. Consider the following reality distortions:

1. Some spouses need stimulants or depressants to face sexual or other marital responsibilities. One patient admitted that her drugs so reduced her sexual needs that she was able to marry a man she knew to be a homosexual.
2. A special type of malignancy is frequently observed in which the ego feels that it becomes more potent and is able to function better under the influence of addicting drugs.

However, this increase of fantasied efficiency is not credited to the drug itself. In a strange, self-deceptive way, the addict physician is convinced that the drug provides an opportunity to work more effectively or creatively. In other words, the addict may rationalize that he or she is more effective not because of an addiction—which is frequently denied—but because the addicting drug has released locked-up potential. This type of reality distortion was demonstrated by a physician addicted to large amounts of Demerol who, following successful treatment, stated that

> When I was on Demerol I was convinced that I could diagnose and treat my patients much better than I ever could before. In fact I was convinced that I was keeping better medical records and doing more effective work during this time. Later when I looked at my records, I was ashamed and humiliated to see how lousy my work had been. If anyone had told me how terrible my work was when I was taking Demerol, I wouldn't have believed them. I would have laughed at them.[18]

Finally as part of this reality distortion, there is a magical quality that the addict imparts to the addicting agent. As one patient stated: "I can't explain it, but I definitely feel better as soon as I take my Miltown. I know it hasn't had time to work. It's just like magic the way it makes me feel better.[18]

**Social**

Considering the social causes of substance abuse in physicians and their families, the dynamics of the family constellation are an important factor. Considerable evidence indicates that the risk of alcoholism is increased by family conditions that impair or disrupt the emotional bonds between parents and children. Children of alcoholics show a high frequency of alcohol and drug misuse, antisocial behavior, neurotic symptoms, and psychosomatic complaints. Parent alcoholism may also be related to delinquency and hyperactivity in children. One puzzling question yet to be answered is why one child in a family develops an alcohol or drug problem and another does not. Family research has traditionally focused on the wife of the alcoholic male. However, as public awareness of alcoholism in women increases, more emphasis is being placed on the alcoholic wife, her husband, and her children. In fact many therapists now treat the whole family rather than just the alcoholic. Information now accumulating on the alcoholic family makes the future of family therapy seem promising, although additional research on the efficacy of this approach is needed.[1]

Earlier studies emphasized the family unit as the place where lifelong drinking practices are formed. This was probably true when families exerted a considerable influence on adolescent development. It may be somewhat less valid at present. The parents' drinking behavior remains an important predictor of teenagers' drug-taking habits. Drinking parents ordinarily will have drinking children, with the degree of usage usually reflecting parental patterns. Abstinent parents are more likely to have abstinent children, though of course many exceptions exist. Some children are so upset by a drunken parent that they react by abstaining. Overly strict teetotaling parents may alienate a child, causing the complete rejection of the parental prohibition towards alcohol and drugs. Such children seem prone to use all substances intemperately.[17] This particular factor is exceedingly important in relation to the professional family. Since the professional is frequently under a great deal of stress and pressure, as indicated above, this stress cannot help but be transmitted to other family members. It is a rather common occurrence to find varying degrees of marital and family disruption in the home of the professional.

Other social factors thought to influence substance abuse include peer influence, which appears in the lives of both the parents and the children. There are pressures to use various substances in a social setting which introduce the physician (or family) to the use of these drugs.[17] Culture and one's particular subculture are also thought to determine whether one will drink and how one will behave if drunk by providing cues (via family, friends, and mass media) as to what is permitted or what is expected.[1]

## Substance Abuse and the Health Care Industry

Many of the programs that have been developed to deal with the problem of substance abuse have not helped physicians because they have failed to meet the needs of most professional abusers and their families. Some have failed because they were rigid in their outlook and restricted in their approach to treatment, using limited therapeutic modalities and providing care only for acutely ill patients. Other failings include poor clinical organization and administration, inadequate *referral* procedures and follow-up, limited knowledge of the resources and procedures of other health organizations and agencies, institutionalized inefficiency, and a general insensitivity to the psychological need of the substance-abusing people they have tried to help. All these circumstances have sapped the resources and vitality of too many substance-abuse programs.[5]

Mistaken attitudes and practices of professionals are reflected in the hospital and health insurance systems. Until recently, 50% of the nation's hospitals did not admit patients with a primary diagnosis of alcoholism, so the patient had to be admitted under the cover of some other diagnosis. Many health insurance plans do not cover alcoholism or drug dependency as illnesses. This situation has improved somewhat, but many institutions still adhere to traditional rejection of chemical dependency. This is a disservice to the patient, the hospital, and society, for it perpetuates the misconception that neither alcoholism nor drug abuse is an illness. This encourages the patient in the symptomatic denial or rationalization of the abuse, further obscuring the illness. The result is often inadequate or incomplete treatment.[5]

All these attitudes and practices add up to a massive denial of responsibility for a massive social health problem. In those cases where the responsibility is unavoidable, the medical professional is generally more than anxious to refer people to Alcoholics Anonymous or other similar types of self-help organizations. These organizations are to be commended for their efforts on behalf of substance-abusing persons. It is interesting to note, however, that substance abuse is one of the few conditions for which the medical professional is quite willing to have nonmedical personnel assume leadership in treatment.[5]

In addition to late diagnosis and unrealistic treatment, a third element reinforced is therapeutic nihilism. This is analogous to a situation where 300,000 units of penicillin were needed to treat pneumonia, and only 6000 units were available. When treatment failed we assumed that pneumonia was untreatable and penicillin was ineffective against pneumonia. This is the heart of the substance-abuse tragedy: we have perpetuated an epidemic not by lack of ability, but by our own ignorance and unwillingness to face the situation as it really is.[19]

It is time for the medical profession to stop turning its back on substance-abusing professionals who want help. They have no desire to be alcoholics or drug addicts or any reason to be ashamed of their illness. Likewise, those concerned with the alleviation of human suffering have no reason to make them feel ashamed or guilty; but that is precisely what we do when we systematically withhold the treatment that they need. Failure to recognize the wide range of factors that contribute to substance abuse is directly reflected in the way we treat those substance abusers whom we do recognize. The underlying attitude of many health care givers is that the alcoholic or drug addict is hopeless and unmotivated for treatment. Such persons are tacitly considered responsible for their illness, unable to control their drug-taking behavior only because they lack the necessary will power. As a result, substance abusers are typically refused treatment until they give up their symptoms—which makes about as much sense as withholding penicillin from pneumonia patients until they give up coughing. Labeling these patients as unmotivated is a convenient device to avoid treating the problem or to transfer the failure from the care giver to the patient. Underlying all diagnostic and treatment attitudes is a fundamental misconception that alcohol and drug abusers are untreatable. Nothing could be further from the truth. We have forgotten that in the practice of medicine and the delivery of care there is one basic overriding attainable goal: to help people hurt less. We should reject the unfair "all or nothing" view of substance-abuse treatment that labels less then total cure as total failure. Above all, it is time that we stopped blaming the affected person for the illness and for our own inability to provide appropriate treatment.[5]

## IMPACT OF THE PROBLEM

Because statistics are sketchy it is impossible to assess accurately the societal impact of professional substance abuse. We can only obtain approximations from some of the information we have available to us. Bissell found that 54% of the physicians in one study did not experience obvious changes in job status as a result of drinking. This, of course, did not take into consideration the quality or volume of work performed. Of the 46% who did report work difficulties, 40% suffered periods of unemployment and 10% were forced to work outside the medical field altogether. Of those who remained in medicine, each reported a decline in status, and several said that their careers had been dramatically affected. A chief of medicine in a medical school took a series of *locum tenens* positions for general practitioners. A famous pathologist worked as a lab technician for another physician. A neurosurgeon, deprived of staff privileges, supported himself by doing routine physical exams. Many of these doctors experienced difficulty with the law. Others stated that, although they had never been arrested, they felt that they should have been; but the police often had been lenient when an erratic driver or a boisterous individual was identified as a doctor. Forty-eight of these subjects (49%) had been arrested, 38% had been jailed, and 19.4% had lost their driver's license. The 48 physicians who had been arrested had a total of 219 arrests and 170 jailings.[2]

In Jones' study of 100 physician psychiatric inpatients, 21 were identified as having alcoholism and drug-dependence problems. Of those, 12 had multiple hospitalizations with an average length of stay of 29 days, compared to 36.5 days for the other physicians who suffered from emotional problems other than substance abuse. It should also be noted that whereas five of the 12 cases had a primary diagnosis of alcoholism, 12 additional cases revealed noteworthy alcohol abuse. Similarly, drug addiction was the primary diagnosis in seven cases and the secondary diagnosis in six. Additionally drug abuse was recorded in the history of nine other cases. Finally, combined alcohol and drug abuse was described in six more cases that did not carry the diagnosis of either type of dependency. Thus although only 12 of the 100 physicians carried a primary diagnosis of substance abuse, 52 (more than half) actually had an alcohol or drug abuse problem. In this substance-abusing group, four of the physicians had suffered falls and two had had automobile accidents after drinking. Eleven had staff privileges revoked by their peers and two had their medical licenses removed. In only one instance was it recorded that a patient had complained that the physician had been intoxicated, and there is no mention in these records of malpractice that might be attributable to substance abuse.[9]

In his study of 51 physicians who had been treated for alcoholism at Lutheran General Hospital, Goby found that 88% of the patients reported that their job performance and family relationships had been affected prior to entering treatment. Following treatment 80% said that they were able to meet all of their work or family responsibilities once they were abstinent and their health improved. However, 35% said they had a change in marital status following hospitalization. Sixteen percent said they were living alone following hospitalization, 72% were living with a spouse or family, and one (2%) was living with a friend.[15]

### Physical Effects

Physicians' substance abuse led to increased incidence of physical problems, especially cirrhosis. Alcohol and drug abuse are related to other kinds of physical problems in addition to the liver: the gastrointestinal tract, brain and nervous system, heart, muscles, and endocrine system are all affected. Alcohol abuse is associated with cardiomyopathy and diseases of the coronary arteries such as angina pectoris and myocardial infarction. Atrial fibrillation is seen commonly in what is emerging as the "holiday heart syndrome"—a cardiac arrhythmia noted in individuals free of overt heart disease who would appear in emergency rooms after drinking on weekends or over holiday periods associated with high alcohol consumption. Alcohol abuse is also incriminated in cancer: heavy drinking has been associated with an increase in the risk of cancer of the tongue, the mouth or oropharynx, hypopharynx, esophagus, larynx, and liver. Alcohol and tobacco have a synergistic effect that increases the risk of head and neck cancer for heavy drinkers who smoke by a factor of 6–15. Although rare, primary liver cancer is often associated with cirrhosis which is nearly always associated in this country with alcohol consumption. Studies in other countries have shown that as many as 90% of the victims who had suffered from either condition had suffered from both. Alcohol abuse is also associated with a variety of inflammatory and bleeding lesions of the stomach, with deficiencies in body thiamine, iron, and vitamin B-12, and with increased incidence of pancreatitis.[1]

In a sample of 98 alcoholic physicians, Bissell and Jones found 44 had suffered from gastritis, 19 from peripheral neuropathy, 16 from severe malnutrition, 14 from fatty liver, 14 from gastrointestinal bleeding, ten from peptic ulcer, five from pancreatitis, four from sclerosis, and one from esophogeal varices.[2] Considering such data, we cannot underestimate the effects of substance abuse on the physical health of colleagues who are so affected. In addition we should not overlook the secondary physical complications related to alcohol and drug interaction.

## Drug Interactions

During the past decade increasing attention has been paid to the physical and behavioral effects of drug and alcohol use in combination. Of the hundred most frequently prescribed drugs, more than half contain at least one ingredient known to interact adversely with alcohol. Most adverse affects due to alcohol and drug interactions are accidental, but the medical toll is high, including an estimated annual 2500 deaths and 47,000 emergency room admissions. Unfortunately, we frequently do not stop to think about the effect that alcohol and other drug use have upon the therapeutic agents which we or our patients are using for various maladies. Some of these alcohol–drug interactions occur only in the face of chronic heavy alcohol use (such as an increased metabolic rate for Dilantin in the chronic alcoholic, which requires larger than normal doses to maintain a therapeutic effect). In the case of tolbutamide, the occasional consumption of a large amount of alcohol increases tolbutamide's half-life, whereas chronic abuse causes a significant decrease in the half-life. Even a previous history of alcohol abuse in a currently abstinent individual can affect the dose level required for certain drugs as compared to those for nondrinkers. The half-lives of warfarin, phenytoin, tolbutamide, and isoniazid are all 50% shorter in an abstaining alcoholic than in nondrinkers. The kinds of drug–alcohol interactions that occur may be antagonistic, additive, supra-additive, or cross-tolerant. Alcohol can interact with salicylates and predispose a patient to delayed clotting and possible hemorrhage. Alcohol can cause a supra-additive interaction with various anesthetics and cause a deeper narcosis to develop than is desired. It may also increase the blood-pressure-lowering capabilities of some antihypertensive agents leading to postural hypertension, faintness, and loss of consciousness. It may even interfere with the metabolism of oral anticoagulant drugs and thus lead to hemorrhage.

Alcohol can have varying effects in connection with antidepressants. With monoamine oxidase inhibitors, certain alcoholic beverages may cause a hypertensive crisis. The combination of alcohol with some antimicrobial drugs may cause a disulfram reaction with nausea, vomiting, headache, and possibly convulsions. Finally the combination of alcohol with barbiturates, major and minor tranquilizers, and narcotics is known to lead to possibly fatal depression of respiratory centers and impaired hepatic functions that may lead to toxic manifestations. Considering the possibility of these various alcohol and drug interactions, it is impossible to believe that we are able to estimate accurately the physical impact of substance abuse on the lives of the physicians and their families.[20]

### Psychological Effects

A more clear-cut, direct effect of substance abuse in the lives of physicians and their families is that of suicide. Epidemological studies have shown an increased incidence of suicide in substance-abusing individuals. Additionally, a number of studies have shown that physicians have a relatively high suicide rate. Rich, in a study of suicide by male physicians during a 5-year period, found that physicians had a much higher rate of suicide by poisioning than other groups based on ready access and knowledge of drugs.[21] One study found that 249 physicians listed in the American Medical Association obituary columns between May 1965 and November 1967 had died of suicide. Suicides exceeded the combined deaths from automobile accidents, plane crashes, drowning, and homicide. An additional 56 deaths were reported as possible suicides. The total for all these kinds of violent deaths was 534—5% of all the physician deaths during that period. The mean suicidal age for these physicians was 49, at or near the usual productive peak for a physician. Substance abuse was an important factor in 40% of the cases and depressive illness was very common. Suicides ranged from a low of 0.01% in pediatricians to a high of 0.6% among psychiatrists. It is estimated that approximately 100 physicians commit suicide annually—a group the size of the average medical school graduating class.[7]

Fifteen of the 98 alcoholic physicians in the Bissell and Jones study reported that they had made overt attempts at suicide: ten had made a single attempt, one had made two attempts, and two had made three and six attempts, respectively. There is probably also some underreporting among these subjects.[2] Blachly and associates studied 80 physicians who killed themselves during 1965–1967 and found that 39% were involved in alcohol abuse and 19% were drinking at the time of their death.[21a]

Jones, in a study of 100 physician psychiatric inpatients, found 15 had attempted suicide before admission and one did so immediately afterward. Four others had attempted suicide on previous occasions. Seventeen more described suicidal thoughts that had prompted their admission. Of the 16 suicide attempts, 14 were by overdose, one by shooting in the chest, and one by laceration of the neck. Thirteen of the 16 entered the hospital with a diagnosis of depression, and seven had a history of substance abuse. Thus 37% of the hospitalized physicians had previous histories of suicidal thoughts or attempts and two had made serious attempts after admission to the hospital.[9]

## Social Effects

As scant as our information is concerning the effects of substance abuse on the lives of physicians, we have even less information on its effects on physicians families. No accurate records are kept of the rate of marital disruption and/or divorce that affects physicians, although in professional marriages it is frequently high. It is also impossible to attempt to assess the incidence of problems in the children of the physician with any degree of accuracy. We do know that the incidence of substance-abuse-related problems in women and teenagers in this country is increasing; we must infer that it is similarly affecting the families of physicians.

Numerous reports in recent years have discussed the impact of teenage drinking in this country. The following trends have been well documented:

1. Drinking during and out of school has extended down to grammar school students and is more frequently encountered than in the past.
2. Girls are more frequently involved in regular drinking. (By the time they have graduated from high school, as many girls as boys use alcoholic beverages, although they do not drink as often.)
3. The combined use of alcohol and other drugs is often observed. Juvenile polydrug use with alcohol as the basic intoxicant is a growing problem.

Not only are there more youngsters trying alcoholic beverages, but larger numbers are drinking heavily and consistently. Pubescent alcoholism has been diagnosed in a number of pediatric psychiatric clinics and has become of increasing concern to those involved in pediatric medicine.[17] Statistics from the FBI in 1975 show that nearly 106,000 young people under the age of 18, including 145 children age 10 and younger, were arrested for violation of liquor laws in this country. More than 41,000 youths under 18 were arrested for drunkeness. Seventeen thousand people under the age of 18 including 51 children under the age of 10 were arrested for driving under the influence in 1975. Approximately 8000 young Americans a year are killed in drunken driving accidents, most of them caused by people their own age. An aditional 40,000 are disfigured.[22] One survey performed by the Institutes of Alcohol Abuse and Alcoholism in 1974 indicated that 93% of boys and 87% of girls in their senior year of school had experimented with alcohol while more than half of the nation's seventh graders had tried drinking at least once during the previous year.[23] It has been suggested that the decreased use of hard drugs during the past decade was paralleled by increases in alcohol abuse by teenagers: they found that alcohol abuse was more acceptable and got them into less trouble with school officials, their parents, and the law.[24] Considering such data and the fact that alcohol and various kinds of psychoactive drugs are usually available in the home of physicians, it is probable that many children of physicians commit various kinds of substance abuse.

During the past several years, studies of the effects of alcohol and drug use on the developing fetus have been published. In 1977 the National Institute of Alcohol Abuse and Alcoholism issued a warning to all physicians in this country on the effects of the fetal alcohol syndrome which causes abnormalities in the offspring of drinking women. The NIAAA reported that the fetus was at risk with the ingestion of as little of three ounces of alcohol a day or six drinks. Children showed various physical abnormalities such as characteristic flattening of the face and shortening of the nose, along with other major abnormalities such as pre- and postnatal growth deficiencies, delay in development, and disruption of fine motor function. Again, it is impossible to know how many children of physicians have been thus affected, but we can assume that some have.[25]

## SOLUTIONS TO THE PROBLEM

Why has substance abuse been able to extract such a heavy toll from our profession? What can we do about it? Goby and colleagues have alluded to some of the special problems of treating alcoholic or chemically dependent physicians.[15] Among these problems is the propensity for the alcoholic physician to refuse or to ignore treatment. In addition, once physicians enter treatment, they are often treated for illnesses other than alcoholism, although the latter is often the primary problem. Some authors have noted that with proper diagnosis and treatment the outlook for successful recovery among physicians is satisfactory. However, physicians have a difficult time forming an effective doctor–patient relationship. In addition, a larger proportion of physician-patients leave the hospital against medical advice than other patients: in one study a third of the physicians hospitalized for substance abuse left prior to completion of treatment and against medical advice.

In some research projects physicians have not been cooperative in responding to followup letters. However, Goby found that few doctors were willing to identify or recognize their alcoholism prior to treatment. They suffered physically, mentally, and professionally and were viewed by many treatment staff as having a poor prognosis, often being unaccepting of professional help. In spite of this, approximately two-thirds of these physician patients reported no use of alcohol or drugs at the follow-up interview. Twenty percent reported use with associated problems and 14% were deceased. Goby concluded that it is possible to have reasonable results in treating alcoholic physicians.[15]

## Obstacles

The Physician's Committee Report of the New York State Medical Society[26] in 1975 listed a number of problems that relate to difficulty in dealing with the substance-abusing professional. Among them are the following:

1. Confusion as to whether the sick physician should be regarded as "ill" or "bad"; treatment plans often combined two opposing views in such a way that neither approach could be taken consistently.
2. Unclear responsibility in New York State where the public assumes that physicians determine the right to practice of other physicians but where, in fact, the power to grant or revoke a license is held by the Department of Education. It does so poorly because of a small staff and inadequate budget.
3. Reluctance on the part of physicians to report a colleague for fear their attempt might result in punishment instead.
4. Concern that intervention in a colleague's personal affairs might lead to unpleasant social, legal, and professional consequences for the would-be helper.
5. Dissatisfaction with the speed and efficiency of available methods for intervention so that these methods are not regarded as

reliable, rapidly responsive, and worth taking except in extremely clear-cut cases.
6. Ignorance of actual reporting and procedures available.
7. Lack of consensus among physicians as to what course of action should be followed; ambivalence thus waits hopefully for unanimity and is rewarded instead with indecision and delay.[26]

Bissell and Jones found that the substance abuse of physicians was probably clearly visible to the general public and their colleagues. Public response to their behavior, indicated by arrests, jailings, and loss of driver's license, occurred more often and with a larger number of formal indications of disapprobation than did professional response as represented by warnings from medical societies and licensing boards, loss of hospital privileges, and actual loss of medical license. That the public is more aggressive in its response than the medical profession raises issues about the self-regulation of colleagues by a professional group. Arrests and jailings are not actions lightly undertaken by police in response to transient actions by physicians. Police are frequently reluctant to arrest more prominent respected citizens of a community. Several of the subjects stated that although they had not been arrested, they felt they should have been.[2]

**AMA Recommendations**

What then should the response of the profession be to the substance-abusing colleague? The Council on Mental Health of the American Medical Association[7] in 1972 issued its first report dealing with this problem. The Council made a number of observations and recommendations:

1. It is a physician's ethical responsibility to be aware of a colleague's inability to practice medicine adequately by reason of physical or mental illness including alcoholism and drug dependence. Ideally, affected physicians should seek help themselves when difficulties arise. Often, they are unable or unwilling to recognize that their problems exist. When exhortations by family or friends are ineffective and when the physicians are unable to make rational assessments of their ability to function professionally, it becomes the responsibility of their colleagues to decide for them and to advise them as to whether they should obtain treatment and curtail or suspend their practices. In carrying out this task, advising physicians should begin informal talks and proceed to more formalized approaches only as necessary according to the following sequence:

a. Discussion of the problem with other physicians who are in close working relations with the affected physician so that they may exert their influence in a positive and beneficial manner.

b. Referral of the problem to the medical staff of the hospital to which the affected physician serves.

c. Referral of the problem to a specific committee of the state or county medical society if the physician is not a member of a hospital staff or if the staff is unable or unwilling to act. This should be a committee reserved exclusively for this purpose, not an existing one such as an ethics or grievance committee. Its function should be to determine whether physicians are suffering from disorders to a degree that interferes with their ability to practice medicine. The committee should comprise examining physicians including, but not limited to, psychiatrists and neurologists. In carrying out its functions, the committee should be guided by procedures that are appropriate to the local situation as worked out by the state or county society.

d. Referral of the problem to the appropriate licensing body in the state if the physician is not a medical society member or if the medical society is unable or unwilling to act. The licensing body should have a committee comparable to the one established by the Medical Society.

2. Spouses can be helpful in bringing physicians into treatment and should become as fully informed as the society's members about the overall problem and the society's approach to its solution. The Women's Auxiliary should be asked to take an active part in this educational program.
3. The AMA's Office of the General Council should be requested to draw up a model law to deal with physicians who have such problems and to disseminate that model to state and county medical societies for legislative action in their jurisdictions.
4. Educational programs should be developed for medical students and the physician in training, emphasizing their vulnerability to psychiatric disorders, alcoholism, and drug abuse.[7]

### State Programs

The AMA Council sent a letter to all state medical society executives noting its interest in drug dependent, alcoholic, and psychiatrically impaired physicians and inquiring whether any state or county medical society had established an outstanding and effective program for handling difficult and serious problems in such physicians. Of the 54 societies canvassed (including Puerto Rico, the Virgin Islands, the Canal Zone, and the District of Columbia), 37 responded. Seven indicated that there was an active state committee charged with the problem and that the state either had or has pending a "sick doctor statute." Another seven reported having no active program, but indicated that some related action was pending or that they had been stimulated into initiating action on the basis of the inquiry. The remaining 27 states responded that there was no county or state society program directed at such a problem, and three went so far as to deny that any such problem even existed in their state. It could only be surmised that the nonrespondents (almost one-third of the number of states associations) were indifferent about these problems or denied their existence.[7]

At the AMA National Conference on the Disabled Doctor (San Francisco, April 1975), at least 13 states had revised their Medical Practice Acts and at least 10 state medical societies had embarked upon or were contemplating organized programs. By 1977 the laws had been changed in at least 26 states, and there was a similar number of medical society programs in operation or formation.[19]

Pioneering efforts in the development of a "sick doctor statute" came in 1969 in the Florida Legislature which revised grounds for professional discipline under the Medical Practice Act of that state to protect the public further against the imcompetent or unqualified practice of medicine. A similar "sick doctor statute" became law in Texas in 1971. Prior to the passage of legislation in these two states, as is the case in most states still, disciplining a practitioner of the healing arts was predicated on the commission of misconduct on one or more of a variety of specified grounds, provided that fault could be proved against the practitioner. In most states, even though a physician's fitness or ability to practice may be substandard, no violation of Ethical or Medical Practice Act occurred unless the alleged misconduct violated a specific standard of behavior. Such a law leaves a board of medical examiners impotent to protect the public against a physician's incompetence unless the physician has also committed an act predicated on fault. Many state laws have a provision automatically suspending the license of any physician judged mentally incompetent or committed for psychiatric care; but, as is well known, such a last resort legal action rarely occurs in the case of a physician-patient.[7]

The "sick doctor statute" defines the inability of physicians to practice medicine with reasonable skill and safety to their patients, because of one or more illnesses. It eliminates the need to allege or prove the physicians' clinical judgment was actually impaired or that they had actually injured a patient. The defined inability can be the result of organic illnesses, mental or emotional disorders, deterioration through the aging process, or loss of motor skills. Further, the inability can arise from excessive use or abuse of narcotics, drugs, chemicals, alcohol, or similar types of material. The act provides that, prior to board action against physicians, there must be probable cause of their inability to practice medicine with reasonable skill and safety to their patients. The intent of this provision is to protect physicians from harrassment by capricious accusations.[7]

If probable cause is shown, physicians are required to submit to diagnostic mental or physical examinations. Implied consent for such examination under the statute has been given by the physicians' using their licenses to practice or by registering annually. The doctrine of implied consent is further used in the law to remove privileged communications that ordinarily exist between physicians and patients. Physicians so ordered to examination waive their legal privileges, thus making available to administrative trial records the examiner's consultation and diagnostic tests and testimony. Accused physicians have the right to receive copies of the examining physician's reports and diagnoses, and there is provision for taking the deposition of the examiners. Furthermore, their own medical experts may present testimony.[7]

Following the hearings, physicians who are determined by the board to be indeed unable to practice, may have their licenses suspended and be placed on probation. The board may compel physicians to seek therapy from someone designated by the board, or it may restrict their areas of practice to those in which they are still believed to be competent. Suspension of licensure privileges is specified to be only for the duration of the impairment, and the "sick doctors" are guaranteed the opportunity to demonstrate to the board that their licenses should be reinstated when they are competent to practice again.[7]

A further provision, again protecting ill physicians, is the guarantee that neither the records of the proceedings nor any unfavorable order entered against them can be used against them in any other legal proceeding, such as a malpractice action, divorce proceeding, or a suit to challenge their testamentary capacity. During the first year after its enactment in Florida, the statute was frequently used for physicians manifesting incompetency due to excessive use of drugs or alcohol. These are the most common disciplinary problems coming before most medical boards.[7]

A departure from the usual centralized medical board approach is found under the Medical Practice Act of Delaware. About 12 years ago, a Medical Censor Committee was created in each Delaware county, consisting of three members of the county medical society appointed by the medical council or board from a list submitted by the medical society. The powers delegated to the committees included those of subpoena and discipline of the allegedly incompetent physician, subject only to the approval of the medical council. It seems doubtful that this decentralization, though closer to a peer review mechanism, would be entirely desirable, since it places considerable power in the hands of persons who might be inexperienced in such matters, however well they might know the ill physician.[7]

A desirable feature for inclusion in the Medical Practice Act of all states is found in the existing codes of Arizona and Virginia. In both jurisdictions it is mandatory that any licensed physician report to the board of medical examiners any information acquired that tends to show that any physician is unable to practice medicine safely. It also provides for criminal immunity under the law for any physician so reporting in good faith. In the cases of drug-dependent physicians, all state Boards of Medical Examiners would be wise to mandate supervised rehabilitation programs of sufficient duration to give the physician every opportunity to remain drug free. California has pursued such a course and has found the affected physicians fairly cooperative. With a first offense, the board takes away the doctor's narcotic stamp and revokes his or her license, and places a stay of execution on the revocation. The sword of impending revocation is very effective—much more so than the seemingly more charitable approach of issuing warnings or reprimands for first offenders. After a second offense, the violator's license is immediately suspended or revoked. A recent study by the California board showed that rehabilitation was successful in 85 of 100 physicians on probation for the use of narcotics. Of the remainder, ten returned to the use of drugs and five committed suicide.[7]

Several states have established programs for dealing with the impaired physician which are of note. The Medical Society of the State of New York in 1973 developed a plan whereby there would be three approaches to dealing with the impaired physician. The first was noncoercive, involving a lengthy confidential procedure for both reporting and approaching the impaired physician, who had the right to refuse to be treated. This was implemented in 1974. They also recommended a coercive approach in which monitored treatment would be required by the Division of Professional Conduct of the State of New York Department of Education to ensure that the sick physician was, in fact, receiving treatment even if it had been refused on a voluntary basis. In 1975 a law was passed in New York which gave the investigation of professional misconduct and the initial recommendation for appropriate licensure restriction authority to the New York State Health Department. This law broadened the basis of professional misconduct as well as the diversity of options which could be recommended for therapy and punishment. The greatest problem that the Board of Medical Conduct has to deal with is inadequate funds to process the large number of complaints that have come to it. The intent of this board is primarily for rehabilitation rather than punishment of the sick physician. However, there are a number of unresolved legal, ethical, and social legislative issues that have appeared to hamper its work.[27]

An innovative approach from California is that of a "physician's hotline," developed by a recovering alcohol and drug abusing physician and one of his colleagues. When this 24-hour service originated in 1973, it was limited to a few specific counties. It received calls and questions concerning the nature of alcohol and drug abuse, the effects on physicians and their families, and requests for referral for treatment. With its initial success the "hotline" concept spread throughout the State of California. In August 1976, the California Medical Association began a confidential phone service for physicians who were having problems that impaired their ability to practice medicine—alcohol or drug dependence, mental or physical illness. The cost of this service was exceedingly low for the Association. When a physician calls the service, an on-call physician returns the call, providing the kind of input appropriate to the particular problem.[28]

Ohio developed its Physician's Effectiveness Board as part of the Ohio Medical Association in 1975. The program is motivated by humanitarian concerns for the public and the impaired physician. It attempts to recognize that substance abuse and mental illness among physicians is often ignored or untreated and that these, in fact, are treatable conditions for which there is a good rate of success. The program encourages all impaired physicians to seek help and to cooperate in treatment as soon as possible, in order for them to retain or regain full effectiveness in practicing medicine. It also attempts to use constructive coercion, if a physician refuses all offers for assistance, when practical impairment poses a threat to reasonable delivery of medical care. If all efforts fail and the physician's impairment threatens the public or the physician's health, the program becomes more coercive. A District Liaison Physician is the contact person for the troubled physician in need of help. The Ohio law, passed in July 1975, makes the operation of the physicians effectivness program the same as a peer review or professional standards review committee. The law also give the Ohio State Medical Board the power to revoke or suspend a physician's license for an inability to practice according to acceptable standards of care by reason of illness or excessive use of alcohol or controlled substances. Thus the Board, upon showing a possible violation, may compel any individual licensee to submit to an examination and ultimately to treatment.[29]

Georgia was one of the first states to initiate and implement a plan for disabled doctors. During the first year of its operation, the statewide program sponsored by the Medical Association of Georgia was returning more than one physician a month back to practice. The Disabled Doctor's Program utilized four basic components: identification, motivation, treatment, and aid to reentry. The identification phase of the program utilized a vigorous educational effort by the medical society's Physician's Consultant Committee who publicized their efforts through medical journals, numerous talks to local medical societies, and presentations to the medical auxiliaries throughout the state, the hospital administrators, the state pharmacy associations, and the nurses' association. The Physician's Consultant Committee made itself available through a 24-hour telephone hotline which was also widely publicized throughout the state, with two members of the committee on call at any time. Following the identification of a troubled physician, two members of the Physician's Consultant Committee from a different part of the state contact the physician to offer help. The committee is able to take no punitive action and operates according to an advocacy model only. The Consultant's Committee makes as many visits as necessary in an attempt to motivate the physician to enter treatment; most of the physicians contacted have indeed done so. Treatment includes an inpatient phase at a rehabilitation treatment program for one month followed by three months of outpatient and follow-up treatment. After four months, the patient returns to practice and continues in contact with the Disabled Doctor's Program for at least a year. The physician and the Disabled Doctor's Program complete an informal contract which spells out their respective commitments to the other. During the first year of its program, Georgia's medical society was able to return 14 doctors to practice and had another 18 involved in treatment or starting contracts. A total of nine doctors declined contracts. The only time that the Board of Medical Examiners becomes involved is when the Disabled Doctor's Committee believes they have failed in involving the physician in treatment, at which time the executive committee of the medical association would notify the Board of Medical Examiners so that they could monitor the physician's practice and take whatever action they deemed appropriate.[30]

The Michigan Medical and Psychiatric Associations formed a joint committee on the well-being of physicians in 1978 to deal with seriously impaired physicians, troubled but still practicing physicians, and medical students and residents. The seriously impaired physician is usually on the brink of professional ruin and requires a major rehabilitative effort including the following:

1. Crisis teams with psychiatric direction to plan and implement intervention.
2. Financial advice and emergency loans.
3. A *locum tenens* roster (perhaps of recently retired but still effective physicians) to serve as interim replacements for impaired physicians.
4. A national network of residential treatment centers for impaired physicians with free services for those unable to pay.

5. Health insurance adequate to cover both inpatient and outpatient therapy.
6. Emotional support and guidance for the physician's family.

The troubled but still practicing physician requires the following:

1. Improved case finding and highlighting of the availability of voluntary confidential help for the physician and family.
2. Information and assistance to the spouse who may be the key in obtaining diagnosis and treatment for the physician.
3. A roster of physicians in each state who are willing to consult with impaired physicians and their families. (Physicians recovered from such a disability could be uniquely useful in this effort.)
4. Self-awareness experiences and mutual support groups to explore stresses of medical practice on families and to enhance the family's effectiveness as *the* support group.

Medical students and residents should be exposed to these principles throughout their training by having medical schools (1) improve students' stress-handling techniques and increase awareness of the physician's vulnerability to emotional disturbances and available help; (2) provide readily available psychiatric consultation and treatment; and (3) teach doctors to ask for help.[31]

Considering the long-term treatment of the alcoholic physician, Bissell and Mooney have pointed out that success depends on both the physician's acceptance that alcoholism is present and the management of this condition as the primary problem. It is crucial that the physician patient and those involved in the recovery process accept that physical, emotional, social, domestic, financial, and even legal problems are all worsened, if not created by, the primary disease of alcoholism. Too often these consequences of a doctor's well concealed drinking are presented as the reason for the alcoholism. Treating these problems alone rather than the alcoholism itself will offer only a temporary reprieve. Bissell and Mooney believe that if these two conditions are met there are several treatment alternatives.[13] The need for recovery must be recognized as taking precedence over the stress and strain of practice, the demands of a family, and the financial obligations and anxiety of other commitments. They emphasize that joining Alcoholics Anonymous is one of the most direct steps towards achieving sucessful treatment. This neither necessitates hospitalization, relocation, or any physical separation from the usual environment nor incurs any financial obligation. More organized initial treatment experience may be provided by a local alcoholism treatment center. Again, treatment should be sought from those experienced and effective in dealing with this problem rather than from colleagues who may know little or nothing about it. Too often, alcoholic physicians have graduated from medical school where alcoholism was only mentioned in terms of its late physical sequelae; they are lost and bewildered once having developed this illness themselves. If appropriate help is not sought, they may easily fall into the hands of other doctors who are equally unprepared. Inpatient treatment in a specialized setting is particularly indicated under the following conditions:

1. If there is hesitancy in getting involved in AA or a local outpatient treatment center.
2. If a family situation is not conducive to this commitment.
3. If medical practice cannot take a temporary back seat to alcoholism treatment.
4. If outpatient treatment has failed to provide prolonged or relative sobriety.
5. If local treatment facilities are nonexistent.
6. If the patient is pharmacologically addicted.

If inpatient care is in order, a minimum of four weeks is indicated. Mere "drying out" is frequently ineffective. If a physician has been self-prescribing other drugs, no matter how seemingly innocuous, residential treatment is usually necessary.

Bissell and Mooney divide recovery into three periods:[13]

1. First is the pharmacological withdrawal, which may require skilled hospital medical care.
2. Next comes the phase of less acute withdrawal. There is no longer danger of convulsions, delirium tremens, or the like, but sleep patterns are often disturbed. Mood swings and emotional lability are common. Thought processes are superficially intact, but judgment and memory are often unreliable. This phase is best handled in a controlled environment that provides protection against the impulsive return to the use of alcohol or other drugs, distance from the problems of the everyday world, education about the disease of alcoholism, and ego-supportive therapy. This is when the alcoholic physician may be encouraged to be a little selfish and demand the time needed to adjust to a sober living experience and to learn or relearn how to deal with ordinary situations without the use of drugs. The duration of the second phase varies widely, but is usually 1–9 months, and obviously continues beyond the time when the physician is in residential treatment, and may include a return to work and family.

3. The third phase begins when the alcoholic physician is able to handle life effectively enough without chemical support to return to full practice and normal daily routines while continuing the designated treatment plan. Some investment of time and effort on a continuing basis is usually necessary to maintain a comfortable sobriety.

Bissell and Mooney are conservative in their use of psychotropic drugs emphasizing that since alcoholics are used to taking alcohol and other drugs, the use of therapeutic doses of tranquilizers, sedatives, narcotics, or analgesics may well lead them to continue drug use following treatment.[13] The alcoholic tends to seek chemical answers to human problems rather than looking elsewhere. Bissell and Mooney have also said that psychiatric treatment is frequently unnecessary; if it is considered, Bissell (an internist) does not even order an evaluation until the patient has been free of drugs for several weeks and is able to participate in treatment. She believes that alcoholics often use well-intentioned psychiatric help to reinforce the denial of alcoholism, preferring to accept another diagnosis that would allow continued drinking while searching for its cause. Apparently her approach is successful.

Jones, studying physician psychiatric inpatients, found that there was a need for more effective and supportive mechanisms to care for sick hospital staff members. Therefore, his institution developed a Committee on Staff Health—a group of experts who offered confidential nondisciplinary help to staff. Physicians or their families were thus able to consult this group about a staff member's disturbed behavior. The group recommended proper care while safeguarding the potential patient's staff position, thus preventing rejection and humiliation from fellow staff members. Jones recommended that the staff members not be afraid to use peer pressure. On the basis of his studies, peer leverage in the form of discontinuance of admitting and operating privileges, for example, was an effective mechanism for prompting hospital admission for the disturbed physician. He believed that the kindly and compassionate use of this mechanism was much better than legally revoking a license later on.[9]

A critical moment occurs once the medical staff has decided to compel a colleague to obtain treatment. The potential patient is most likely depressed and probably using alcohol and drugs. In addition to having marital and family difficulties and being faced with the loss of income during hospitalization, there is a loss of prestige because of revoked staff privileges. The person may develop suicidal thoughts or make a suicide attempt (which Jones found in 15% of the cases.) Therefore, once the medical staff has decided to recommend hospitalization, it is essential that they exercise maximum care of the patient until he or she is safely in professional hands. Jones also found that direct confrontation of the substance-abusing patient by concerned members of the family and medical staff was appropriate. The family members need to be carefully prepared ahead of time about the method and goals of confrontation. Jones also stressed the necessity of follow-up care to ensure successful treatment.[9]

An interesting aspect of the two-week physician training course developed by the Long Beach Naval Regional Medical Center and described by Dr. Pursch, is that of the first 475 physicians who came to the course, 9% turned themselves in for treatment and stayed for an additional six or seven weeks. Of the first 838 medical department officers, which included physicians, nurses, dentists, physician's assistants, and health care administrators, a total of 202 people identified themselves and are now recovering alcoholics within the Navy Medical Department.[12] This experience underscores the importance of educational efforts for case finding and outreach to impaired physicians and their families. By helping people learn about alcoholism, the Navy has been able to make them become aware of their own need for help.

### Summary

How then, do we deal with the alcoholic or drug-abusing physician or family member? This first step is to help the affected person recognize the fact that the problem exists. Experts seem to agree that some type of benign confrontation is usually necessary, along with educational efforts to help the afflicted individual understand the nature of the problem. The second step is to become an "objective clarifier," to help the person understand the ramifications of the problem, its various causes, and factors that are related. The third step is to assume the role of "consultant stategist," to figure out a game plan to deal with the problem. This includes inpatient treatment, if necessary, outpatient follow-up, attendance in AA or some kind of substance-abuse self-help organization if one is available, and involvement of the family for family therapy and/or support. If the physician-patient is then willing to participate in a treatment program, the chances of success are very great.

## CONCLUDING REMARKS

Two relevant and noteworthy points have been made in the professional literature in recent years. Dan Beauchamp, an epidemiologist at the School of Public Health at the University of North Carolina in Chapel Hill, suggested that the per capita consumption of alcohol is an index of the adequacy of existing public and private controls. These controls or limits, especially when they encourage minimal or infrequent exposure to alcohol, are crucial policy variables. When these limits or controls are weakened, the general level of consumption increases and the rate of exposure to damaging levels of alcohol tends to increase. Thus Beauchamp believes that the availability of unlimited quantities of alcohol is the true cause for alcoholism rather than the individual's inability to control his or her drinking: most individuals who have drinking problems do have an inner capacity to control their drinking; anyone exposed to enough alcohol is likely to develop the problem. Furthermore, he believes that blaming alcoholics is a way of shifting the focus so that political pressures for unlimited alcohol availability in this country can continue to be successful.[32]

In order to reduce the rate of unsafe drinking, then, we must create stricter public and private controls over the availability of alcohol to society at large. These more stringent controls will necessarily impact upon the alcohol industry and ultimately upon all drinkers, and entail lowering the overall general consumption level as a start. One goal that public policy for alcohol might have is zero growth of per capita alcohol consumption. Although we may never eliminate alcohol problems or even reduce them significantly, we can at least try to contain them. Alcohol problems are a predictable consequence of the widespread availability of alcohol in this country. By banishing the "myth of alcoholism" from our midst, says Beauchamp, we may be able to help alcoholics everywhere by sharing with them some of the responsibility for their plight.[32]

In a similar vein, Dr. Marvin Block of the School of Medicine at the State University of New York in Buffalo wrote an article suggesting that large sums of money are being spent to determine why some people become alcoholic and others who consume the identical beverage do not. Further research is being carried out all over the world to find out what physiological and psychological factors if any contribute to the development of alcoholism. It is generally conceded that both the psyche and the soma are involved in the disease process, but no specific cause of the effect has as yet been identified. Hence, this comparatively new research trend seems to him to be destined to cause more damage then it may ever hope to repair. He believes that such studies confuse the issue. They start with the premise that alcohol use cannot be separated from certain ways of life and must, therefore, be looked upon as necessary. It is almost as though we cannot live successfully without the necessity for a drug effect within our lives. Block questions whether our society is so standardized that membership in it must depend on proof of one's ability to accommodate to a known addictive drug. Thus we find, on the one hand, our educational programs focused on teaching our children and young people how to live in a difficult and complex world and how to meet problems in a rational and orderly way. Such teaching helps them to mature. Unfortunately, other forces intrude and interfere with such teaching. Escape from life's problems through the use of various substances is offered as a "less arduous" alternative. Much advertising in this country is devoted to emphasizing the ease with which a person may be relieved of discomfort through drugs or alcohol. According to Block, our youth are learning through television and other media to use drugs and alcohol to avoid problems and skip responsibilites in a wanton search for relief or pleasure. He contends that rather then spending money on research to find out ways of enabling concerned alcoholics to go on drinking, and spending money on advertising to help more people become alcoholics, it would be better to allocate funds for preventive education, teaching our young people how to meet problems of living and enjoy life without resorting to extraneous drugs, the most common of which is alcohol.[33]

His message is clear. We should stop placing alcohol on a pedestal and start thinking about ourselves.

## REFERENCES

1. Summary of the Third Report on Alcohol and Health, NIAAA Information and Feature Service, No. 53, November 30, 1978.
2. Bissell L, Jones R: The alcoholic physician: A survey, Am J Psychiatry 1976, 133(10): 1142–1146.
3. Lee FI: Cirrhosis and hepapoma in alcoholics, Gut 1966, 7:77–85.
4. Small IF: The fate of the mentally ill physician, Am J Psychiatry 1969, 125:1333–1342.
5. Chafetze M (ed): Alcoholism and health professionals, Psychiatr Ann 1976, 6 (3): 47–55.
6. Modlin HC, Montes A: Narcotics addiction and physicians, Am J Psychiatry 1964, 121:358–363.
7. Council of Mental Health of the AMA: The sick physician, J Am Med Assoc 1973, 223 (6): 684–687.
8. Vaillant GE, Brighton JR, McArthur C: Physicians use of mood altering drugs, N Engl J Med 1970, 282:365–370.
9. Jones R: A study of one hundred physician psychiatric inpatients, Am J Psychiatry 1977, 134(10): 1119–1123.
10. Welner A, et al.: Psychiatric disorders among professional women, Arch Gen Psychiatry 1976, 36: 169–173.
11. Levine D, et al.: The historical approach to understanding drug abuse among nurses, Am J Psychiatry 1974, 131(9): 1036–1037.
12. Pursch J: Physicians' attitudinal changes in alcoholism, Alcoholism Clin Exp Res 1978, 294: 358–361.

13. Bissell L, Mooney A: The special problem of the alcoholic physician, Md State Med J 1976, 25(3):79–80.
14. Little R: Hazards of drug dependency among physicians, J Am Med Assoc 1971, 218: 1533–1535.
15. Goby M, et al.: Physicians treated for alcoholism: A followup study, Alcoholism Clin Exp Res 1979, 3(2): 121–124.
16. Rado S: Narcotic bondage, Am J Psychiatry 1957, 114:165–170.
17. Cohen S (ed): Teenage drinking: Bottle babies, Drug Abuse Alcoholism Newsl 1975, 4(7): 1–4.
18. Pierson N, Little R: The addictive process and unusual addictions: A further elaboration of etiology, Am J Psychiatry 1969, 125(9): 1166–1171.
19. Steindler E: Help for the alcoholic physician: A seminar, Alcoholism Clin Exp Res 1977, 1(2): 129–130.
20. Alcohol–drug interactions, FDA Drug Bull 1979, 9(2).
21. Rich C, Farris P: Suicide by male physicians during a five year period, Am J Psychiatry 1979, 136(8): 1089–1091.
21*a*. Blachly PH, Disher W, Rodner G: Suicide by physicians, Bulletin of Suicidiology, Dec 1968, pp 1–18.
22. Mounting encounter attack against child alcoholism, US News World Rep 1977, July 11: 33–34.
23. Young people and alcohol, Alcohol Health Res World 1975, Summer: 2–10.
24. Faigel H: Where have all the junkies gone?, Clin Pediatr 1975, 14: 703–705.
25. Drinking and pregnancy: The government is concerned, Med World News 1977, April 18: 25–26.
26. Physicians Committee Special Report, New York State J Med 1975, 75(2): 420–423.
27. Gitlow S: Disabled physician—his care in New York State, Alcoholism Clin Exp Res 1977 1(2): 133–134.
28. Newsom J: Help for the alcoholic physician in California, Alcoholism Clin Exp Res 1977 1(2): 135–137.
29. Clinger R: Help for the alcoholic physician in Ohio, Alcoholism Clin Exp Res 1977 1(2): 139–141.
30. Talbott G: Disabled doctors program in Georgia, Alcoholism Clin Exp Res 1977 1(2): 133–145.
31. Sargent D: Treating the impaired physician, Am J Psychiatry 1978, 135(12): 1573–1574.
32. Beauchamp D: The alcohol alibi: blaming alcoholics, Society 19xx, xx:xx–xx.
33. Block M: Don't place alcohol on a pedestal, J Am Med Assoc 1976, 275(19): 2103–2104.

# part three

# The Minority Physician

# The Woman Physician

Until 12 years ago, more than 90% of American physicians were men. With such a preponderance of males in medicine one might have been forgiven for thinking that the initials MD stood for male doctor. However, times have changed and females now comprise close to a quarter of all the physicians in the country.

The title "Doctor of Medicine" first came into use about 1000 years ago at the famous medical school of Salerno, Italy. There, on the Gulf of Salerno in a town about 30 miles south of Naples, eminent physicians began to substitute scientific medicine for more traditional healing. They replaced Pater Nosters and votive offerings, the standard medical practices of the day, with pulse evaluation, bloodletting, and purging. Most of the doctors who led this transformation from mystical to more scientific medicine at Salerno were referred to as "brillant men"; but several women were among them. Four of these "Ladies of Salerno" were named Trotula, Abella, Rebecca, and Constanza.

Not much is known about Abella and Rebecca, but Trotula authored a watershed textbook on obstetrics. Constanza suffered from the same problem that besets some of her modern-day medical sisters; she was renowned more as a "stunning beauty" than a great healer.

In this chapter, Dr. Carol Nadelson provides incisive observations into the role of women in medicine from earliest history to the present.

*J.P.C.*

# 13

# The Woman Physician: Past, Present and Future

*Carol Nadelson*

## EARLY HISTORY OF WOMEN IN MEDICAL CARE

Women have historically been the pharmacists, nurses, abortionists, counselors, midwives, and "wise women," as well as witches. There have *also* been women physicians, although they were rarely permitted to perform in the same capacities and positions as men.

As early as 1500 B.C., women studied medicine in Egypt. In fact, Moses and his wife Zeporah were students at Heliopolis. In 1000 B.C. women physicians in China had medical roles which encompassed activities other than traditional midwife and herb-gathering ones. Medical roles were also reported for women in Greek and Roman civilizations.

Throughout history, women have functioned as special attendants for women, assisting with labor and delivery, advising women on the functions and disorders of their bodies, and tending newborns. This involvement, however, was not considered to be part of the discipline of medicine, since childbirth and symptoms related to it were considered physiological or normal processes, and not related to illness or dysfunction.

Formal medical learning was first consolidated and established with the founding of a medical school at Salerno, in Italy, in the ninth century A.D.. Prior to this medical training existed as an informal apprentice system. By the 10th and 11th centuries, women apparently studied at Salerno. Although several names are mentioned in early histories little is known about most of these women. Records in the eleventh century, however, do reveal the existence of a woman "physician," Trotula who made important contributions. She wrote texts on obstetrics and gynecology, and also headed a department of diseases of women.

Trotula, and other women "physicians," were not M.D.s since the degree itself was first awarded in the 12th century. It was, however, awarded only to men at that time. A special diploma was offered to women until 1430, when Constanza Calenda became the first woman to obtain the degree of Doctor of Medicine.[1]

In the late medieval period, women of wealth practiced a kind of medical care, particularly in Italy where the universities were not closed to them. They were also permitted to practice in France, England, and Germany if they qualified. The role they had generally included bleeding, administration of herbs and medicines, reducing fractions, and midwifery.

By the end of the 15th century, as medicine became established academically in various centers in Europe, the movement to exclude women from formal involvement in medical care gained momentum and women were specifically limited to functioning as midwives. This reflected a wider societal trend and occurred in the context of the ideology of misogyny as encapsulated in the *Malleus Maleficarum* (1486 A.D.). Witch hunting at this time was active and focused the restlessness and discontent of the population. It capitalized on the "spiritual and mental" inferiority of women. Even when active witch hunts subsided, however, their aftermath placed women in a seriously compromised position and eliminated them from roles in medical care other than traditional caretaking ones or those that involved the care of women and their reproductive functions.

## WOMEN IN U.S. MEDICINE IN THE 18TH AND 19TH CENTURIES

In colonial America, the healing role of women was critical to survival. At this time, there were relatively few university-trained physicians since the first American medical school was not founded until 1765 (the University of Pennsylvania—and it excluded women). Prior to that time medicine was practiced by those who appeared to be particularly talented, and they were trained in an apprentice system.

In the 19th century, since women were barred from "regular" medical training, many were often trained in the homeopathic or eclectic traditions and set up flourishing practices without diplomas. In 1847, Elizabeth Blackwell (1821–1910) became the first woman to be admitted to a "regular" medical school in the United States. She was awarded a degree from the Geneva Medical School. The New York State Medical Association promptly censured the school, and when her sister, Emily, applied a few years later she was rejected. Emily subsequently received her M.D. from Western Reserve.

In 1850, Harriet K. Hunt (1805–1875), who had established herself in an "irregular" practice in Boston in 1835, applied for admission to Harvard Medical School. She was admitted, as were several black men, however she was denied her seat when the all-male class threatened to leave if women and blacks were admitted. It was not until almost 100 years later, 1946, that Harvard Medical School began to admit women.[2]

We cannot be surprised about this resistance to women in medicine if we consider the prevailing views about them. An 1848 textbook on obstetrics said, "She (woman) has a head almost too small for the intellect but just big enough for love."[3] In 1905, F.W. Van Dyke, President of the Oregon State Medical Society, noted that "hard study killed sexual desire in women, took away their beauty, brought on hysteria, neuroasthenia, dyspepsia, astigmatism, and dysmenorrhea." "Educated women," he added, "could not bear children with ease because study arrested the development of the pelvis at the same time it increased the size of the child's brain and therefore its head. This caused extensive suffering in childbirth."[4]

By 1850, three all-female "irregular" medical colleges were founded in the United States: one in Boston (now Boston University), one in Philadelphia (now Medical College of Pennsylvania), and one in Cincinnati. The Boston Female Medical College was originally designed primarily to prevent male midwifery.

The road continued to be difficult even for those women who managed to obtain training both in the United States and in Europe. Medical societies refused admission to women and hospitals denied them appointments. In general, however, those women who graduated were from middle- or upper-class backgrounds and often had fathers or husbands in medicine. They entered to join their families in practice. The patients of the first generation of women physicians were largely poor women or children.

The effect of exclusion by medical societies and hospitals was to spur many female physicians to open their own hospitals and clinics. In 1857, Drs. Elizabeth and Emily Blackwell founded the New York Infirmary and College for Women, where they cared largely for indigent women.

Between 1880 and 1900, however, 18% of physicians in Boston were women; by 1900 over 50% of the class at Boston University and over 40% at Tufts were women. Despite these numbers, the role of women in medicine continued to be hotly debated. The productivity and lifestyle of female physicians were questioned then as now. In 1881, Rachel Bodley, Dean of the Women's Medical College of Pennsylvania, surveyed the 224 living graduates of the school and found that the overwhelming majority were in active practice. In fact, those who had married reported that their profession had no adverse effect on their marriages, nor had marriage interfered with work.

## WOMEN IN 20TH CENTURY MEDICINE

After the Flexner Report of 1910, medicine became an established discipline with high standards for training and practice, and a number of medical schools were closed. Among these were those that admitted women. The number of women entering medicine thus began to decrease. Some schools, however, were persuaded to admit women by other means. Johns Hopkins, for example, received a sizable endowment from women provided that women be admitted on the same terms as men. Despite this history, however, Johns Hopkins has never had a female department head.[5]

Flexner presented an interesting view of women in medicine, stating that "medical education is now, in the United States and Canada, open to women upon practically the same terms as men. If all institutions do not receive women, so many do, that no woman desiring an education in medicine is under any disability in finding the school to which she may gain admittance." He went on to state, "now that women are freely admitted to the medical profession, it is clear that they show a decreasing inclination to enter it."[6]

Indeed, the number of women physicians remained relatively stable and then slowly decreased, so that while women comprised 6% of physicians in 1910 and 5% in 1920, they comprised only 4% in 1930, the lowest point. The percentage climbed to 6% again in 1950. The reasons for this persistent low figure in the United States, compared with European countries where the percentage increased, cannot be as clearly understood as related to motivation alone. This is suggested by the fact that between 1970 and 1975, when overt efforts were made to attract and admit women, the number of women entering medical school more than doubled.[7,8] In fact, within a decade women made up over 30% of the freshmen class.[9]

Medicine has been a paradoxical profession for women in the United States. The caretaking functions do not inherently contradict "traditional" views of women and female roles, but the technological and instrumental aspects do, as does the status of the physician. Thus, while 70% of health workers in the United States are women as are 98% of nurses, the number of physicians has remained low. The shift began with affirmative action programs as feminism reemerged. Thus broader societal changes have had an important influence.

This view is corroborated by increases in other career choices for women. As these changes have been occurring in medicine, higher female enrollments have also been reported for other traditionally male dominated professions such as architecture, engineering, the sciences and law. Despite this increased female participation there is a wide gap between the proportions of men and women in professional training to those who have attained positions of prominence and responsibility in their fields.[10–12]

From one perspective this is to be expected since those women entering have not yet attained positions of prominence. Lest we become too sanguine, the lessons of history must be understood. When women have had a significant influence on the health fields, external factors have often been influential, including wars, physician shortages, or major cultural reorganization. Attitudinal changes were often related to expedience or pragmatism.

In the Soviet Union, when midwives proved themselves to be effective as doctors in the Russo-Turkish War of 1870, the influx of women into medical schools began. But, after the 1917 revolution, when the prestige of medicine was reduced, women were admitted to medical school in even greater numbers. Recently, however, as medicine has attained a slightly more prestigious position in the USSR, the number of women physicians has fallen sharply. Moreover, the number of women physicians in the Academy of Medicine has always been exceedingly small (<10%). The *feldscher,* the medical intermediary akin to a nurse practitioner, has emerged to perform more routine work. Almost all feldschers are women, as are the "barefoot" doctors in China.

## DOES THE EXPERIENCE OF MEN AND WOMEN IN MEDICINE DIFFER?

Evidence collected before the current increase in numbers of women in medicine suggests that women have a different and probably more stressful psychological experience than men. Phelps, in 1968, reported that dropout rates from medical school for male and female students for academic reasons were similar.[13] However, of those leaving for nonacademic reasons (usually personal), 8% were women and 3% were men. This gap is closing, and the difference in attrition between male and female medical students is less than 1%.[14] Attrition rate, however, is only one indicator of stress and does not describe the entire experience.

Although there has been a belief that women do not perform as well as men in medical school, there is no definitive confirmation of that view. Rooney and Weinberg did find that, in their first years, the women in their sample did less well than the men.[15] They cited "problems in adjustment" as the reason. Clearly what constitutes or determines these "problems" is an important variable and must be understood. Further, differences seem to be eliminated by the clinical years in medical school.

Adsett reported that a greater percentage of women medical students than men sought psychiatric counseling.[16] He commented, however, that it was not clear whether this is related to a greater ability for women to ask for help, or to the role conflicts or environmental pressures which he indicated were greater for women. We do know that women in the United States generally use psychiatric facilities more than men, and the same questions have been raised about this difference.[17] It is even possible to speculate, however, that asking for help appropriately may be preventive and an indication of strength and good judgment rather than a measure of extreme difficulty. This is reinforced by looking at the numbers of male physicians, who may be reflecting the stress they experience, involved in substance abuse problems.

Evidence for the particularly stressful experience of women physicians is supported by the data of Steppacher and Mausner who reported that, while the suicide rate for male physicians was 1.15 times that of the overall male population, the female physician rate was three times that expected for women.[16,18] Furthermore, of the group of women who killed themselves, 40% were under age 40, while less than 20% of the males who committed suicide were under age 40. More suicides occurred among women than among men during the training period and a substantial proportion of these women were single. Although it has been noted that access to the means to suicide may be an important factor explaining the lack of sex difference for physicians, it does not explain the age difference.

Another indicator which contributes to the view that there are greater stresses for women in medicine can be seen in the differential divorce rates for male and female physicians. While the divorce rate for male professionals, including physicians, is lower that that for the general population, the divorce rate for female physicians is higher than for both male physicians and the general population.[19] In dual-career couples in other occupations as well, the rate is higher than that for "traditional" couples. Since 80% of female physicians marry either physicians or other professionals, their marriages do appear to be vulnerable; but this does not suggest that medicine is specifically a more problematic field than any other.[20]

On the other hand, women physicians who do not marry professionals are also likely to experience marital stress. Often their growth in status relative to their husband's strains the relationship. Discrepancies in interests and lifestyle and the husband's expectations of the role of a wife may come into conflict with the wife's aspirations, needs or capacities.[21]

Data on mental illness, divorce and suicide are dramatic but they do not deal with the pain and distress which is reported clinically; nor do they speak to the problems and frustrations of individuals. These do not necessarily produce frank symptoms, or overt failure of performance, but they may reduce satisfaction, ambition, and success.

While the amount and character of academic work is the same for men and women; other aspects of the medical school experience are not necessarily similar and may speak to the sex differences reported. The social environment is often perceived differently by male and female students. For example, students learn how to function, in part, by identifying with people who act as role models, particularly those who are seen as successful.[22] These include teachers, peers, and others who care for patients.[21,23–27] Since most medical school faculty members are still predominantly men, the male student can identify with other physicians and maintain consistency with his own masculine identification. This is not possible for the female student. She may have difficulty finding a female physician who can be a role model, since there may not have been any in her past experience, nor are they currently readily available in medical school.[11,27–33]

## CURRENT STATUS OF WOMEN IN MEDICINE

The number of women on faculty remains low, particularly in the highest ranks. Women in academic medical positions are more likely to be part-time and to have less prestigious assignments. They are also underrepresented in administrative and leadership positions. Until 1982 there were no female deans and there are still no vice presidents for medical affairs, and few women serve on specialty boards or chair departments. While in the late 1970s 15.8% of medical school faculties were female physicians, women comprised 3.5% of professors, 5.2% of associate professors and 7.8% of assistant professors.

Although the numbers of women in medicine nearly tripled between 1968 and 1978, there was a gain of only 1.9 percentage points in the size of the female faculty. Further the distribution of female faculty members among the various departments remained relatively stable. The largest number of female faculty members continued to be in psychiatry and pediatrics and the fewest were in orthopedics.[34]

More recently there has been some upward movement in the academic ranks of women and, among the newly hired there was also a slight increase in the numbers of women. The 1980 faculty data reveals that, although women constituted only 5.7% of the 1960 graduating class, 14% of those women and 9.6% of the men had faculty professional positions. Thus, there are indications that women will be more prominent in academia in the future.[34]

With regard to department chairs, there are also some, but few, changes. In 1978, 33 women chaired academic departments out of approximately 2,400 positions. In 1980, 56 chairs were occupied by women. Women, however, continue to occupy 2% of the total number of chairs. In pediatrics more women hold chairs than in any other department—7%—although 27% of the pediatric faculty are women. Other departments with substantial numbers of women faculty but few chairs include anatomy, microbiology, physical medicine, anesthesia, and psychiatry.[34]

Farrell, et al. pointed out that the professorial title with the highest percentage of women was professor emeritus.[35] In 1965–1966 women were best represented in the oldest age group of medical faculty since they may have entered during an earlier "golden age," at the turn of the century when, as we have seen, a larger number of outstanding women were swept into medicine by the tide of the first feminist movement. Thus, the dramatic change which occurred after the Flexner report, is perhaps a lesson well worth learning.

Although there are no hard data to indicate that women on medical school faculties are not competing with their male colleagues in terms of sustained scholarly productivity, some evidence does support this view: female scientists publish fewer papers than their male colleagues.[34]

Women have also not involved themselves actively in formal medical oranizations; when they do they are rarely leaders. In 1979 the percentage of women physicians in the AMA was 18%.[36]

Within fields of specialization there are also differences with regard to board certification. In 1978 only 38.4% of all female physicians who finished residencies held specialty board certificates compared to 57% of male physicians.[37] Furthermore, of the 364 officers and directors of the medical organizations of the American Board of Medical Specialties only 3%, or 11, are women.[34]

The explanation for these data on productivity and involvement has generally focused on the conflicting demands of family and career. These conflicts lead women to choose less intensely involving, more flexible pursuits and to compromise their plans for specialty certification and career development. Women often choose fields or pursue paths for pragmatic reasons rather than because of true interest or talent.

There are other differences in the experience of men and women which may contribute to data on performance, success and involvement. Women trainees continue to report that they feel excluded, isolated, or not regarded as seriously, particularly when there are special rewards, like fellowships.[27,38–41] While the changing peer culture promises to alter this picture, we must be cautious. Those women who are training and practicing continue to describe an absence of peer support and negative attitudes towards female physicians, especially in leadership positions. Furthermore the subtle effects of institutional practices which were set up without women in mind, particularly those that do not account for the timing of training with regard to childbearing, are important factors.

Unless there are very real changes in the organization of medicine or in family styles, expectations, and practices, there will continue to be active participation in leadership positions only by "superwomen" and by women of exceptional energy, commitment or talent. The large number of women physicians who are competent, dedicated and creative will not be able to make the kinds of contributions promised by their capabilities.

In the past, female physicians who have had demanding career aspirations have chosen not to marry or to have children, or they have limited their professional commitments.[13,33,40–45] Since current pressures are for women to pursue their careers and also to have children, male as well as female roles and expectations must change, both philosophically and pragmatically, for women to be able to do this. In a dual-career family, a structure which fits most women in medicine, traditional models of family interaction often change to some extent; but regardless of career demands, women do more often limit their aspirations to enable their spouses' to be fulfilled. This has important implications for women physicians. Several studies have indicated that among the factors correlating with professional performance in women, the number of children was inversely related to medical activity.[17,32,46]

Role proliferation and consequent role strain have also been described in high career women.[47] This phenomenon has been repeatedly reported in women physicians as well. Heins et al. have found that, despite the fact that the women physicians in their sample spent 90% as much time as men in medical work, they tended to assume full reponsibility for home and family.[48]

Women physicians marry in the same proportion as women in general, but tend to marry later in life and to have fewer children. Over one-half are married to physicians. They clearly report problems in integrating career and marriage and perceive family commitments as interfering with their optimal functioning, whereas men rarely do.[31,38,39,49] Despite this, however, few women physicians report more than a one-year interruption in training or practice. While it is possible to conclude that there is no evidence that the stress is excessive since they do perform, as indicated there is evidence of lower female achievement in medicine.[32]

A recent survey of current activities and concerns of Harvard Medical School graduates revealed that a larger number of women were working part-time, or in positions they viewed as compromised, based on family considerations.[50] It is interesting that 45% of the men when answering a question about arrangements for the care of children simply stated "wife" and another 10% reported that their wives "had help." Obviously this solution is not an available alternative for women physicians, and it implies a clear belief about who has primary responsibility. When asked about conflicts related to marital or family situation, women overwhelmingly reported their problems related to time pressures and desires to be with children, obtaining suitable jobs for both partners, and other dual-career issues.

Although these data derive from one alumni group of physicians, it is important to note that this group was chosen for high achievement, leadership and motivation, with a good history of adapting to challenges. There may be greater difficulties predicted for those who are less highly competitive and achieving.

## WHAT ABOUT THE FUTURE?

As the current cohort of medical students from the 1970s mature into practicing physicians and potential faculty members, it is not clear what male/female differences will emerge. A study by Harris and Conley-Muth (1981) noted that although the practice preferences of women and men differed somewhat, with men preferring group, individual, and academic practice and women preferring salaried work in a hospital, clinic, government, or industry, there were no significant differences between males and females in the number of hours they expected to work or the mean annual salary they expected to earn in five years.[51]

Despite expectations, however, it is important to consider the reality of current practice patterns and their future implications. Women currently tend to be in salaried positions, working regular hours, fewer in number than their male colleagues, and earning less than what men in medicine earn. Only about 2% of women M.D.s never work in medicine.[52]

In 1976, 43% of women and 64% of men were in office-based practice and 46% of women and 28% of men were in hospital-based practice. Also in this year, the specialties of pediatrics, anesthesia, pathology, and psychiatry had the highest proportion of women physicians, 23%, 14%, 14% and 15%, respectively.

Further, the popular specialties for women had the lowest income. In 1972 the net income for medical practice for men was almost $48,000 and for women it was almost $28,000. The differences are related to differences in hours worked and specialties. Data from 1977 indicate that female physicians continue to earn about 40% less than male physicians. When adjusted for differences in hours practiced per year the net income of women physicians per hour of practice is four-fifths that of men. About one-third of women physicians have fixed salary, fixed hour appointments compared to 15% of men. Lack of board certification may play some role in the salary differential.

The average time spent in practice by women is 32.6 years and for men 35.8 years. If this calculation is extended over a life span it suggests that women spend 40% less time in active practice over their careers than do men. This, however, must be measured against other data which suggest that women work nearly 90% as much as men.

If we assume the same number of years of practice for women and men and apply 1977 data to hours practiced per year, women physicians would spend only about 25% less time than do men in active practice over their careers. The AMA data suggests that the number of hours practiced per year for a woman is about four-fifths of that for a man. The implications of this for predicting the number of physicians needed in the future must be taken into account. Of course, if men take more active family roles and balance career and family as women now do, they will practice less as women practice more. Thus, the total number of physician-hours and years are potentially the same.

The Association of American Medical Colleges' 1981 data from 10,000 medical students reporting all areas of specialty interest indicate that there is very little difference between males and females in career choice decisions based on medical school faculty, positive clinical experience, negative clinical experience, type of practice or schedule, financial advantages, and the needs of society.[53] There were some differences in weighing of influences. For example, women more often marked financial advantages as having no influence and positive clinical experience as having more influence than did men. The differences, however, were very small, and the current economic situation may well change this picture. Women have characteristically entered pediatrics, internal medicine, psychiatry, and family practice. Very few have entered the so-called surgical specialties including obstetrics and gynecology. Although this appears to be changing, it is not yet clear exactly how much will change. Internal medicine and obstetrics and gynecology have increasing numbers of women entering these specialties, and even the surgical fields show some increase. Pediatrics and psychiatry continue to show increases in the numbers of women entering residency.

Of the residency positions filled during the academic year 1979–1980, women held 23.1% of residency positions, but they filled only 8.3% of the surgery training positions. The number of women residents in general surgery has remained at 5% since 1977 despite the total number of women in graduate medical education increasing from 15% in 1977 to 24% in 1979. In 1977, more than one-half of practicing women physicians clustered in pediatrics, psychiatry, or family practice–general practice. Men most frequently specialized in surgery, internal medicine and family-general practice.[37]

The implications of these data are interesting since these are the lowest income specialties in medicine. Further, it has been suggested that as the numbers of women in a field increase, the prestige of the field decreases.

The impact of women has also been interesting in terms of patient care. The presence of women physicians in primary care facilities has an important effect on women's health care. In the National Medical Ambulatory Care (NMAC) Survey of 1977, 71.5% of the patients of women general practitioners and internists were women as compared to 60% women in the practices of men physicians in these specialties. Moreover, female general practitioners and internists also average about 21% black and other minority patients in their practice as compared to male physicians who see about 9% black and minority patients.[54] These data probably reflect the location of women physicians in many organized facilities in underserved areas.[55]

Further, changes in the political and economic arenas affect women physicians in major ways. Women are the highest users of health care services in all settings and all specialties, thus the adequacy of reimbursement affects them and their physicians.[56] As women have increasingly entered the work force, they have been eligible for better health benefits as workers, but because they still predominate in low paying, low status jobs, these benefits are lower than for men. Moreover, since women over 70 outnumber men of that age by more than two-to-one and most of these women are living on subsistance incomes with no Social Security benefits or pensions, any change in functions or reimbursement will disproportionately affect them and the physicians who care for them.[57]

The reimbursement system affects women physicians in another way. All third-party reimbursement is higher for subspecialties than for general care. Sixty-one percent of women physicians are in the primary care specialties.[54] Organized settings for primary care, especially in underserved areas will be very hard hit by funding cutbacks and women physicians will be at high risk for losing their jobs. The practice style of women physicians also puts them at a disadvantage in the current financing system. Higher reimbursement rates are available for procedures than for personal care. The National Medical Ambulatory Care Survey indicated that women physicians are slightly less likely to order lab tests and diagnostic procedures than their male counterparts.[54] Furthermore, women M.D.s working the same number of hours per week as men tend to see fewer patients and spend longer time with their patients, especially their female patients, which is less financially rewarding.[54] Finally, there is little or no reimbursement for health maintenance and prevention which places the pediatricians and public health M.D.s (over 20% of whom are women) at a disadvantage.

Another important area for consideration is research. The involvement of women scientists in research and peer review of research efforts is increasing, but is still small. As research investigators from the NIH women have been awarded an increasing proportion of research grants, from 7% in 1974 to 9% in 1978. For a special group of research grants for new investigators the proportion awarded to women increased from 5% in 1974 to almost 15% in 1978. With regard to research proposals women have fared as well as men for approval and the amounts of money have been the same. Fellowship awards for women accounted for one-fourth of the total in 1978. With regard to career research awards, those provided in recognition of research and teaching careers, the number of women receiving such awards increased dramatically from 66 in 1974 to 147 in 1978, 12% of all awardees. The changes, however, have been for women with Ph.D.s.[12]

With regard to the membership of NIH grant contract review committees, women represented 17% of the professional consultants in 1978 and 15% five years earlier. For all NIH advisory councils' review committees and other boards, women comprised almost 18% of all professionals in 1978 which represented a 37% increase over this same committee in 1973.[12]

## CONCLUSION

Where then does this take us? If we return to our history we must view the changes of the past decade with cautious optimism. We have trodden the path before, but we have turned around or we have been driven off of it. Unless there are major changes in the attitudes, expectations, and experiences of those entering medicine we are in danger of repeating our history. Current realities fly in the face of deep societal changes. Only the forward movement of women as active participants, in their fields, as collaborators and colleagues, will enable them to contribute to their full potential, and will allow society to enjoy the benefits of their activity. While men and women may or may not have similar or different innate or intrinsic personality traits, and we are far from conclusive definition of what these are, or what their limits and scope are; we have not yet begun to encompass human potential in its full range and possibility.

## REFERENCES

1. Corner GW: The rise of medicine at Salerno in the twelfth century. *In:* Lectures on the history of medicine: a series of lectures at the Mayo Foundation and the Universities of Minnesota, Wisconsin, Iowa, Northwestern, and the Des Moines Academy of Medicine, 1926–1932. Philadelphia: W.B. Saunders Co., 1937, pp 371–399.
2. Nadelson C, Notman M: Women and biomedicine: women as health care professionals. *In:* Reich W, ed. Encyclopedia of bioethics. Vol. 4. New York: Macmillan, 1978, pp 1713–1720.
3. Shryock RH: Medicine in America: historical essays. Baltimore: Johns Hopkins University Press, 1966, p 184.
4. Bullough V, Voght M: Women, menstruation and nineteenth-century medicine. Bull Hist Med 1973, 47:66–82.
5. Turner T: Women in medicine: an historical perspective. J Am Med Wom Assoc 1981, 36(2):33,34,37.
6. Flexner A: Medical education in the United States and Canada: a report to the Carnegie Foundation for the Advancement of Teaching. New York: The Carnegie Foundation, 1910.
7. Dube WF: Medical student enrollment 1972–1973 through 1976–1977. J Med Educ 1977, 52:164–166.
8. Dube WF: Women students in U.S. medical schools: past and present trends. J Med Educ 1973, 48:186–189.
9. Turner K: Memorandum #81–7 to the Women's Liaison Officers of the Association of American Medical Colleges. Washington, D.C., December 14, 1981. (unpublished)
10. Suter LE, Miller HP: Income differences between men and career women. *In:* Huber J, ed. Changing women in a changing society. Chicago: University of Chicago Press, 1973.
11. Epstein C: Encountering the male establishment: sex-status limits on women's careers in the professions. Am J Sociol 1975, 15:6–9.
12. Kilson M: The status of women in higher education. Journal of Women in Culture and Society 1976, 1:935–942.
13. Phelps C: Women in American medicine. J Med Educ 1968, 43:916–924.
14. Crowley AE, ed: Medical education in the U.S. JAMA 1975; 234:1338.
15. Weinberg E, Rooney J: The academic performance of women students in medical school. J Med Educ 1973, 48:240–247.
16. Adsett C: Psychological health of medical students in relation to the medical education process. J Med Educ 1968, 43:728–734.
17. Gove W, Tudor J: Adult sex roles and mental illness. Am J Sociol 1973, 78:812–835.
18. Steppacher RC, Mausner JS: Suicide in male and female physicians. JAMA 1974, 228(3):323–328.
19. Rosow I, Rose KD: Divorce among doctors. Journal of Marriage and the Family 1972, 34:587–598.
20. Berman EM, Sacks S, Lief HI: The two-professional marriage—a new conflict syndrome. J Sex Marital Ther 1975, 1(3):242–253.

21. Lief H: Doctors and marriage: the special pressures. Medical World News 1977, 18(3):38–50.
22. Lucas CJ, Kelvin RP, Ojha AB: The Psychological health of the pre-clinical medical student. Br J Psychiatry 1965, 3:473–478.
23. Kimball P: Medical education as a humanizing process. J Med Educ 1973, 48:71–77.
24. McGuire FL: Psycho-social studies of medical students: a critical review. J Med Educ 1961, 41(5):424–445.
25. Miller GE: Teaching and learning in medical school. Cambridge, MA: Harvard University Press, 1961.
26. Mudd JW, Siegel R: Sexuality—the experience and anxieties of medical students. N Engl J Med 1967, 281:1397–1404.
27. Notman M, Nadelson C: Medicine: a career conflict for women. Am J Psychiatry 1973, 130(10):1123–1127.
28. Bowers J: Special problems of female medical students. J Med Educ 1968, 43:532–537.
29. Campbell M: Why would a girl go into medicine? New York: The Feminist Press, 1973.
30. Hilberman E, Konanc J, Perez-Reyes M, Hunter R, Scagnelli J, Sanders S: Support groups for women in medical school: a first year program. J Med Educ 1975, 50:867–875.
31. Roeske N: The quest for role models by women medical students. J Med Educ 1977, 52:459–466.
32. Westling-Wilkstrand H, Monk M, Thomas CB: Some characteristics related to the career status of women physicians. Johns Hopkins Med J 1970, 127:273–286.
33. Williams P: Women in medicine: some themes and variations. J Med Educ 1971, 46:584–591.
34. Braslow JB, Heins M: Women in medical education: a decade of change. N Engl J Med 1981, 304(19):1129–1135.
35. Farrell K, Witte M, Holguin M, Lopez S: Women physicians in medical academia: a national statistical survey. JAMA 1979, 241(26):2808–2812.
36. American Medical Association, Council on Long-range Planning and Development. Women Physicians in Organized Medicine. 1979, 43:729–731.
37. Rinke C: The economic and academic status of women physicians. JAMA 1981, 245(22):2305–2306.
38. Edwards M, Zimet C: Problems and concerns among medical students, 1975. J Med Educ 1976, 51:619–625.
39. Lopate C: Women in medicine. Baltimore: Johns Hopkins Press, 1968, pp 27–35.
40. Matthew E: Attitude toward career and marriage, and development of life style. Journal of Counseling and Psychiatry. 1969, 11:375–384.
41. Matthew MPH: Training and practice of women physicians. J Med Educ 1970, 45:1016–1024.
42. Cosa J, Coker RE Jr: The female physician in public health conflict and reconciliation of the sex and professional roles. Sociology and Social Research. 1965, 49:294–305.

43. Rosenlund M, Oski F: Women in medicine. Ann Intern Med 1967, 66:1008–1012.
44. Shapiro CS, Stibler B-J, Zelkovic AA, Mausner JS: Careers of women physicians: a survey of women graduates from seven medical schools, 1945–1951. J Med Educ 1968, 43:1033–1040.
45. Cohen ED, Korper SP: Women in medicine: exigencies in training career. Conn Med 1976, 40:103–110.
46. Thomas CB: What becomes of medical students: the dark side. Johns Hopkins Med J 1976, 138:185–195.
47. Johnson CL, Johnson FA: Attitudes toward parenting in dual-career families. Am J Psychiatry 1977, 134(4):391–395.
48. Heins M, Smock M, Martindale L, Stein B, Jacobs J: A profile of the woman physician. JAMA 1977, 32(11):421–427.
49. Scher M, Benedek E, Candy A: Psychiatrist-wife-mother: some aspects of role integration. Presentation at the Annual Meeting of the American Psychiatric Association. Honolulu, Hawaii, May 1973. (unpublished)
50. Nadelson C, Notman M, Lowenstein P: The practice patterns, life styles, and stresses of women and men entering medicine: a follow-up study of Harvard Medical School graduates from 1967 to 1977. J Am Med Wom Assoc 1979, 34(11):400–406.
51. Harris M, Conley-Muth M: Sex role stereotypes and medical specialty choice. J Am Med Wom Assoc 1981, 36(8):245–252.
52. Heins M, Smock S, Jacobs J, Stein M: Productivity of women physicians. JAMA 1976, 236:1961–1964.
53. Turner K: Memorandum #82–1 to the Women's Liaison Officers of the Association of American Medical Colleges. Washington, D.C., February 1, 1981. (unpublished)
54. U.S. Department of Health and Human Services. Characteristics of visits to male and female physicians. *In:* National Medical Ambulatory Care Survey (NMACS). Washington, D.C.: U.S. Government Printing Office, 1977. (DHHS-PHS publication no. (PHS) 80–1710).
55. Boufford JI: Women and health issues. Presentation to the Women's Liaison Officers of the Association of the American Medical Colleges. Washington, D.C., November 3, 1981. (unpublished)
56. U.S. Department of Health and Human Services: Health—United States, 1979. Washington, D.C.: U.S. Government Printing Office, 1980, p 168. (DHEW publication no. (PHS) 80–1232).
57. U.S. Department of Health, Education and Welfare. The older woman: continuities and discontinuities. *In:* Report of the National Institute on Aging and National Institute of Mental Health Workshop, September 14–15, 1978. Washington, D.C.: U.S. Government Printing Office, 1979, p 16. (U.S. DHEW-PHS-NIH publication no. 79–1897).

# The Female Surgeon

Traditionally, surgeons have been macho and male. Until recently, women were not encouraged to apply for surgical training because they were considered by their male colleagues to be unsuited for its long hours and dedicated commitment. The occasional female surgeon encountered prior to 1970 was considered an oddity rather than a true representative of her sex.

While the number of female surgeons has more than doubled from 2129 in 1971 to 4953 in 1981, the relative number continues to remain small. The 5000 women surgeons comprise a mere 5% of the total number of surgeons in the country and represent less than 10% of all women doctors in America. By comparison, about 25% of male doctors are surgeons. Only 20% of women surgeons practice general surgery and more than half, 2882, are firmly entrenched in the time-honored female specialty of obstetrics and gynecology.

Now, as increasing numbers of women embark on surgical careers, they are finding it easier to pass through doors which were once tightly bolted to women. Several determined women doctors including Susan Adelman, author of this chapter, have blazed the way.

As one female assistant professor of surgery tartly recalls "My residency in general surgery was a series of large hurdles, each topped with a nasty set of spikes that had to be overcome at any cost. Upon entering surgical training in the early 1970s I was told I was the second female to be admitted to the program. When I contacted the first, I learned she had survived only two months. In spite of a brutal call schedule, unpleasant facilities, and a stone wall of prejudice against women in training, I endured the experience until I could begin a university-affiliated residency."[1]

The customary picture of a surgeon as a *male* in *his* white coat, or pastel colored scrub suit in the burnished glow of operating room lights, will take a long time to be eradicated. Television has reinforced this concept, time and again, as it aggrandized male images and egos. A generation of Americans grew up with the resolute Ben Casey, his two top buttons perennially undone, performing neurosurgical miracles weekly. Americans today are no less impressed with the intractable Hawkeye Pierce's surgical prowess or the reflective Trapper John and his uncanny diagnostic ability.

In this chapter Susan Adelman, a pediatric surgeon, recounts in poignant detail the acrimony and disrespect she was subjected to and the occasional sympathy she was afforded, when she was being trained as a surgeon, less than a decade ago.

*J.P.C.*

# 14

# The Female Surgeon

*Susan Adelman*

## DECIDING

The decision to become a female surgeon is an emotional one; it had better be, because practical considerations today stongly argue against anyone rationally deciding to go into surgery. According to the GMENAC study, surgery is one of the most overcrowded areas in medicine today. It is interesting to note that, in recognition of this, fewer men are now applying to surgical residencies. In contrast, the number of women entering surgical training programs is rising. Interesting. The number of women actually entering surgical residencies is not great, but it does reflect a noticeable increase in both the actual and relative numbers of women, right at the time that surgical practice is becoming more competitive, and less desirable to men, than ever.

Even 15 years ago, when the percentage of women graduating from American medical schools was still the traditional 7%, women were already visible in pediatrics, anesthesia, pathology, family practice, and psychiatry. The population of female surgeons across the country at that time was virtually restricted to a very few women averaging from 50 to 60 years old. In 1972, I finished general surgery residency; two other women also finished other surgical residency programs in town, and one woman had preceded me the year before from my program. As far as I know, we were the beginning of the new generation of female surgeons. When I finished my pediatric surgery residency two years later, six other women throughout the country graduated either that or the following year, representing the new generation. Since then, one or two of the 15–20 pediatric surgery programs in the United States have graduated women each year. What each of us has to reveal about our experiences depends on which generation we represent.

A woman's experiences in a surgical residency depend also on the personalities of the dominant men in the program, on her personality, and on their interaction. After residency, her survival, growth, and success depend on the same factors, as well as the market factors of supply and demand. Now we come back to the GMENAC study: graduates are going to have an increasingly hard time breaking in now because there is more competition.

Men and women appear to make career decisions in different ways. This difference may be diminishing now that women make up a quarter of today's medical school graduating class and consequently feel more at home in the medical world than they did before. Men considering my field have asked me, "Will there be jobs?" Women have asked, "Will I like it? Can I do it?" Men seem to understand from the very beginning that they will have to live with their career choice for a lifetime, support their families with this career, and measure their own worth by their achievements in their career. They pick and choose careers guided by information about where opportunities for financial or academic success are greatest, and where the probability of advancement is strongest. Women traditionally pick what they "like best." They seem to pick careers that will appear compatible with being womanly, most easily allow them to combine job and family, and afford them at least some protection against the more brutal pressures of competition, or of running their own business. Another contemporary factor has now entered the picture: the desire to prove that a woman is as proficient, strong, and hardy as a man even in a traditionally male career.

This last factor has great potential for harm if it is the sole reason, or even if it is the major reason, why a woman chooses surgery. Probably today the graduating surgeon is doomed to greater frustration in finding a satisfactory position than his or her peers in other medical fields or surgical predecessors. Thus there are fewer and fewer "practical" reasons to choose surgery. If she chooses it, she had better love it.

I realized in medical school that I loved surgery. I had not planned to love it; I had not previously considered it, and I was not necessarily pleased to find that I was attracted to it. It sounded like a very hard life. The first colleague in whom I confided was a convivial former college athlete who later became an orthopedic surgeon. Since he intended to enter a surgical residency too, I felt emboldened to talk to him. "Oh yeah? What residency are you thinking of? Do you think you will stay in town for residency? Have you heard anything about the Henry Ford hospital program? I was thinking of applying there. What kind of surgeon do you want to be? You know, being an artist you'd be a terrific plastic surgeon. Have you thought of that?"

Quite possibly it was this conversation that solidified my resolve to go into surgery. I wonder what would have happened if I had talked first to the second person I picked to confide in. This was a general surgery staff man, of foreign origin, with a smile in his eyes and an intelligent manner. He drew himself up, frowned fiercely, and said, "Surgery? A woman cannot be a surgeon. A woman can cut and sew nice little stitches, but be a surgeon, never! I worked with a woman surgeon once. She could cut all right, and she could stand there and put in sutures, but once she got in trouble she was finished. I saw her get in trouble once, and she had to leave the room. The first-year residents had to take over. Then, when everything was under control, she came back into the room and went back to putting in stitches, nicely, nicely. A woman surgeon? Impossible."

## GETTING ACCEPTED

Whether a woman will be accepted in surgery seems to depend primarily on whether the woman is secure with her choice and with her ability. An eminent senior surgeon will usually be better able to accept and encourage a young woman than will a young man in his 30s: the supportive senior man is long past the danger of feeling threatened and has seen enough young male surgeons make mistakes or get in trouble to know that a woman's early fumbles and errors are just par for the course, not a consequence of her being female; the younger man is still nervous about creating his own professional reputation and future and will be more reluctant than the older man to take risks with residents, less forgiving about pre- or postoperative care problems, and more frightened at the possible graduation of a young attractive woman who will become a competitor. If she is unattractive on the other hand, he will also resent her for that.

An older eminent mentor can play a crucial role in starting a young woman out properly in surgery. In my experience, a woman does not usually search for a mentor; she simply knows when she has identified one, because of common interests, similarities in approach, or personal compatibility. It is like a marriage, but the parties do not have to live with each other. The best surgical mentor is probably still a man, unless it could be a woman who has been around for a long time and who is clearly professionally successful. Conventional behavior, style, and interaction among surgeons is unequivocally male, and it is unlike the style of most women. After a woman's period of trial and error—mostly error—it helps immeasurably for her either to study a mentor or to be able to ask him how to appropriately respond when conflict between peers arises, or even when patient management problems occur. What may appear to be discrimination against the woman may be just that, but it also may be the normal way that men in the field are accustomed to treating each other. Here is where a mentor would help. A family of brothers would help, too.

Surgeons have to cope with fear constantly. Surgical training involves unusually long hours and stern staff–resident interaction—part of its "macho mystique." In the most "high-powered" general surgical programs, every single resident has to fight exhaustion and terror while attempting to acquire a new set of skills. A woman in this position is in great danger of feeling that only she is having a hard time—that the men in her program are mostly doing well, and that they are self-confident, tireless, poised, and far better at handling the strain than she. She is tempted to see herself as anomalous, less well suited to the job than her male compatriots, more easily fatigued, more emotional and excitable than the men, and highly conspicuous. As a result, the woman puts far greater pressure on herself than the men do, creating a self-fulfilling prophecy. Certainly a female surgical resident has to have far more basic endurance than a man, because she burns up far more calories to get the energy to deal with the added pressures.

Whether or not a female surgical resident is actually subjected to explicit discrimination in ward work, assignment to surgical procedures, call schedules, or senior residency appointments depends entirely on the program and the surgeons who run it. Another female surgeon told me the story of a woman who was moved up through her program to the level of senior resident, kept on year after year waiting to be appointed chief resident, then finally told that no woman would ever be a chief resident in that program.

Today, some of the old niggling inconveniences that plagued women in surgery are vanishing, but even up to 12–14 years ago the problems still remained to be identified. Then, there were often no arrangements for a woman to sleep in the hospital while she was on call, because the men on call slept dormitory style and shared a bathroom. When I started, I had to beg for an empty bed in the hospital. I found that the beds reserved for rooming-in mothers were usually unoccupied, and I often slept there. There were two locker rooms in the operating suite, one marked "Doctors," the other marked "Nurses." I used the nurses' locker room. The surgeons' lounge could initially be entered either directly from the outside hall or from the doctors' locker room. One day, the outside door was locked to prevent the internists from eating all the donuts and drinking all the coffee. This only left the door from the mens' locker room. Nobody remembered me. One of the high points of my residency came the next day when I appeared in the surgeon's lounge, flushed and triumphant, after running the gauntlet of the showers in the mens' locker room. At first, nobody thought about how I had come in, then light dawned, and the room burst with gasps, roars of laughter, then applause.

The door was then permanently locked and I ran that gauntlet every day for the rest of my residency, sometimes twice a day. It also contributed to the men's feelings of insecurity when they wanted to take showers, so I took pity on them and at least shouted a warning that I was coming through before I appeared. The men found my locker room appearances so amusing that they even included me in a couple of informal locker room "sitting rounds" sessions, discussion sessions about problem patients on the service. My attendance at these sessions ended abruptly one day when the steward of the mens' locker room indignantly chased all of us out.

In some operating rooms, the dictaphones for operative dictations were located only in the mens' locker room or in an adjacent lounge. Times have changed so much however, that other operating suites now even have tiny locker rooms for woman doctors, separate from the nurses locker rooms. That is status!

In my program, the men could exchange their soiled white lab coats for clean ones by going to the steward in their locker room. I had to trek down to the laundry, during the limited hours that the laundry was open, to exchange my coats for fresh ones. Sometimes I was too busy to make the trip for days, and I had to work in a coat stained with blood and excrement. The men I worked with all seemed to sport coats whose whiteness practically blinded me.

When the hospital did build female doctors' sleeping quarters, they were placed on the corridor just outside of the operating room and were innocent of sink or mirror. Therefore, I faced another ordeal when I got up the morning after being on call: I had to dash to the nurses' locker room to wash up and fix my hair before anybody would recognize the disheveled mess coming around the corner.

A woman's major initial worry is whether she will be accepted by peers and patients. Fortunately, whether she is or is not well accepted in the beginning, any woman who finishes a surgical residency successfully has earned her acceptance from other surgeons, hospital staff, and patients. Patients are the easiest: they are very sensitive to the doctor's bearing, her manner, her apparent concern for them and their problems, her attention to detail, and her manifest competence. If the doctor seems unsure of herself, however, patients will pick it up; *then* they will become nervous about her and about her being female. If, on the other hand, the surgeon or surgical resident shows confidence in her own abilities, not by blustering but by projecting calm inner certainty, the patient will pick this up too, feel confidence in the physician, brag about the smart lady doctor, and swell with pride having suddenly become so liberal. The female patient will not only feel confidence, but also be proud that one of her sex is doing so well. Incidentally, it is not that easy to project a calm confidence when you are a surgical resident, overworked, and scared to death.

Naturally, patients vary. It is hard to forget the man who smiled benevolently at me when, as chief resident, I came to his bedside leading the junior residents on rounds, and he greeted me with "You stay with these smart men here, young lady. They'll teach you a lot." There was also a memorable old lady on a ward which happened to have a male nurse on one shift. When I told her that I did not want the head of her bed elevated, she reassured me, "The doctor was just here, dear, and he rolled it up. I'm sure it's O.K. Don't you worry." I can also still see the face of the lady who gave me a maternal smile as I came into her room to remove her stitches after I had taken out her gallbladder the week before. "Are you going to take those stitches out all by yourself?" she asked incredulously.

Of course, there are times in a busy residency when the "knife and gun club" patients from the emergency room try one's patience, and one's response to loud obnoxious behavior from these patients can get short and to the point. After several such encounters on one ward, one night, a new gunshot victim appeared on the ward, just hurt badly enough to make him contentious. He began to bait me, and a protective chorus of advice rose up from the men in the surrounding beds: "Hey, you better cut that out. You can't do her like that. You gotta watch out for her, you hear me. She's mean."

## ROLE OF THE RESIDENT

Fun as the men might be on the wards, there is no question that my bugaboo in the clinic was hernia examinations. My staff surgeon was a hernia expert, and large numbers of young auto workers with hernias were referred to him. As a junior resident, I had to do all the initial examinations when I rotated on his service, and as a senior resident on his service I had to check all the junior residents' examinations. Not only did the young men look shocked to see me when I walked in, but they also frequently found that they were afflicted with an uncontrollable physiologic response during my examination which mortified them and made me blush and try to hurry my examination. The solution ultimately lay in a deftly manipulated crushed-up sheet which I placed strategically and moved aside a little bit one way, then the other way while I checked for hernias. Inside a multitude of sins could be hidden.

My surgical service was also responsible for most of the screening proctoscopic examinations in the hospital, including those done for the executive physicals. Again, my appearance in the room was always greeted by male patients with dismay. I soon learned simply to commiserate with those who signified their distress and to concur that it was just not their lucky day, but that there was nothing more to do about it than to just get on with the examination. One rather elegant executive turned, looked around at me in the middle of the examination and asked, "Does this mean that we have to get married?"

If generalizations could be made—and they can be made gingerly—elderly patients have the most trouble accepting a female surgeon, children have the least, the highly educated have little or no trouble, and the very ignorant often do not care. Blue-collar workers, especially first-generation Americans, may at first be skeptical, but their final opinion depends on how the doctor conducts herself, on the wisdom of her advice, and on her results. Almost no patient ever refuses treatment by a female surgeon, unless perhaps the question is posed as one of my referring doctors posed it; "How would you like to go to a woman doctor?" Today many patients, not only women, beam happily at the lady surgeon, proud of her for "being so smart." Paternalism and maternalism may be difficult, but they are better than hostility. The whole issue fades away with the passage of time and with increasing experience and confidence on the part of the surgeon.

The most important acceptance is that from the female surgeon herself. At first, she will only say that she is a surgical resident, while her male contemporaries are already introducing themselves as surgeons. When she starts in practice, she will tentatively share an office in case she fails, whereas her male colleague, if he can afford it, will fully equip an office of his own. It is harder for a woman to believe that she will really be a surgeon until she is one. The female resident and the young female surgeon just starting practice also waste more time and energy than a man would worrying about what people will think when they do something wrong. They share these fears with minority graduates and anyone else who has reason to believe the barriers to acceptance will be higher.

In my residency, as long as I worked as hard as my male peers, complained less than any of them, asked for no special concessions, and generally behaved in exactly the same manner as my male fellow residents, I enjoyed comfortable working relationships with almost everyone. Tasteless comments were extremely rare, although one senior resident of mine, encountering me on a ward at two in the morning did say, "Tell me. What are you doing here at this hour, when you could be at home making somebody happy?"

I concluded that I had to swallow my disgust for cleansing enemas, disguise any fear I might feel about putting chest tubes in on awake patients, and suppress my embarrassment about catheterizing male patients. I also learned never to complain, never protest that I was tired, never answer back, and never say "I can't," "I won't," "I'm afraid to," or "I never did it before." Residency was a crash course in "macho" behavior, some of which stood me in good stead later on, and some of which proved to be just as disastrous for me as it sometimes is for men. After finishing that program, it took a long time before I was able to admit that I did not know something, that I needed help, that I was too tired, or that I was afraid.

A woman can earn the animosity of her male co-workers by constantly asking for alterations in her call schedule, work hours, and assignments on account of her home responsibilities. Her co-workers may acknowledge that she has these responsibilities, but they will resent the fact that they receive no special concessions. It will appear suspiciously like she is taking advantage of being female.

Another type of female surgical resident is the one who is obsessed with the need to prove herself, to everyone, all the time, to the extent that she not only thinks about it constantly but she also talks about it constantly. She will repeatedly recount in detail a long story of a skirmish with some staffman who impugned her competence by some chance remark but against whom she retaliated gloriously. She will be hated by everyone. She apparently needs to accentuate the drama of being the lone woman in her surgical program, and she likes to create constant conflict between herself and her male oppressors so she will feel even more heroic. The surrounding males, however, find it very tiresome to constantly be cast in the role of oppressors.

The whole issue of when, whether, and how to project a feminine image is a major problem for the woman in surgery: a surgical scrub suit is drab, baggy, and sexless, and lately the shirt and pants have become a unisex costume in many hospitals. In some hospitals, female surgeons wear pants to differentiate themselves from nurses, but in other operating rooms nurses wear pants too. A female resident looking at herself in the mirror sees a woman who is tired, drawn, and has circles under her eyes; she wonders if she will ever be attractive again. She also finds herself and hears herself imitating masculine speech patterns, attitudes, posturing, and sometimes a masculine walk. She notices the way in which the successful males around her assert their authority, and she wonders if anyone will ever trust her if she tries to assert herself in a feminine way. She may also wonder what that way would be.

There are various ways to handle this problem. In the past, it was a cliché that women in surgery acted just like men: they became "butch." Several of those I have met actually did, though most did not, but this is still the conventional image. Some young women even today go this way. Others react strongly against this image and dress in a manner that is frankly sexy. The major reason is to differentiate themselves clearly and definitively from the "butch" lady surgeon image, and to prove that they are "normal" women, and attractive at that—so there.

This image can also lead to conventional male–female interactions in the work place, which will even further complicate the woman's interpersonal relationships, as well as drain off the precious energy that she should be so judiciously rationing just to get through her ordinary workday. It can also result in male-baiting behavior, in which a man is encouraged to make a conventional pass only to find that she considers his pass further proof that men just think female colleagues are good for one thing.

The relationships between a female resident and the staff nurses again seem to depend on the personalities involved. If a woman attempts to imitate the swagger and the bombast of her male colleagues, the nurses will cut her down to size fast. If the resident, or the staff surgeon, adopts an "us girls" attitude with the nurses, commiserates with them about their treatment by her male colleagues, laughs at their stories about the more obnoxious men, and makes the nurses proud that another woman has "made it," they will not resent her. They will feel that they finally have an ally on the surgical staff. Of course, in order to do this, the woman has to get over her initial needs to show them that she is the doctor, to hide her ignorance in front of them, and to show the world that she is a doctor, not a nurse. She also has to learn not to be afraid to have male colleagues see her talking with nurses and lump her with them, as "You girls," instead of with themselves as "One of the boys."

## STARTING PRACTICE

Entry into practice can be especially crushing for a woman, especially if she tries to start out in an area where competition is vicious. Some women retreat into research or into academic medicine just to avoid this conflict. While this is not the only reason for women to join university faculties, certainly a large percentage of graduating female surgical residents end up staying on in their university or accepting other full-time appointments. These seem safer, more sheltered. If women do go into practice, they usually join partnerships and avoid setting up their own business arrangements. They are sometimes willing to work for years as poorly paid and overworked junior partners, for the same reasons.

A woman subjected to a campaign by her competitors to drive her out of town has many of the same reactions as a man does, but she wonders how much of the hostility is directed at her womanliness. When men are subjected to harassment, hounding, and insults, they usually understand right away that their problem is that they are competitors, and they become angry, stubborn, and doggedly resistant to the pressure. The typical female thinks, "What is wrong with me? Why do they hate me? What did I do? Which of my weaknesses or deficiencies have they discovered that they want to keep me out, keep me off the hospital staff, or cut off my business?"

A man who trys to injure a woman professionally has all kinds of extra material available to him to use in defaming her reputation. His reasons for wanting to hurt her may be no different from his reasons for doing the same thing to a man, but when his rival is female he can cast aspersions with an entirely new twist. A young man in surgery may be complimented by being called "aggressive"; it sounds quite different for a woman. A letter, describing her as "having a mind of her own"; might be translated as "bitch." In locker room conversations, allusions may be made to "problems" that a woman may have had getting along in her residency. This may be true, in part because of the added pressures on her, but translate as "she is a bitch."

One chairman of a surgical department in a hospital to which a female surgeon applied for privileges shook his head and said that he had heard that she had an awful lot of trouble getting along with her colleagues, nurses, and the operating room staff during her residency. Translation: bitch. He said that he had a close, friendly staff and that his was a close, friendly hospital. He could not afford to take on a liability like her. Since she had left the hospital where she did her residency under the warmest and friendliest possible circumstances, she was surprised and hurt. She went around for months asking everyone she knew what was wrong with her, as if suddenly her best friend might break down and admit that she had bad breath. It turned out that a powerful competitor in town had been in a position to write a letter to this man and to make a personal contact with him in which he skillfully conveyed the impression by innuendo that she was a bitch.

One woman started a research project with colleagues in her hospital, only to find that word had been passed to the chairmen of the other departments involved that no project with this woman's name on it would ever be approved by the surgical department. Another woman has related the tale that a friend in the emergency room began to send her cases, and notes flowed into the emergency room insisting that a strict protocol be observed in making all emergency room referrals—a protocol which excluded her. One woman was passed over—in favor of a man finishing residency several years after she did—when staff coverage for the resident service was assigned. Still another tells the story of her application for a university clinical appointment, which was almost squelched by a note to the university from her department chairman saying that there were no plans now or in the future for her to teach residents or students.

A female surgeon reports that whenever a case of hers went bad, it became the star case on the next Morbidity and Mortality conference. She lived in fear of seeing herself featured in that conference. Her colleagues handled the situation in the conference with a lovable sheepishness or a rough bluster which seemed to get them off the hook. She stammered in terror. The residents were also encouraged to bring their complaints about her to the department chairman. When she complained about his encouraging residents to complain about her, she was told that the chairman had instructed the residents specifically to "treat her just the same as you would anybody else."

An anesthesiologist in one hospital observed that when a certain woman had a big case, a senior staff man would always find an excuse to look in the room. He even noticed that the woman surgeon's colleagues would not look her in the eye in the corridor when they passed her, and would fidget and smirk when she said something in the lounge.

It is gratifying to report that for me almost all of this type of harassment has now gone by the boards and that even a department chairman who turned me down from his staff is now effusively polite. Time helps. The surgeon who just stays put, toughs it out, and does her best will eventually establish her reputation, independent of what her detractors may say. Activity which enhances the community perception of her helps considerably. This could comprise visibility in a specialty society or the county medical society, research, writing, lecturing, or participation in community or religious organizations.

There are still problems, but they become fewer each year that a woman is in practice. Referring doctors still may send a woman their routine cases, then reserve their most heoric, dramatic cases for male surgeons. Doctors may try to protect a female surgeon by not calling her at night or on weekends, when they would think nothing at all of calling a male surgeon. Chivalry still lives. Female referring doctors may not be able to imagine themselves doing a particular operation, so they cannot imagine a female surgeon doing it either and send it to a man. On the other hand, a referring doctor may be downright embarrassed about assuming that a woman surgeon has to be brilliant.

It is delightfully comfortable for me to talk with the young mothers of my patients, and my babies are a delight when they survive and thrive. Mothers seem to feel more comfortable themselves when they deal with me, rather than with a man. I am glad therefore that I chose this field, but I have to admit that I chose it because I am a woman. I thought people would think it sounded right "for a woman." Throughout general surgical training, I was told that I would never be able to establish a practice, that I "would starve." I felt that to be competitive I would need a gimmick. Pediatric surgery sounded like a field in which my being female might be an advantage, especially since so many of my referring doctors would be female pediatricians. When I told a fellow general surgery resident what field I had chosen, he chided me, "Why are you copping out? You are stepping backwards. You have already proved yourself in general surgery. Why are you giving up and going into pediatric surgery?"

## SURGEON AND SPOUSE

Less than half of the female surgeons that I know are married. Far less than half of these women have children. At least two women I knew had children during their general surgical residencies. One woman married and had a child when she was in her early 40s. Most have none. This is in distinct contrast to female pediatricians, many of whom practice part-time or take salaried positions while they have and bring up children. Surgeons seem more unwilling or more afraid to make the same compromises.

For one thing, it is very difficult to imagine going through a general surgery residency with children at home. It could be done, but it would mean scarcely seeing the children for five years. Women can easily combine a surgical career with marriage. Many of us have done so, though the man has to be very secure, independent, and understanding. Some female surgeons marry other doctors, but these seem to be in the minority: with conflicting call schedules, the partners might seldom see each other for weeks at a time during residency. The same thing happens with other medical couples, but surgical call schedules are particularly arduous.

A woman in a solo practice of surgery can never plan a party, cook a dinner, or entertain without worrying about getting an emergency call in the middle of her preparations or in the middle of serving her dinner party. This can seriously inhibit her social life and that of her husband. The husband must be able to understand and to handle it. A woman and her husband both must be prepared to abandon weekend plans, to be awakened in the middle of the night, and to stop in the middle of projects at home at the ring of a beeper. Both she and her husband have to adjust their lifestyles to her job.

The husband must be able to stand intimidating competition in social status, income, and titles. It helps him if he is proud of his wife and if he identifies with her work to some extent. This makes it easier for him to make sacrifices for her job. It does not help if he resents the large amount of time his wife spends working and the little time she spends with him. It does not help at all if the husband wants or expects his wife to cater to him or to be subservient. It does not help either if he shows an excessive interest in the income she generates. This can make her feel that she is killing herself just to support him. Men may have resented doing this for years, but women are just now learning how unpleasant this may feel. If both spouses have roughly comparable incomes, much jealousy is avoided.

The most difficult years come early in the surgical residency and early in practice. Not only does the husband have to put up with a woman who has adopted "macho" manners and aggressive ways, but he may be shocked to discover that he also periodically has a crying crushed woman on his hands who has not stood up for her rights that day at work and who is exasperatingly unassertive. The type of highly assertive man who would be likely to marry a female surgeon would have to be frustrated on hearing how his wife handled a situation which he would have handled by telling off everybody concerned.

Many a male surgeon carries himself as if the adulation of hundreds of admiring patients has risen to his head. The general surgeon's bravado and his arrogant facade have made him the butt of jokes within the medical field. Everyone has a story about surgeons like the one who entered a patient's room, peered at an arteriogram, looked up at the patient and said on the way out of the door, "The vessels in your leg are blocked. It will have to come off."

The woman surgeon feels vulnerable herself, and she can more easily understand patients' needs for her to sit down with them, answer their questions, and give them detailed explanations. A woman is motivated to try harder, like Avis, to head off any doubts that her patients or her peers may have about her competence. If her feeling of vulnerability leads to greater preoperative preparation, improved patient work-up, more meticulous surgery, and more attention to therapeutic details, it means better patient care and greater patient satisfaction. If this causes enough anxiety to distract and sidetrack her while she is trying to take care of her patients, it will have a deleterious result.

## ONGOING PRACTICE

Possibly also because of concern about peer criticism of their results, women are often less willing than men to delegate surgical procedures to residents, and they may need to take care of more details of pre- and postoperative care themselves. Because of concern about criticism and lack of cooperation from residents, they also may delegate too much. A young surgical staffman will have these same problems too, but a woman stays at this stage longer than a man does. Women have more trouble initially in striking just the right tone when teaching male residents, both in and outside of the operating room. Part of this too is because it is trickier for women to reach the right note of firmness with anesthesiologists, residents, and other hospital personnel. Sometimes women frankly overreact and become arbitrary, and sometimes they are much milder than male surgeons, more open to suggestions, and more willing to entertain opposing points of view.

When a woman in surgery does face what seems to be professional discrimination, she has to check herself constantly to make sure she is neither being paranoid nor letting something go by for fear of being paranoid. A referring doctor may or may not have deliberately failed to call her for a certain case because she is a woman. A surgical competitor who has stolen a case from her may or may not have done the same thing to a man. The referrring doctor is a special problem, because as long as the woman does not antagonize him over this incident he still remains a potential referring doctor for the next case. On the other hand, she knows that he must have figured that she would not shout or scream as a male surgeon would, and if she says nothing this time he will do the same thing again. If she does shout and scream as a man would though, he will probably think that she is volatile, excitable, and would not be able to handle a case like the one he just sent to someone else anyhow. If he really did not think that he acted through prejudice, her vociferous complaints will just sound paranoid to him.

Similarly, the surgical competitor, senior partner, or department chairman who may steal a case from a woman, see that a woman gets only lesser cases, or pass over a woman for an appointment may do so either unconsciously or deliberately. If the discrimination was unconscious, the man confronted by an angry, accusing woman often will maintain that *he* helped her when she started out, *he* trained her or *he* hired her, and he will feel aggrieved and unfairly treated. If the discrimination was conscious and deliberate, he probably calculated that the woman would not dare protest, would be too uncertain of her ground to protest effectively, or would be vulnerable to the charge that she was being paranoid.

A male superior will be resentful if he anticipates that any action of his will have to be defended against a charge of prejudice. A woman will be resentful if she anticipates that her protests will be seen either as paranoia or as sly accusations. Such a sequence may leave everyone wondering who is paranoid. The sequence is devoutly to be avoided, and it will be avoided if the woman neither shirks from confrontation nor allows herself to be drawn into confrontation when she is beside herself. If takes a long time to learn that before any such confrontation, she has to find herself, organize herself, set the time for the confrontation herself, and spell out her point effectively. Done properly, this will nullify whatever advantage the man may otherwise have.

Many of the barriers that were still up only ten years ago are now broken down. Many of the old attitudes have already changed, and senior surgeons in many programs now point proudly to their women surgeons, reacting defensively on their behalf when their ability is questioned. Such facilities as sleeping rooms for women residents are now usually adequate. Women in surgical programs are less frequently alone today, and they no longer lack female surgical role models. Unfortunately, now the country has too many surgeons, and surgery has started to become a less attractive career for women as well as men, just as things are looking up.

# The Afro-American Physician

The first American-trained black physician was probably Dr. James Denham who was born around 1762. He learned *materia medica* from Dr. John Kearsley, Jr in Philadelphia. Later, he gained experience under Dr. George West, a British military surgeon. Following the Revolutionary War Dr. Denham worked for Dr. Robert Dove in New Orleans. Dr. Dove was so impressed with Dr. Denham's medical knowledge and obvious skill that he permitted Dr. Denham to purchase his freedom. Dr. Denham then became a renowned medical practitioner throughout Lousiana.

But a black doctor such as Dr. Denham was rare in early America. Throughout the 18th and first half of the 19th centuries black doctors were few and far between. The first Afro-American to graduate formally from medical school was Dr. James McCune Smith. He was a New Yorker who obtained his medical degree from the University of Glasgow in 1837. Shortly afterward, Dr. David K. McDonough became the first black to graduate from an American medical school. He attended the College of Physicians and Surgeons in New York. Although three blacks were admitted to the Harvard Medical School in 1850, the number of black physicians remained low until Howard University started its medical school in 1868. Thereafter the number of black physicians began to increase. Howard's first class consisted of "seven colored and one white" students; it graduated its first woman doctor, Mary Dora Speckman, in 1872.

A second black medical school, Meharry Medical College, opened its doors in Nashville, Tennessee in 1876. The school was named after a white family, the five Meharry brothers, who provided the funding. With two schools producing medical graduates the number of Afro-American doctors in the country gradually increased to 909 in 1890. Less than 100 of these had graduated from "white" medical schools. Five years later, Drs. Robert F. Boyd, Miles V. Lynk and twelve colleagues gathered in the First Congregational Church in Atlanta to found the National Medical Association. They committed the association "to fight for better care and medical opportunity for all Americans." Though small in numbers at the turn of the century, its membership now exceeds 8000.

Throughout the first half of the 20th century the number of black physicians stablized at 3500. In 1942 there were 3810 blacks out of a total of 180,496 physicians in the country, or 2.1%. About 100 of these Afro-Americans were women. The number of black doctors continued to grow in the 1950s, 60s and 70s. In 1960 the figure was 4706, in 1970, 6106, and by 1980 it exceeded 10,100. However, that number is low when one considers that black Americans comprise more than 11% of the population as a whole.

Such underrepresentation of Afro-Americans in medicine should be a matter of concern to all physicians. "Can anything be done about it?" and "Are there special difficulties that blacks experience in medical school or as physicians?" are questions that come to mind. Black physicians tend to work primarily with blacks and provide the bulk of medical care delivered to the black population. A National Center for Health Statistics[1] survey shows that 87% of patient visits to black doctors are made by blacks, and that whites make only 10% of the visits to black physicians.

In this chapter, Dr. Augustus A. White III, professor of orthopedic surgery at Harvard Medical School, provides an overview of the Afro-American physician. He also discusses other issues pertinent to both black and white physicians. His observations are balanced, philosophical and pragmatic; they spring from a unique combination of southern American roots tempered by northern American educational experiences. Clearly, Dr. White is a talented teacher who is also a remarkable Afro-American physician. His cogent advice on career development and personal advancement in medicine is lucid and persuasive and can be utilized to good effect by all physicians, regardless of race.

*J.P.C.*

---

1. United States Bureau of the Census: Bureau of the Census Catalog, Washington DC, GPO, April 1980.
2. National Center for Health Studies: National Ambulatory Medical Care Survey. Washington DC, Dept HEW 1977.

# 15

# The Afro-American Physician

*Augustus A. White, III*

## INTRODUCTION

> "Get over on that table! Okay, now lie down, we don't have all day!" The black, moderately emaciated, white-haired woman, shivering and dazed from a combination of fear, hostility, medication, and air conditioning, slid from under her thin white sheet off the stretcher and onto the operating table. The white surgeon who had shouted the commands stormed out of the operating room to the scrub sink and the black orderly looked around for a blanket. The scene was in a new small private hospital for blacks in a large southern city, summer of 1957. I should not have been shocked or surprised; after all, I had grown up in the South. I had sold black newspapers. Several times a year, somewhat like the patient above, I had experienced that strange combination of intense rage and fear when the front page carried headlines and several graphic photographs of a black man who had been lynched. I should not have been shocked by a few harsh, hateful words from a middle-aged white surgeon to a frightened elderly black about to have major surgery for suspected malignancy.

The dramatic impact of that little scene in the operating room was based on my naive idealism. The highly romanticized idealism that we traditionally attribute to physicians was foremost in my mind. I thought that all doctors were kind, compassionate people. I still believe that most are and I guess it's even possible for a generally compassionate doctor, in some kind of schizophrenic way, to display racist attitudes and behavior. In any case, this was the experience that greeted me on my first day of work in a hospital. I had just finished college, been accepted to medical school, and been given a job as a surgical technician for the summer.

By 1957 lynchings had become rather rare; yet this 300-bed facility was the first modern hospital, in a city of about 500,000 blacks, where blacks could be patients. You could have your own private physician, black or white. However, if you were a black, patient or physician, you were not allowed to be a patient in or practice medicine in the very best major hospitals in that city. In a sense, America had come a long way yet still had a long way to go. Today, the same generalization is valid. In this chapter, I cover briefly some of the history of medicine as it relates to Afro-American heritage and suggest the current status of that heritage. I then discuss my personal view and make some suggestions that are intended to accentuate the positive and eliminate the negative aspects of coping as an Afro-American physician.

## IN THE PAST

Imhotep, who lived about 3000 B.C., was physician to King Zoser of the Egyptian Third Dynasty. This man was the first identifiable figure in medicine. His numerous contributions to and genius in a broad variety of disciplines resulted in his becoming a demigod 500 years after his death. We know that the Egyptians were dark-skinned Africans. Dr. W. Montaque Cobb, a world authority on Afro-American medical history states, "if Imhotep were strolling about any street in the United States today he would be classified as black. Therefore, we claim him and note that we started at the top of the medical profession [five] millennia ago. Though we have not been there since, we have been contributing all along and are on our way."[1]

It is important to mention here briefly some of those "contributions all along." The use of a live virus as an inoculation providing immunity against smallpox was brought to America by Onesimus, an African slave. Medical historians rarely mention this, however, but the story of Onesimus is an important narrative well presented and documented in Cobb's work.[1] Two Afro-American physicians, Dr. Absalom Jones and Dr. Richard Allen, distinguished themselves by their contributions during the yellow fever epidemic in Philadelphia in 1793, when that city was the nation's capital. Government leaders including George Washington, John Adams, Thomas Jefferson, and Alexander Hamilton left the city; Matthew Clarkson, the mayor, was desperately in need of help. Drs. Jones and Allen volunteered their services and those of the African Society. They organized and led the society's members and others into what was essentially a modern-day Red Cross. Citizens were trained to provide some of the medical and nursing care. The sick were transported and the dead were buried. Under the leadership of Drs. Jones and

Allen, over 2000 blacks were mobilized and led in public service during this major epidemic.

All of the following distinguished Afro-Americans are significant contributors to the medical field nationally and internationally:

- Dr. Charles R. Drew was a pioneer in research which led to the founding of blood banks. He was also a renowned Professor and Chairman of the Department of Surgery at Howard University. As of 1980, Dr. Drew had trained more than half of all the black, board-certified general surgeons in the United States.
- Dr. LaSalle D. Lefall, currently the Professor and Chairman of Surgery at Howard, is an Afro-American and Past President of the American Cancer Society.
- Dr. Charles Epps, a black physician, is an author of a major orthopedic textbook and a member of the American Medical Association's prestigious judicial council.
- Dr. James Comer is Dean of Yale Medical School.
- Drs. Mitchell Spellman and Alvin Poussaint are Deans in the Harvard Medical School.
- Dr. Joseph Henry is a Dean at the Harvard Dental School.
- Dr. Jane Wright is Professor of Surgery at the New York Medical College and a cancer chemotherapist.
- Dr. Levi Adams is a Vice-President of the Medical School at Brown University.
- Dr. Maurice Clifford is the President of the Medical College of Pennsylvania.

There are many others who could be included here, but this list is enough to provide a sense of the progress and activity of black physicians.

For the reader interested in the history of people of color in medicine, I recommend the highly scholarly, astute, and interesting work of Dr. W.M. Cobb,[1] which ought to be required reading for all Afro-American physicians and recommended reading for all American physicians.

## STATUS OF BLACKS TODAY IN MEDICINE

It is useful to consider contemporary history regarding the issue of recruitment and production of black physicians in the 1970s and 1980s.[2] As a result of demands made by a black minority, consciousness-raising within the dominant group, and external and internal pressure on the federal government to make its democratic ideals more real, substantive programs were developed to increase the number of black medical students who matriculated to and graduate from predominantly white medical schools. When one reviews the figures, a trend is apparent. The percentage of blacks in all medical schools at the end of 1969 was 2.2%. A sturdy increase continued up to 6.3% by the end of 1975, about the time of the Bakke case. Between 1975 and 1980, there was a gradual decline in the percentage, down to 5.6% in 1980. For the academic year 1980–1981, the percentage was 5.7%, and for 1981–1982 it was 5.9%.

This stabilization probably results from a number of factors: a possible loss of committment on the part of the various institutions and individuals involved; a possible decrease in the pool of applicants; and definite significant economic strains on the resources of black applicants and of the institutions. Nevertheless, the considerations that stimulated this movement are every bit as cogent and urgent now as they were at the time of their inception.

Research shows that the most powerful predictor of first-year enrollment and graduation of black students from professional schools is the presence of black faculty. Although some programs have increased the number of black faculty, it appears that their presence has declined in the past 2 years. At present, only about 2.5% of the 444,000 physicians practicing in America are black, whereas the black population in our country accounts for 11.7%.[2a]

How the black physician fares after graduation is not a topic about which there is a great deal of information. We know that there have been problems in obtaining staff privileges at various institutions. The National Medical Association has taken a leadership role, focusing mainly on black physicians, in ensuring fair policies for obtaining privileges in hospitals and in speaking out on issues that relate to medical care as it effects Afro-Americans.

## COPING IN MEDICINE

Almost any way you look at it, medicine, today, is a stressful profession.[3] The suicide, divorce, and addiction rate is high among those in the profession: our work demands a great deal of us, as we do of ourselves. Moreover, today's society is quite stressful for most people.

Against a background of a highly stressful profession in a highly stressful society, we must also deal with the problem of racism. Comedian Richard Pryor describes the situation essentially this way: He's struggling along, just marginally able to cope as a sensitive human being and suddenly, out of nowhere, someone comes along and puts "nigger" into the situation. Now he's totally decompensated and must regroup, reorder his priorities, and change his tack significantly. He must now allot a great amount of emotional, intellectual, spiritual, and physical energy as well as time to combat, defend, adjust to, avoid, or ignore that powerful variable called racism.

The extent to which Mr. Pryor or any American black can minimize, eliminate, ignore, or use that thrust of racism to advantage depends on his or her self-confidence, life experience, and coping skills. This chapter speaks to that individual; I have not emphasized calls for social, political, and group action, although these are, of course, equally if not more important. However, in terms of solving the *immediate* problems and needs of the individual, I prefer to offer suggestions for attitudes, thoughts, and actions that will be helpful at work tomorrow.

I am aware that most people, especially doctors, do not like to be told how to behave even if they are reading a book about modifying their behavior. I am not writing as a representative of anyone other than myself and in no way am I attempting to speak for all black physicians. I am not setting myself up as an authority or claiming special credentials for criticizing white physicians, or for advising white physicians on how to behave. I am, however, planning to present some coping mechanisms for white and black physicians as they interact with each other in their Aesculapian travels. These are my best shots and they are coming right from the hip. They seem to work well in minimizing the negatives of racism and maximizing the positivies of humanism.

## TO MY FELLOW AFRO-AMERICAN PHYSICIANS

I am assuming that most of your skills lie primarily in the area of medicine and its related activities rather than in politics and social action. (We should remember, however, that there have been a number of outstanding physician—social activists and leaders, such as Drs. Montague Cobb, Frank Clement, and Benjamin Spock. Still, most of us do not possess their talents in this area.) It is extremely difficult to control the thoughts, feelings, and behavior of others, but you can and must be able to master your own behavior, thoughts, and (yes, to a great degree) feelings. This is critical for survival. You can immediately begin to affect your own actions, but it is very difficult to get others to behave the way they ought to or the way you want them to. I am also assuming you possess a certain amount of inner strength or you would not be coping as a *doctor*. If you have elected to become a physician and have survived the competition, challenges, and difficulties thus far, then you do indeed have the necessary inner strength to cope with the racial contingencies you may encounter. The skill will be to use that strength in the most effective manner.

### We Are Black Physicians and We Are Physicians

For survival, success, and happiness in your personal life this seems to be among the most important ideas we can explore: unless you have elected to function in your professional life totally in a segregated black setting (which is virtually impossible, I might add), then do not allow yourself to function exclusively in your profession solely on black issues; instead, expand into the overall problems and activities of medicine. My recommendation is that you allocate time and energy to make a definite contribution in your profession beyond your own personal professional activities. The contribution does not have to be Nobel-prize-winning research: it can be in the organizational aspects of medicine, in teaching, in clinical research, by serving on committees, or through membership and participation in societies. This kind of activity has considerable value to your professional and personal development. You make new friends and contacts, and become known for your capabilities and respected for your views on many issues. You also learn more about how the system works and how to use it effectively to achieve worthwhile goals. Simply put, you participate more fully, make a contribution, and influence activities in the mainstream of your profession.

### You Can't Just Call Him a "Whole Bunch of Bad Names"

In confrontation and disagreement, many of us exhibit cultural differences. In black culture, for the most part, confrontations and disagreements are dealt with very frankly, forthrightly, and vociferously. There is even some tendency toward inflation and exaggeration of the hostilities. In the medical world, for the most part, these confrontations are managed in the context of deflated hostility, unstated "real bases" of disagreement or argument, and subtle glib types of verbal warfare, much of which is behind (or between) the lines. For black physicians, this cultural difference can provide an astonishing clash and significant problems.

There are two kinds of problem that we as blacks may experience from this: (1) we may underestimate the level of hostility involved or expressed on the part of an adversary and (2) we may shock or frighten the hell out of colleagues who may question our sanity or fear for their lives if they do not understand. Frankness and a forthright confrontation on "the real problem" has advantages for all concerned and our cultural patterns have a contribution to make here. Exaggerations and marketing "wolf tickets"* may however be unnecessarily inflammatory and counterproductive.

**The Mentor Phenomenon**

Several years ago I had the very educational and intellectually stimulating pleasure of participating in a seminar course on the campus of Harvard Business School. During free time one afternoon and as part of a relaxing stroll about the campus, curiosity took me into a major lecture hall. This huge lecture room was full: students were sitting in the aisles and on the edges of their seats listening to a man in his late thirties or early forties. He wore an appropriately executive three-piece blue pinstriped suit, and lectured eloquently with obvious charisma, control, authority, confidence, and wisdom. The essence of this scene was that this dynamic man radiated success and was in fact heir apparent for the leadership of one of the biggest and best-known corporations in the United States and the world.

During this dynamic and multitopical speech, the business executive began to describe his formula for success. The message that he emphasized was that he always sought advice for decisions of importance. People with more experience and knowledge were able to help him with decisions and thereby sharpen significantly his judgment and ability to carry out these decisions.

In medicine we learn in many different ways from numerous sources—from books, from our own experience, and most of all directly from others. I have always believed that the only kind of mistake that is excusable is one that is thoroughly and truly original; one for which its perpetrator had no warning whatsoever. Most banalities generally make a good deal of sense and are relatively valid and true, but one of the most uncharacteristic banalities is the following: "You gotta get out there and make your own mistakes in order to learn." Truly original mistakes, if we survive them, are definitely great teachers and provide us with something to teach others; unoriginal mistakes are for the dull and uninformed. We must therefore make a distinct effort to learn from others.

Implicit in this is the fact that one has a great deal to gain from having one or more mentors. If you wish to view this mentor phenomenon in a utilitarian sense, you can consider that you are not taking anything that you are not going to give back. If you have a positive experience with a mentor, you can be sure that when your time comes you will be able to pass on your experience and wisdom effectively to some new person who has chosen you as a mentor.

*"Wolf tickets" are false threats.

One may have the good fortune to find oneself on a purely spontaneous basis under the influence of a gifted mentor; however, things do not always happen on their own. We must make some effort. When you come in contact with an individual whose style, achievement, integrity, leadership, or any other characteristics attract you, you can seek some substantive opportunity to get to know that person and to work with him or her. Sooner or later you will find someone with whom the rapport is good and a productive positive relationship will develop. Mentors obviously have some opportunity to be of help, not only in sharing knowledge and experience, but in many other ways that contribute to career development. Certainly there have been numerous successful people who did not have mentors. However, there is no doubt that such a relationship is significantly helpful and enriching.

### "Are You Really Standing There with Your Colored Self and Criticizing My Intellect?"

Face it: many white Americans grew up with the conscious or unconscious idea that they are intellectually superior to blacks. For those whose education is dominated by television and films, this is not at all surprising. A look at what our youth are taught and not taught in our schools will further substantiate this assertion. Students are rarely exposed to the intellectual achievements of blacks. Moreover, several recent (1982) surveys reported in the news media showed that the majority of Twenty-Fifth Year Reunion graduates of highly regarded Northeastern colleges thinks that blacks are intellectually inferior to whites.

Put this "educated" white person, who thinks blacks are intellectually inferior, into a stressful situation such as Vietnam. In the military one's rank is based primarily on longevity and performance. During the Vietnam war, 2-year volunteers came under the medical draft laws. The non-career physician was invited either to volunteer and come in as a captain under the Doctor's Draft or not volunteer, be dealt with under the Non-Doctor's Draft, and enter as a private. With these options I found myself an enthusiastic volunteer, working vigorously as a captain and orthopedic surgeon in Vietnam. There were a number of physicians in the Army who ranked significantly higher than captain. There is also a de facto rank within the Army which is found almost anywhere in medicine: on issues of medical leadership and decision making, the individual with the most training and competence in the area in question really outranks everyone else.

> We are on orthopedic rounds at the 85th Evacuation Hospital in Qui Nhon, Vietnam, 1966: the bedside of a young white combat injured trooper. The entourage at rounds is comprised of several doctors, nurses, and health assistants. The patients are being presented to me, the lowest-

> ranking officer (captain) in the group who happens to be an orthopedic surgeon (and black). I had just completed my residency training at Yale Medical Center and successfully studied for and passed the first part of my orthopedic board exams. Consequently I knew most of my orthopedics and "thought" I knew it all.
>
> During surgical rounds, with good meaning and in the interest of maintaining the highest quality of medical care for these patients, I found it necessary to disagree with, change, and therefore criticize some of the decisions and practices of my higher-ranking white colleagues. There was discussion and the alternative points of view appropriately had to be explained, justified, and documented. This was not done disdainfully or with disrespect, but in a way that was tactful yet matter-of-fact. However, I am a strong believer in the attitudes that Medgar Evens expressed when he said "We shouldn't be scratching when we don't itch and we shouldn't be shuffling and dancing when there's no music." Although I was aware of the possible mind-set of these white physicians in this tragic, stressful, military, multiethnic setting, I did not bend over backwards to apologize or protect their egos in these not terribly infrequent bedside situations. In reflecting on this situation, I realize that it must have been extremely difficult for some of these people to accept my criticisms, whether implicit or explicit. We know that many physician's egos cannot accept criticism even from their white professors; from a young black man, it must have been devastating. Even though I was not the least bit arrogant in this activity, I am sure that it cost me something, either through ill will or covert uncooperativeness.

This story reminds ourselves that the impact of our professional criticism feels more like a wallop for many of its recipients. It is up to you to determine how many layers of sugar coating, if any, you wish to put on your criticisms. Female physicians are obviously in somewhat of an analogous situation, although the white male recipient of your criticism has at least been criticized by many of his elementary school teachers, his mother, wife, or some other special female person. However, seldom has he been criticized by a black person in an intellectual setting. For them it is a new and unsettling experience.

The white physician has, through education and socialization, come to think something like this: "Black folks may be able to run, jump, play basketball, and dance better than I; but how can it be that this black person is not only teaching me medicine but is criticizing me for not doing something for my patient in the best possible way?" Many of you black readers have been or will be in the position of the teacher-critic. Why not give your white student or colleague the same respect you would give a patient? You can make your point through your teaching without creating an enemy. It will not only make you look good but often save you some trouble. Most of us do not have quite enough time to do what we have to do medically, so there is little benefit in adding to our inevitable list of detractors or creating non-medical problems to solve. Make your point as teacher or critic (if necessary), but do it gently and respectfully so as to the recipient's possibly racist attitude as their problem and not yours too. Of course, it would be nice to reeducate that person, but you must ask do you have the time and is it possible?

**Anticipated Responses**

One of my best psychiatry professors told us the following true story to drive home a point. When he had been a psychiatric intern, there was an extremely hostile patient in the corner of a cell who refused to eat for several days. Most everyone was afraid to approach the man with a food tray, because he had smashed a few trays, dishes, and personnel at meal times. Our good teacher expressed the opinion to all who were near that if the man were approached with warmth and concern, he would not behave with hostility but would simply accept the food without incident. The tray was prepared, our teacher walked up to the cell with a group of nurses, took off his glasses, and got the tray from the nurse who waited outside. He then walked slowly toward the patient speaking in kind warm, reassuring tones. The patient waited as the doctor approached and things seemed to be going very well. When the young intern got just within reach of the inactive patient he received a beautifully directed right cross to the left eye. Before the tray hit the floor, our teacher was out of the cell.

The point was that he had sent a signal to the patient that he anticipated violent behavior and he got just that. When he took off his glasses to enter the cell, he in essence said to the patient: "I know you're violent and I expect that you might hit me."

What does this have to do with coping and surviving as a black physician? When dealing with white persons or institutions *always* treat them initially as though they are good, fair, just, moral, and concerned. Continue to relate to them in that way until proven otherwise. This will help you tremendously to get on with problem solving and engender their cooperation and respect. This approach was used frequently with great success in the South by black people during the very difficult years of racial segregation and oppression when we did not have the kind of power that we do now.

When you approach a potentially adverse relationship with an individual or institution, do not assume that the individual or institution is going to treat you in a racist manner. Remember also that people do, in fact, tend to behave in the way that they perceive they are expected to behave. Assume that the individual or institution is just, fair, and reasonable and will behave in that manner; things will probably work much better. There is plenty of time to shift gears if that assumption proves wrong.

### What Color Is Your Jersey?

Learn to recognize your friends. Particularly in times of stress, do not allow yourself to fall into the error of assuming that there are not some loyal and supportive friends out there, black or white. They are willing to help you either because of their personal commitment to you or because of their personal philosophy about what is right and wrong and what to do about it. You must learn to discern who those people are and avoid the mistake of completely turning them off by assuming they are prejudiced against you. This prejudice is just as unreasonable and inappropriate as the prejudice that you may be battling.

### He Whom the Gods Would Destroy They First Make Mad

This is a quotation that was taught to me by my mother in Memphis, Tennessee, years ago. I think it is one of the most true and wise aphorisms that one could incorporate into one's life philosophy.

Take an example of outright prejudice and racism involving your career in a significant way. Fighting this with anger and hostility is not going to be in your best interest. If you can harness your anger and hostility and redirect it in a carefully worked out plan of attack, you are more likely to win. For instance, if that energy can be used to gather the necessary data to document your opinion and point of view thoroughly, then you are going to do much better. There are now a number of laws on the books and a number of established institutional mechanisms for the evaluation and appropriate rectification of similar wrongs. If you have the background and the track record to be fighting a battle within the medical context, you can fight with well designed and executed strategies. In other words, "don't hate, calculate."

### Affirmative Action: The Double-Edged Sword

The black physician says to him- or herself, "This sure is a great position. Did I get it just because I'm black?" Try this one: "That sure was a great position. Did I *not* get it just because I'm black?" If you are black and did not chuckle with sincere amusement at the irony of those lines, you are in a certain amount of trouble.

Take the first case: you do not want to work 25 hours a day at 110% effort to prove to everyone that you are five times as good as anyone else in that position. If you survived at all with such an attitude, you would be sick, divorced, or at least frustrated (in more ways than one). The obvious response is "what difference does it make?"

Get on with the business of doing your work in a thorough and competent way that satisfies your level of self-expectation.

In the second case, you have to make a simple judgment: How important is this position to me? What is the chance of getting a similar position in the near future? Can I *prove* that I'm more qualified than the person who got the position? Do I have the time, energy, and resources to fight this through the necessary legal and activist mechanisms? When you carefully, honestly, and objectively answer these questions, perhaps with a good and reasonable friend, your course will be clear. Then you can either fight or move on to develop your next opportunity.

Even if you think it through and decide not to sue or challenge, I believe you should persevere and keep working toward your goal and the position you deserve. My conviction is that, in the medical profession, those who have the abilities and do the work will sooner or later be rewarded by the system. The reward may not come the first time, and it may not be as full as it ought, but do not give up. If you give up completely and withdraw, or carry the hostilities and frustrations from one situation to the next, you have already penalized yourself.

Remember that you decided to be a doctor and not a civil rights leader. You should feel no more guilt and responsibility for not waging a civil rights battle in your professional life than Jesse Jackson should feel guilty for not treating patients. This is not to say that if Jesse Jackson can offer some first aid to a patient along the way during his outstanding work as a civil rights leader he should not do it. Nor is it to say that you should not speak up at appropriate times or organize appropriate kinds of "first-aid" or "emergency" civil rights activities from time to time. However, my suggestion is that you need not try to wage the social–political reorganization and reeducation of society within the context of your medical and health care team or your research environment. Concentrate on your work—that is challenging enough.

### Am I Having Trouble Because This Person Doesn't Like Black Folks or Doesn't Like Me?

How do you separate hostilities, disagreements, or outright conflicts that may be personal or situational with no racial prejudice from those that are truly racist? One can ignore the question and perhaps inappropriately assume that it does not matter, or that the conflict is due to racism when it is not, or that it is personal when in fact it is racial. On the other hand, you may agonize over which situation really exists and waste a great deal of time and energy trying to determine motivations.

Perhaps neither of these approaches is advisable. It is important, where possible, to determine which is best because your course of action will vary. If the problem is racism, then there will be no real solution: that is something that does not change easily, if at all. If the hostilities or conflicts are on a personal basis, they can sometimes be resolved either by compromise, adjustment, or change. When in doubt as to the type of conflict, sometimes exploring the very question of race with those whom we are in conflict can answer the question, or even help partially resolve the question. My suggestion is that we *ask* those with whom we are in conflict: not accuse them, but ask them. The answer, as well as the overall response, will go a long way toward helping you determine your most appropriate course of action.

**You're Good but You're Not Perfect**

This is addressed primarily to students, residents, and young people starting a medical career in practice or in the academic world. Sometimes we encounter Afro-American colleagues who seem to be pressured by an intense, almost pathologic desire always to have an answer and always to be right. Obviously, no physician of any ethnic or racial origin truly possesses these characteristics, albeit no small number may think they do. You should not allow yourself to become either defensive or depressed when this inevitable occurrence—being mistaken—comes to pass. Neither you nor anybody else knows everything. Your blackness does not require that you be more concerned than another about incidents, mistakes, or gaps in knowledge.

**Are We the Only Ones With Any Culture?**

Black doctors should not get caught up in thinking that we are the only people in the world with ethnicity, culture, or even "soul." Acknowledge and be respectful of the cultures of others, just as you would appreciate their acknowledgment, interest, and respect for our culture. If a Japanese friend likes Count Basie or Duke Ellington and you have the occasion to express your appreciation for Seiji Ozawa, do so. If an Indian friend likes Dizzy Gillespie and you like Ravi Shankar, do no hesitate to let that person know it.

Our goal is to live productively and harmoniously in a multiethnic society. To the extent that there can be mutual sincere appreciation expressed among the various cultures, that goal can be achieved.

**The "Sam" Incident**

The following story is an example of the kind of mistake one can make. Happily, due to sheer luck, I was spared the ultimate culmination of the error.

> I had a somewhat surly classmate in medical school. Although we were not the best of friends we certainly had no problems between us. How-

> ever, he referred to me over a 1- or 2-day period as "Sam." "Sam" is not my name. I had heard the name "Sam" used in a generic ethnic way when I lived in the South. (Need I say more to have you understand what I mean by a "generic ethnic" way?) In the South, years ago, blacks were called by their first names and expected to respond to the white caller as "Mister" or "Sir." If the black man's first name was not known he was conveniently called "Sam." Well, since I do not have a quick temper, my classmate was allowed several "Sams" while I contemplated both my defense and offense on this issue. (I shall not excite you with the options that were under consideration.) Just before my offensive was to begin and as a bunch of us were getting up to leave the lunch table, this particular classmate's girlfriend appeared. He greeted her with "How ya doin', Sam?" I had been taking offense at a totally innocent, albeit not the most clever or intriguing use of a slang expression. I believe that my classmate was in no way attempting to express a racist attitude toward me, but was simply using this appellation for all of his acquaintances. Somehow, I had not noticed it to be general, which it was, but taken it to be specific to me, which it was not.

If there is a moral to this story, it is that we must try to be sure that we do indeed have an enemy before we attack. None of us, black or white, can afford to create any unintentional enemies, particularly those based purely on our own errors in judgment.

**What About Our Patients?**

Of course, some of our patients are prejudiced. I do not know what it is about medicine—whether it is the service aspect of the job, the societal mystique, or an ingrown respect that physicians are still allowed—but all things being equal, patients are the least likely to express any prejudice overtly; there are exceptions, of course.

A number of friends and colleagues over the years have been the first black to show up in some given medical setting, either as the first intern or medical student; even under those circumstances there was a relative paucity of difficulties. I remember well a conversation years ago at Stanford with our esteemed colleague, the late Professor Sam Kuntz, who was the first black medical student to be admitted to the University of Arkansas Medical School. One of the points that he emphasized about his experiences there was that, although there were a few racial incidents involving patients, they were extremely rare. He recalled that by far most of the difficulties he had experienced had come from colleagues, including nurses and other hospital personnel. It has certainly been my experience throughout the years that patients who are approached in a forthright, professional, and empathic manner have rarely expressed any racial bigotry.

## Are Our Prejudices Better Than A White Person's Prejudices?

The answer is no. One prejudice that we sometimes have is mentioned because I believe that it can frequently be very counterproductive. Avoid this error in judgment whenever possible.

Do not allow yourselves to assume, consciously or unconsciously, that all whites are racists. Of course they are not, and perhaps only a minority is. You need not always wait for the other person to take the initiative to be friendly; this is used as a screening mechanism to rule out the possibility of having such a friendly gesture on your own part be rejected by a racist. If you do try to be friendly and your gestures are rejected on some kind of racial basis, there is very little lost. From your own individual ego and pride you should remind yourself that it is the rejector's problem and loss, not yours.

## Sensitivity, Compassion, and Empathy

One of the realities of the Vietnam war was that, all other things being equal, most blacks in the military got along a little bit better with the Vietnamese than did their white countrymen. This is not to be explained on the basis that people of partial African heritage and Afro-American culture "naturally" get along better with the Vietnamese who are of Asian-French culture; nor is it at all reasonable to assume that it's a matter of similar pigmentation.

My hypothesis is simply that it was because of the sensitivity, compassion, and empathy that oppressed people tend to develop. I think this may be a factor in the tendency for Jewish people to be compassionate and charitable and for women, for the most part, to be sensitive. Oppressed people become more cautious and are much more likely to be carefully attentive to the importance of paying adequate respect to the worth of other humans. Of course, there are exceptions on both sides of this sizable generalization; but my point is that the black physician can and should develop this potential and utilize it fully in dealing with patients. Treat them with kindness and respect and do not look down on them as inferior. There is a very important study (which ought to be required reading for students and residents) by a group of physicians which shows that patients treated for backache by physicians and chiropractors tended to like their chiropractor better: they treated them more as equals and with more empathy.[5]

Black physicians take note: your socio-political disadvantage has a potential advantage. Make the best of it. Draw on your sensitivities and concern for basic respect and equality of all human beings and transfer that generously to your patients.

**Brief Note on Begrudging Praise**

We praised and congratulated ourselves for our compasison and ability to express respect for all humankind. We glibly attributed this virtue to the psychology of an oppressed or colonialized people. Frantz Fanon[4] and others have described the in-group hatred and the tendency of colonialized or oppressed people to take on and exaggerate the attitudes of their oppressors. I believe that there may be a subtle form of self-deprecation that creeps into our behavior pattern. We, as black physicians, seem to carry a very high threshold for being able to recognize and lavishly praise, either in the written or spoken word, the talent and ability of our own. I have become aware of both poles of the continuum. On the one hand, the letter of recommendation from a black professional for a black student or professional offers such begrudging praise. The person or student may have done everything and may be a scintillating person, but you would never know it from reading the letter of recommendation or hearing a black colleague's description. On the other extreme, however, a Jewish person may tend to describe or recommend "their doctor" with such praise that you want to go to the phone immediately even if you are not sick. These are generalizations of course, but they make a point: when it is deserved, let us give each other a little more credit and respect and not be shy about telling black or white colleagues about an excellent student, resident, or physician, who happens to be black.

**Some Notes on Ethnocentrism**

Never categorically exclude yourself from the possibility of developing a mutually respectful and satisfying friendship or cordial relationship with any other human being. One of the most illogical and disappointing things that I have seen in universities is a black student *actively* deciding to exclude the development of genuine human relationships with individuals from other than black ethnic backgrounds. Often this pattern, developed in school, continues into one's postgraduate, professional, and personal life. To do this may be a reasonable philosophical decision, but it has significant liabilities. If we, as Afro-Americans, do this in the United States of America, we categorically exclude 90% of the population of this country in which we live and work. I believe that people who do this are deluding themselves and living in a fantasy world. If you become a physician in this country, you have made a decision to function somehow within "the establishment." We must use all moral and legal means to improve the society through change, but one cannot be entrenched in the establishment and still be a "revolutionary." Either you are in it or you are out of it. If you are in a profession such as medicine, do not kid yourself—you are in the society and the establishment. To participate in society does not imply that you agree with everything in the establishment. You have nothing to gain, however, by sustaining naive prejudices which prevent you from partaking fully of the fruits and the responsibilities of the established society. Mutually respectful, friendly relationships with people of other ethnic groups significantly enhances your potential to improve and enjoy, live and work in this multiethnic society. Some of your classmates and colleagues may in fact be future presidents, judges, governors, deans, senators, bankers, cabinet members, or newspaper publishers. The first American Pope may, right at this moment, be a classmate of yours: get to know her.

If in the United States there were a Black Gross National Product, Black Federal Reserve system, Black Senate or Congress, Black Military-Industrial Complex, Black Health Care System, and Black State Department, total ethnocentrism would still not be desirable: this Black American nation would have to interact with the ethnic groups of the rest of the world.

My suggestion, in sum, involves three basic points:

1. Respect, embrace, and enjoy your own culture and people as much as you please.
2. In addition, participate in your professional life as a person who will make friends, suggestions, contributions, and criticisms the same way any other good positive citizen would. Strive for excellence: this cannot and will not be ignored.
3. Finally, you participate socially with your professional colleagues and others in the dominant society. It is simply an important part of the way things work, for better or worse; it is no myth that the basis for a lot of "big deals" develops on the golf course. Also there are some people out there whom you will like and who will enjoy and appreciate you.

## The Game, the Rules, and Excellence

This little point is probably self-evident but I feel better expressing it: in your particular professional lifestyle, learn the rules. Look at the successful people in the field, white and black. Observe them and study the rules by which they seem to play. If you are not sure of a rule, ask someone who knows (part of the mentor phenomenon). Then, as you learn the rules, begin to play ball: play it hard, strive for excellence, and play it fair. Once you have won, there is time to try to change some of the rules if you like. If you get too involved and mixed up in trying to change the rules before you begin to play, you run the risk of the game being over too soon before you get into it.

## TO MY CONCERNED WHITE FELLOW PHYSICIANS

### A Note to the White Teacher

One of the most common problems of which I have become aware in speaking with medical students around the country is the old syndrome of the Invisible Man.[6] I am referring to the situation in which consciously or unconsciously the teacher on rounds or in small conferences appears to deny the existence of Afro-American students. Colleagues, let me tell you, this is devastating. Treat the black students the same way you do the other students. Interact with them. If you think they are shy and not speaking up, encourage them. If they are doing a good job, tell them so. If you think they are not working, give them a boot. If they are doing an outstanding job, help direct them into a highly productive career, the same way you would any other student. This is just as gratifying as helping anyone else, if not more so. Do not allow anyone on your service to be "invisible" (as described by Ralph Ellison, an outstanding black writer, in "Invisible Man").

I am aware of a number of white professors or teachers who have identified and encouraged black students. These students are often hungry for encouragement. The inspiration and productivity that is generated per "unit of encouragement" given a black student is tremendous and profoundly gratifying.

### The Beer After Work

You probably have not really thought about it, but much of what goes on at work is impacted by the "drink after work." In other words, you penalize yourself, your unit, and your black co-worker when you consciously or unconsciously exclude him or her from all your "working group" social activities. Your black colleague may well refuse a few times (they should not), but give them a few chances. They hold a position in your working group, so make the situation as productive and pleasant as possible. You may make a new friend and you will definitely improve your "team" by warmly including *all* your players.

### White Ethnocentrism

Fellow humans, guard against judging your Afro-American colleagues and students purely in the context of your own white American culture. Do not allow yourself to judge such a person against the norms of what you have come to know *culturally* as a good or ideal physician. This is simply not fair. It is suggested that in the noncultural aspects of behavior, all physicians should be judged the same: by his or her knowledge, how well it is applied and how carefully, how much concern there is for patients, and so on. We cannot, however, fairly judge the physician by the style of his or her clothes, provided they are clean;

the style of his or her speech, provided it is understandable; how "comfortable" you feel, provided his or her job is being done; how much he or she knows about Western classical music or English literature, provided that knowledge of human anatomy, physiology, and pharmacology is certain. A major problem for some minority individuals in the medical profession is that white colleagues tend consciously and unconsciously, to have spillover of cultural judgments into professional ones. The competitive black physician should be required to meet the highest standards of professional competence, but need not be required to "qualify culturally." For a black physician, who is highly ambitious and wishes to progress in his or her career as rapidly as possible, waiting for all our white brothers and sisters in medicine to read this paragraph and change their attitudes and behavior is not going to be satisfactory. It depends on your personal philosophy and priorities, but it would not necessarily hurt to allow some acculturation on the part of the ambitious black physician.

### In Summary

A few suggestions have been made here for concerned white physicians who wish to resolve some of the problems that presently exist. Obviously, there is a great deal more to be communicated to a concerned person in America who wishes to avoid racist attitudes and behavior. Such information, interestingly, is not in any well-known best seller. There are numerous workshops and sensitivity training programs available. Let me suggest for now, however, that you read this chapter with a goal of projecting yourself in the role of a black physician and attempting to empathize with his or her situation. Finally, on a more practical day to day basis, take care to treat your Afro-American colleagues the way you like to be treated. Work out your mutual problems with the care, caution, and respect that you employ in working with any human problem for which it is very important for you to achieve a just and lasting solution.

## CONCLUDING REMARKS

This chapter has attempted to offer some suggestions for coping in the stressful profession of medicine with regard to the issue of race relations. Race relations involve very intense personal emotional feelings and, of course, to some extent, political realities. However, race relations are very much human relations. Therefore, for the most part, the advice suggested here is based on human more than race factors. I have suggested that the *first* solution to most of these problems is to be approached on a human rather than a racial basis. If that does not work, it may then need to be escalated to a racial or a political level.

An excellent way to deal with the stress or stresses of human/racial problems in medicine is to follow the Oslerian advice, "Do today's work today."[7] This has proven valuable in several ways. Some units of achievement and its accompanying satisfaction continue to accrue. There is the therapy of diversion from frustration, and there is an effective humanitarian mechanism of channeling frustration and hostility into helping your patients. When you elect to fight directly, take the time and energy to design, plan, and prepare thoroughly for your actions. A well thought-out and designed plan of action is most likely to make you a winner.

It is at best very difficult and most likely impossible for you to fully control your environment or the attitudes of those around you. However, if you work at it, you can go a good distance in controlling your own attitudes and behavior. Based on this premise, I've made several suggestions you can work on to help you survive as an Afro-American physician. Strive for excellence. Seek to make a contribution to your profession in addition to your patient care. Participate in the mentor phenomenon. Don't waste time and energy on small scrimmages; save your human resources for the major battles and the wars.

There is another bit of advice that is worth mentioning and I believe it is implicit in much of what this book is about. We must not be reticent to seek counsel and help—psychiatry of course, if you need it, but that is not all I mean. The wise and experienced counsel of faculty members, friends, a person in another field, a classmate, or a colleague can be invaluable. I believe that many people in medicine have strong egos; certainly the public believes this. Sometimes these strong egos block the kind of communication, support, and catharsis that can be so important as we struggle with various problems, be they racial or purely human. Of course, try to solve your problems by yourself if you can, but do not let them fester too long unresolved and without counsel. No matter how composed a person may appear whether it be the Dean, the superstar surgeon, the president of the University, or the *bon vivant* orderly who seems to have it all together, all have problems that they have difficulty with at some time or another. None of them is solid rock; do not assume that you or anyone else has to be that way.

## REFERENCES


1. Cobb WM: The black American in medicine, J Natl Med Assoc (Suppl) 1981; 73:1183–1244.
2. Blackwell JE: Recruitment and production of black physicians in the seventies, J Natl Med Assoc 1981; 73:489–493.

2*a*. United States Bureau of the Census: Bureau of the Census Catalog, Washington DC, GPO, April 1980.

3. Stress: Medicine's occupational hazard? Harvard Alumni Bull 1982; 56(1):18–44.
4. Fanon F: The Wretched of the Earth. New York, Grove, 1965.
5. Kane RL, Olsen D, Leymaster C, Woolley FR, Fisher FD: Manipulating the patient: A comparison of the effectiveness of physician and chiropractor care. Lancet 1974; 1:1333–1336.
6. Ellison R: Invisible Man. New York, Random, 1952.
7. Osler W: "A Way of Life." Address delivered at Yale, April 20, 1913. New York, Paul B. Hoeber, Inc., 1937.

# The Physically Handicapped Physician

Attitudes toward the handicapped have varied markedly from one society to another and from time to time. In general, the handicapped were considered inferior to normals because they were though to have limited potential for contributing to their own or the common good. Fortunately, this is no longer the case and the handicapped, even though they are limited in some ways depending upon the nature of their handicap, are recognized as having the potential to be as productive as most citizens.

The natural progression of aging ensures that, sooner or later, every physician can expect to become handicapped. The handicap may be relatively minor, such as a slight loss in vital capacity where the doctor cannot walk or run as fast as formerly; or it may be that presbyopia at age 45 heralds declining abilities. However, few physicians who experience such physiological changes consider themselves truly handicapped even though they require spectacles or other artificial support. The term "handicapped" is usually reserved for persons with more severe disability. There are many subcatagories of handicapped physicians ranging from those who have been handicapped from birth to those who become handicapped after they graduate from medical school.

In this chapter, Dr. Spencer B. Lewis, founder of the Society of Handicapped Physicians, describes the restrictions placed on the physician with physical handicap and how handicapped physicians are made to feel helpless and vulnerable. He also outlines what can be done to help handicapped doctors.

Two months after he wrote this chapter, Dr. Lewis, a physically handicapped physician himself, died suddenly at age 34. Though he was diabetic and blind, he conducted an active family practice until he passed away.

*J.P.C.*

# 16

# The Physically Handicapped Physician

*Spencer B. Lewis*

It is estimated that there are approximately 18,000 disabled physicians in America today.[1] This represents 1% of all licensed physicians in the country. About a quarter of these are not working currently but with appropriate support could be rehabilitated to active medical practice. Unfortunately, few other statistics are available about handicapped physicians. Most of my information has come from personal contact and a survey of 30 handicapped physicians. Of these physicians the majority (84%) are engaged in active practice and 16% are retired. The income of this group is lower than that of the physician population as a whole because many of these doctors are engaged in part-time practice and teaching. Their age range does not differ from that of the general physician population, though their mean age is higher due to the inclusion of some older physicians who have disabilities caused by aging. Specialties in this group include psychiatry 16%, pediatrics 16%, family or general practice 16%, internal medicine 12%, physicial medicine 8%, occupational medicine 4%, radiology 4%, obstetrics and gynecology 4%, anesthesiology 4%, dermatology 4%, and emergency medicine 4%. The remaining 8% of respondents were medical students with no listed specialty. Notably absent from this group were specialties requiring exteme manual dexterity, keen sense organ perception, complete motor function, and some degree of stamina such as ophthalmologic and ENT surgery, plastic surgery, neurosurgery, and so on. Psychiatry, on the other hand, is probably well represented in our sample because its practice involves primarily the mind as a diagnostic and treatment tool.

The leading cause of disability in this group was visual impairment, which affected 28%. Other disabilities represented were paraplegia 24%, multiple sclerosis 16%, amputees 8%, CVA 8%, deafness 4%, allergy 4%, collagen disease 4%, and impaired physicians 4%. The point in the physician's career where disability was incurred had a significant effect on the type of specialty chosen, full versus part-time practice, and eventual retirement. The earlier the disability occurred, the more likely that psychiatry would be chosen as the specialty. Older physicians were more likely to continue their previous practice on a reduced or part-time basis or to retire. Newly licensed or practicing physicians were more likely to continue their present practice at the same or on a mildly reduced basis or to switch to psychiatry as a specialty.

It is important to remember that this sampling only included those physicians who consider themselves to be disabled. It did not include an even larger number of physicians who probably suffer some minor or unrecognizable disability such as hearing and visual losses which are correctable with aids, chronic diseases controllable with medication, and disabilities in progress of which the physician is not aware or does not acknowledge. It would be enlightening to have these other statistics available because there are few data about such partial physical disabilities. This paucity of information may represent a lack of awareness of the problem by most physicians and an attendant lack of interest.

To understand the problems, needs, and strengths of disabled physicians properly, we need to understand the problems better, and the needs and strengths of the disabled person in society as a whole. It is important to compare and contrast societal attitudes toward the disabled with those they hold toward physicians. It is also important to examine the attitudes of physicians toward the disabled and compare them with physicians' attitudes about themselves. A brief analysis of these varying situations helps to undertand better how the disabled physician is perceived by both society and by his profession.

## ATTITUDES TOWARD THE DISABLED

Society's view of the disabled is generally not a good one. First of all, the disabled person is seen frequently as an unwhole person, someone who through the loss of a faculty or faculties has lost a certain degree of independence and totality. He (or she) is certainly not perceived as the equal of a "normal" person for he is often dependent on others to assist him in the course of everyday living. He is often viewed as a burden on society and considered less productive than others. Consciously or unconsciously, the disabled person is often considered to be mentally retarded to some degree.

Many disabled persons find that others sometimes address them as they would an elderly or retarded person by raising their voices and simplifying their language. A disabled person in the company of a nondisabled person is treated often as a third or nonperson. One cerebral palsy victim reports that when dining out, the waiter asked her friend if it were okay if she had a menu. I am blind and more than one waiter has asked my wife if I wanted coffee or dessert. Worst of all (although it may be a blessing in disguise) was the drug salesman, who after learning I was blind, began to direct his sales pitch to my wife who assists me in my office.

Many people are uncomfortable with disabled individuals because of uncertainty as to how to behave around them, react to their disabilities, or best assist them. Most are sympathetic toward the disabled and often pity them. Unfortunately this sympathy is sometimes misplaced or misapplied when interacting with the disabled. A wheelchair-bound physician tells the story of a lady who dropped a quarter in his lap as she passed him on the sidewalk. This woman thought she had been kind and sympathetic; the disabled physician thought she had been uncaring and insulting.

Physician attitudes toward disabled persons do not vary much from those of the general public. As patients, the disabled represent failures of medical science; they are the people that medicine failed to cure. A physician's contact with a disabled person is usually limited to diagnosis and treatment and ends when the patient leaves the hospital. For reasons of sympathy and perhaps feelings of personal vulnerability, many physicians feel uncomfortable telling the disabled their diagnoses and that their disabilities are permanent. Doctors, however, are quick to encourage the patients with the fact that research is being done to solve their disabilities and that there will probably be cures in the future. They are less concerned about what the disabled are going to do *today* and often do not know where to refer the patients for rehabilitative and vocational training.

Most physicians do not encounter disabled persons outside their medical practice, as friends or social acquaintances. They almost never encounter them as colleagues. In fact, the disabled are placed in a world far removed from that of the physician, who most probably find it difficult to imagine the disabled fitting well into that one.

Society's view of the physician is almost directly opposite to the one held about the disabled. The physician is seen as a person with superhuman powers, perfect in all respects—mentally, emotionally, and physically. What practicing physician has not heard a patient exclaim, "You're a doctor, you're not supposed to get sick." It is an unwritten rule of medicine that physicians do not get tired, do not get ill, and do not become disabled.

Physicians are held up as some of the most respected persons in society. They are considered to be successful, productive, and valuable members of the community as well as respected community leaders. They are also perceived by most as having few emotional or family difficulties.

Physicians' views of themselves do not vary greatly from those just stated. In fact, physicians have often been guilty of reinforcing, promoting, perpetuating, and even enjoying these myths. Physicians certainly feel that they are tough, indefatigable, and indestructable. What medical student, intern, or resident does not remember being chewed out, even after working a 36-hour shift, for being tired, his or her judgment a bit hazy and thinking a little disorganized. Most consider themselves to be of more than average intelligence and economically and socially superior to the community at large. Thus, in spite of the knowledge of various problem areas among physicians (see Part Two), their attitudes toward themselves do not vary much from those expressed by the general public.

Deviations from the above "norms" are generally poorly tolerated. To illustrate this point it is only necessary to mention the current debate over whether the "impaired" physician really exists. This problem has been handled poorly by physicians and most efforts in this area have been punitive rather than supportive.

It is upon such a setting based on myth, ignorance, and prejudice that disabled physicians present themselves. They are disabled persons with all the attendant attributes but also physicians, whom people consider the epitome of independence, responsibility, and intelligence. This combination represents a contradiction in terms—physician who is disabled. I think this combination is more difficult for many physicians to accept than it is for others. It is probably difficult for most physicians to see a person who is supposed to be a patient and not even the equal of a "normal" person taking on the awesome responsibility of being a physician. It is very difficult for physicians to accept the fact that physically disabled persons can be the same as they—healers.

Most do not stop to realize that the physician's work is primarily mental. Most of the physical work in medicine is accomplished by others less skilled than the physician. In fact the physician's training is not directed toward physical development or stamina, but is geared primarily to developing mental skills.

Certain stresses are placed on any individual who suffers a disability and the physician is no exception to this rule. Physical disability has an impact on all areas of a person's life—emotional, physical, and professional, affecting relationships with family and others.

## SUDDEN DISABILITY

When disability strikes suddenly, the disabled person goes through essentially the same stages as anyone who has experienced a loss, be it the loss of a loved one, self-esteem, a faculty, or a limb. There are feelings of denial, anger, depression, guilt, and finally acceptance. Feelings of helplessness and dependence usually accompany the onset of disability. People who have been productive and independent suddenly find that they are less able to care for themselves alone. Their ability to function independently is greatly reduced; tasks performed, without thinking, before the disability occurred become insurmountable obstacles. For example, a person who becomes blind loses independence of movement and he either has to stay home or rely on someone else, a guide dog, or cane. Routine daily tasks such as eating, writing, cooking, and so on become impossible without retraining. One can but imagine how such a disability affects a physician who has previously exemplified the spirit of independence, achievement, and control.

Attendant to feelings of helplessness and dependence comes the feeling of heightened physical vulnerability. A person who has become disabled or has suffered an illness which has taken away a portion of his or her physical being often feels at great risk for further injury. Such feelings of special vulnerability can lead to a state of physical, emotional, and mental inertia which can make one an invalid. Also attendant to feelings of vulnerability is the knowledge that one is not indestructable and that one day one will die.

Shame and guilt are the constant companions of the disabled. One feels ashamed to be less than whole and not as perfect as those who are not so affected. One also feels guilty, responsible for one's disability. These feelings are magnified many times for disabled physicians because they "should have known better" and did not take proper care of themselves. Many may also feel that physicians who cannot take care of themselves can certainly not be relied upon to take care of others properly.

A sense of isolation accompanies most types of disability. The disabled person feels alone, as if the only person in his particular circumstance, though intellectually knowing this is not so. He or she may feel emotionally and physically separated not only from nondisabled people, but also from those having the same disability. The disabled tend to overemphasize their particular disability and put a great premium on the lacking faculty or function: If deaf, on hearing; if blind, on seeing; and if lame, on walking. Physicians probably magnify their disabilities even more, because of their great concern for competence and thoroughness, and feel incompetent in those areas of the physical examination they cannot perform, or perform with diminished capacity. Such feelings of inadequacy in these limited areas may easily extend to involve the entire field of medicine.

Competence presents the greatest obstacle to acceptance of the disabled physician by the medical profession. Other physicians, hospitals, nursing staffs, and licensing boards frown on disabled doctors. As with impaired physicians, these groups sometimes become more of an adversary than an aid. For example, one blind physician recounted that his colleagues wanted him to resign from the hospital medical staff because they could not see how he could perform a proper physical examination on his patients. Many suggested that he change his specialty from family practice to psychiatry. An attempt was even made by some to have his medical license severely restricted or even revoked by the state board. All these actions were taken in spite of the fact that this physician had never shown any incompetence, poor judgment, or questionable practices before or after he became blind. Perhaps the base of this problem of acceptance is the general attitude held about disabled people as well as the myths about physicians discussed previously. The automatic response to disabled physicians is to begin emphasizing those areas where they might have problems instead of noting their strengths and abilities and building on those. All physicians have strengths and weaknesses and tend to gravitate to specialty areas where the former are emphasized. The disabled physician should be expected to behave no differently.

## BARRIERS

The disabled are confronted, both in society and in medicine, with barriers to their independence. In many cases it is the environment rather than their own ability which prevent them from accomplishing certain tasks. Poor physical planning in cafeterias, hallways, nursing stations, bathrooms, and patient rooms serve to make disabled physicians appear even more disabled than they really are. These factors are well illustrated by the paraplegic medical student who had to be placed on a board and stood upright in order to reach the operating table. This was inconvenient for the nurses who had to perform this task, and for the surgeons who had to wait for it to be completed. It was also a source of embarrassment and humiliation for the disabled medical student.

The financial burden faced by disabled persons is staggering. There are hospital bills, expenses for travel and rehabilitative training, bills for assistance aids both for equipment and human aides, time lost from gainful employment, and higher insurance costs. Disabled physicians also face lower income than their colleagues because of the fewer number of patients they will see after cutting back in their practices. They will also have fewer hospitalized patients. Furthermore, there is added time away from practice because of their own need for treatment and rehabilitative training. In addition to the increased cost and difficulty of obtaining all types of insurance, they might also find discrimination from hospital staffs who claim the hospital faces a higher liability insurance because of them, though this fact has never been proven.

The impact on the disabled person's family may also be a great one. In addition to the aforementioned problems of finance are those of role changes that occur. The disabled physician, who has often been the chief breadwinner, most independent, and the leader in the family finds his or her spouse taking a greater role in all these areas. This involves considerable psychological readjustment.

One of the most burdensome problems faced by disabled physicians is the lack of rehabilitative, occupational, and counseling services available to them. Most agencies involved with the training, retraining, and counseling of the disabled are not accustomed or geared to providing these services to highly educated and trained persons such as physicians. A blind physician reports that he was offered training in sewing on buttons, communicating with sighted people, writing a proper business letter, running a vending stand, and keypunch. It was almost impossible for him to communicate to these agencies that he already had a profession and only needed some aid in performing a few of the tasks involved in it. Disabled physicians are often left to figure out for themselves how to perform some of the tasks of medical practice and to discover what aids, if any, are available for doing this. Personal physicians, the AMA, and other groups representing the various medical specialities are of little aid in this area.

## COPING

The means of coping with a disability are as many and varied as there are disabled persons in society. I feel, however, that there are certain common elements involved in all coping strategies. First of all there must be an acceptance of one's own disability and the vulnerability and dependence that comes with it. This is not an attitude of defeat but one of reality. One cannot constantly dwell on what has been lost, but must learn alternative ways of replacing it. Involved in this process is an actual self-accounting: getting to know oneself better, recognizing strengths, weaknesses, and potentials. Knowing this, one can begin to capitalize on the strengths and either strengthen or minimize the weaknesses.

Along with the acceptance of disability comes the acceptance of dependence. This is not a bad word, but something which everyone, especially physicians, should explore and accept more. The disabled quickly learn that life is a difficult road to travel alone and that they will need aids, both human and mechanical, to assist them. They must constantly remind themselves that this is not a sign of weakness: none of us can exist apart from the caring and help of others.

Rearrangements in the immediate environment are often necessary to allow the disabled person maximal independence. Barriers must be removed by widening doorways, installing ramps for a wheelchair-bound person, adding braille lettering on appliances for the blind, and captioning broadcasts for the hearing impaired. Similiar rearrangements in the physicians' office are often necessary.

Readjustments in the number and types of patients seen will also have to be made. Physicians with most types of disabilities find that there are certain portions of the physical examination they can perform only with diminished capacity, if at all. Such patients will have to be referred to or evaluated with the help of an able assistant. Physician assistants, nurse practitioners, and certified nurse-midwives are useful in this area. Someone the physician has personally trained or an assistant trusted completely, both ethically and professionally, is invaluable.

Seeing fewer patients allows a physician more time with each patient to take a more thorough history. A good history can often more than compensate for certain details of a physical exam and concentrate effort on those areas needing exploration. I cannot overemphasize the importance of letting each patient know, either before making an appointment or before being seen, that the physician is disabled and what that disability is. It may be further explained that this may prevent the physician from treating some types of problem and that referral might be necessary. I have found that complete honesty in this area is essential and will prevent further unforeseen problems in the future.

Patient acceptance is a welcome cornerstone in coping. I have chosen to discuss patient acceptance as an aid rather than a problem because I have found the great majority of patients are totally accepting of the disabled physician. Patients choose the disabled physician for the same reasons they choose any physician—caring and competence.

Disabled physicians bring a totally new dimension to medical care, becoming more than passive participants: they are active partners, fellow travelers with the ill. They intimately understand the pain, fear, and the helplessness that goes with illness and are able to bring this empathy into care for patients—in some ways, making them better physicians than their nondisabled colleagues.

The 1980s will see disabled physicians making a greater impact upon the medical field, due in part to the larger number of disabled persons choosing medical careers and more physicians being willing to admit disabilities and identify with the disabled. These new and old disabled physicians will probably be more vocal in demanding that the medical profession respond to their special needs and strengths.

Toward achieving these goals, I propose an organization for disabled physicians. This organization will have the following functions:

1. Promotion of unity, comraderie and support among handicapped physicians.
2. Education of the public and physicians about disabled physicians.
3. A newsletter to serve as a means of communication among disabled physicians.
4. Political voice in organized medicine and society.
5. Liaison with other organizations for the handicapped.
6. Admission, retention and support of disabled medical students.
7. Rehabilitative, counseling, legal and financial aid to disabled physicians.

These and other efforts will have to be made if the disabled physician is to gain full equality and recognition with other physicians. They are an asset too valuable for medicine or society to lose.

# The Homosexual Physician

Physicians are classically conservative and slow to release strongly held convictions. This characteristic has often served them well but on occasion it has impeded progress: almost 50 years elapsed before the value of Mendel's genetic discoveries was recognized; physicians who should have known better chose to ignore his findings. Similarly, in the behavioral sphere, doctors are slow to accept change. During the past two decades there has been a heterosexual revolution which some physicians have yet to accept; but there has also been a homosexual revolution which many doctors and society generally are even less ready to recognize. More "gays" are emerging from the closet and militantly letting it be known that they are homosexual. They have challenged laws that discriminate against them and had considerable success in that area. With these changes it is likely that more "gay" physicians will become apparent and will work, as they have always done, side by side with their heterosexual counterparts. Only now they will be openly recognized as homosexual. How "straight" doctors will relate to them remains to be seen.

To this day, the idea that a physician could be homosexual is anathema to a great many doctors. Although Kinsey demonstrated that 4% of males are hard-core homosexuals who eschew women all their lives, many physicians find it difficult to include doctors in that statistic. Physicians' attitudes toward homosexuality today may not be all that different from those of the doctor who wrote in the *Practioner* in 1954: "These unseemly explorations [homosexual experiences] during growth are better unrecorded; one would certainly get just as high percentages from the obliquities of other appetites, of gluttonies and pilferings. It would have been a cleaner world if Kinsey had stuck to his rats."

Clean or not, if Kinsey's 4% figure is accurate there are about 16000 male homosexual physicians in the country. The rate of overt female homosexuality is much less but also exists.

In this chapter Dr. David R. Kessler discusses the lifestyle of homosexual physicians and the prejudices and pressures that are placed upon them.

*J.P.C.*

# 17

# The Gay and Lesbian Physician: Unique Experiences, Opportunities, and Needs

*David R. Kessler*

## GENERAL BACKGROUND: UNIQUE EXPERIENCES

Gay and lesbian physicians are subject to many of the same stresses as other doctors, involving both the expected changes and unforeseen traumas of life. They are related to such factors as the specific life stage, past life experience and personality, and the particular attributes of the physician's role. For the gay and lesbian physician, however, there are some additional stress-causing factors that are unique to the homosexual's experience in our society. These include:

1. the process of *"coming out"* (the emergence and integration of a homosexual identity);
2. the need to deal with the negative value placed on homosexuality by themselves and by others (*homophobia*); and
3. the need to adjust to particular kinds of *relationship styles* that are prevalent among homosexuals but are viewed with disdain by most others.

### Coming Out

Non-gays generally take their sexual orientation for granted; for gay people this is rarely the case. Nongay people do not have to "come out": theirs is not a minority sexual orientation; nor is it devalued and stigmatized. People would not be surprised, much less dismayed, to learn that they or others were heterosexual.

The same is not true for homosexuality. In Western society homosexual behavior has been considered either a sin, a crime, or an illness.

Heterosexuality is thought of as "natural," homosexuality as "unnatural." There has been almost no cultural support for homosexuality. Instead, harsh punitive attitudes have forced most homosexuals to hide their true sexual preference from public view.

The world of homosexuality has been, and largely continues to be, a secret subculture. Although understandable, this has led to the development of unrealistic myths about homosexuals. The rejection of homosexuality has been exemplified in the phrases "the vice that dares not speak its name" and "the unspeakable crime against nature." The connotations have been so negative that to this day it is still difficult for many people to think about homosexuality, much less talk about it openly. So mysterious and hidden has the world of homosexuality been that most gay people have had a very isolated and lonely experience finding out who and what they are and how to live with the homosexual part of themselves.

***Childhood.*** The development of sexual orientation was studied in 1500 gay and nongay men and women in San Francisco during 1969–1970. Many predominantly or exclusively gay and lesbian adults reported that in their childhoods they already felt different from their peers. The boys were frequently reluctant to engage in the "rough and tumble" competitive team sports of their playmates. They often played with girls or engaged in more individual, less aggressive athletic endeavors, such as tennis, swimming, or track. Many of them came to be regarded as "sissies," or at least as less stereotypically "masculine" than their peers. They also began to regard themselves as nonconformist in their sex-role behavior. Most of the prehomosexual males were aware of homosexual arousal during childhood before ever engaging in any homosexual activities.

***Adolescence.*** Adolescence is the period of frequent same-sex attractions. Preheterosexuals, however, move rapidly toward greater sexual arousal and encounters with members of the opposite sex. Prehomosexuals, though, especially the males, experience ever-greater reinforcement of their same-sex arousal and behavior patterns. Many gay men start having gay sex encounters in their early teens. For lesbians this pattern usually does not become established until later.

Prehomosexuals experience other differences as well during adolescence. Those destined to be homosexuals report that their adolescent sexual feelings were predominantly homosexual. Almost all of them had been sexually aroused by another male before the end of adolescence. They were also much more likely to have engaged in predominantly homosexual activities in their preadult years and were more likely to have enjoyed such sexual encounters. For prehomosexual males the adolescent experience involved a growing sense of difference from their peers. They tended to be more alienated, less happy, and have lower self-esteem. In adolescence the prehomosexual males were also less consistent in their sexual feelings and behavior.

The childhood and adolescent patterns for women exclusively or predominantly lesbian in adult life are similar to those for their male counterparts. Prehomosexual girls, for example, are much more likely than preheterosexual girls to display childhood sex-role nonconformity. They engaged in typical girls' activities less, and preferred typical boys' activities more. More of them had worn boys' clothes or simulated being a boy. More of them thought of themselves as having been very masculine while growing up.

More of the lesbians described having felt predominantly homosexual and many more of them remembered having been homosexually aroused and having enjoyed their first lesbian experience during their teen years. More of them had had such an experience in their teen years, though only about a quarter of them rated themselves as having been predominantly homosexual in behavior, and 70% indicated that in their teen years they had not taken part in any homosexual activities. For many of them their homosexual encounters were presumably in the form of childhood sex-play. Prehomosexual women, then, were more likely to have had some type of pleasurable same-sex arousal and/or encounter while growing up than their nonlesbian counterparts.

Most of the lesbian women studied described their adolescent sexual orientation as predominantly heterosexual, although even more heterosexual women did so. More of the lesbian women reported an inconsistency in that their behaviors (social sex-role) were more heterosexual than their feelings. Adult lesbianism did not correlate with a history of decreased or traumatic heterosexual experience. Rather, as in gay males, homosexual preference seemed to arise with little or no reference to heterosexual feeling or behavior. It was the homosexual feelings that seemed to play the important role in the later development of adult lesbianism.

A few further words of clarification are in order. Not all boys who are "sissies" nor all girls who are "tomboys" invariably grow up to be predominantly or exclusively homosexuals as adults. Nor is it true that these traits are invariably found in the early life histories of all lesbians and gay men. About one-half the gay men were typically "masculine" while they were growing up, and one-quarter of the heterosexual men were not. During this same period in their lives, one-third of the heterosexual, and only one-fifth of the homosexual women, were highly "feminine."

***Fighting It.*** Homosexual arousal and behavior are seen negatively by our society. As individuals become increasingly aware of their own tendencies and impulses in this direction, there often is an understandable desire psychologically to deny the truth about one's sexual interests and avoid homosexual behavior. This stage has been called "fighting it."

There are various manifestations of this phenomenon. To counter the growing recognition of their homosexuality, some individuals attempt to remain celibate. Many men and women, on the other hand, throw themselves vigorously into compulsive heterosexuality. They may continue to date members of the opposite sex, continue to engage in heterosexual behavior, and may even get married and have children. About 20% of men who are predominantly or exclusively homosexual have been married. This figure is even higher for lesbians.

Such individuals may go to extreme lengths to avoid any possible association with whatever they think might remotely associate them with homosexuality. They may retreat from anything that might represent a homosexually arousing stimulus. They frequently attempt to obliterate their homosexual fantasies and impulses by the use of alcohol and other drugs, or by avoiding too intimate a friendship with a member of the same sex. They may seek psychiatric treatment, in the form of psychoanalysis or behavior therapy, for example, in order to be "changed." In extreme cases, a few such people may become outright gay-haters, or experience severe psychotic mental breakdowns. Some have become so depressed, agitated, and desperate that they have committed suicide.

Others in this stage may allow themselves to participate in homosexual acts, but only under circumstances that allow them to rationalize their behavior as not being "truly" homosexual. For example, many such individuals may engage in homosexual behavior only when they are intoxicated, telling themselves later that their behavior was not fully under their control. Men may engage only in impersonal or anonymous gay sex, such as at mens' restrooms or bathhouses, in order to limit the experience to a physical one rather than risking any type of emotional commitment.

Young men may engage in gay sex only in exchange for money, justifying this to themselves as their means of earning a livelihood. They may insist on being either the active partner in anal intercourse or the passive recipient of fellatio, and by means of this "insertor" role retain untarnished their sense of "masculinity." If married, they may have gay sex only when away from their spouses—for example, when out of town on business trips—doing so not only to minimize the chances of discovery, but also to be able to rationalize their homosexual behavior to themselves as being merely "accidental" or "situational."

There are some people, perhaps more so in recent years, who do not experience so much of this "fighting it" stage. These people progress relatively smoothly and effectively into the later stages of the coming-out process, or so it would appear. Others, less fortunate, may spend a lifetime in self-defeating conflict about their homosexuality.

*Coming Out to Oneself.* This is the stage in which there is not only a growing awareness but also acceptance of oneself as homosexual. At first, many individuals harbor the idea that they are the only gays or lesbians in the world, or at least in their locality. They do not know any other gay people or of the existence of any gay organizations. Later there is the growing need to make contact with others like themselves. It is at this point that many gay people leave their homes and families and move to cities where other gay people are to be found. For some, this may result from the rejection they have experienced when their sexual orientation became known to their families and friends. After a while, they became much more settled and consistent about their sexual orientation and interests, but also still feel very vulnerable and alone.

*Coming Out into the Gay World.* With the increasing openness of many gay people, meeting places, and organizations, it is now easier for a gay person to become a member of some type of gay community. He or she may establish a circle of gay friends and/or sexual partners, frequent gay bars or discos, or join any one of a number of gay groups. Once established in some part of the gay subculture, one can quickly gain access to other people in one's own community, and in other localities and countries as well. One can soon become part of an extensive, partly visible, but still largely underground gay network.

There may be a growing sense of being part of a "gay family"; one's interactions, outside of, or even within working hours, may be almost exclusively with other gay people. To the degree that this is true, one may be said to live in a "gay ghetto."

For many gay men, especially, this may be a time of active sexual experimentation. Frequent and varied sexual encounters may occupy a substantial part of one's existence. For lesbians, this is more often a time for seeking a partner and settling into a committed relationship.

*Going Public—or Coming out of the Closet.* This is the last stage in the acquisition of an integrated and positive gay identity. Outwardly, it involves revealing one's sexual orientation to nongay people, such as one's family, co-workers, or even the general public. These steps are best taken when one feels relatively secure and positive about oneself as a gay person, has weighed the advantages and dangers of revealing oneself, and has also considered the possible reactions of the others involved. When accomplished without anger, provocation, or flaunting, this step can be crucial in helping to integrate one's private and public existence and make possible much more fulfilling and intimate contact with others. One no longer has to hide, either inside oneself or inside the "gay ghetto." One is much more able to see oneself as a total human being who incidentally (or importantly) happens to be gay.

Not all gay people complete the entire process by going public. Most people who are generally referred to as "gay" have not necessarily revealed their sexual orientation to their families or in their work situation, although they usually are "out" in the gay world. There is no consistent age at which these various transitions occur. For some lesbians and gay men, it may be only after several decades of heterosexual marriage that they begin to "come out" to themselves.

**Homophobia**

Everyone growing up in our society, gays and nongays alike, is conditioned to have irrational negative feelings, thoughts, and behavior toward homosexuality. This is referred to as "homophobia." The details of the process by which this comes about need not concern us here, but the evidence of gay self-hatred and its consequences are important to our subject, and can be thought of as resulting from a chronic barrage of incorrect perceptions and ideas about what it means to be gay.

Our most powerful societal institutions have promulgated a very unfavorable view of homosexuality. The church warns us that homosexuality is a sin, contrary to nature, and an indicator of the moral degradation of society. The state passes laws making homosexual acts a crime. Medicine and psychiatry teach us that homosexuality is some type of illness or abnormality. Many psychiatrists, having had experience almost exclusively with those unhappy homosexuals seeking psychiatric help, seem to feel that gay people are, for example, emotionally unstable and are doomed to unrewarding relationships. These notions persist even though the American Psychiatric Association, after reviewing the relevant research data, concluded in 1973 that homosexuality per se was not a mental disorder.

Many people confuse sexual orientation (heterosexuality, homosexuality) with basic gender identity (maleness, femaleness) and are convinced that homosexuals really want to be members of the opposite sex. There is also the concurrent idea that homosexuals hate members of the opposite sex. This leads to the belief by some that gay men really want to be women and also hate women! A variant of this notion is that homosexuality is not compatible with gender-appropriate behavior (masculinity, femininity); thus, for example, "a real man" would never allow himself to have any homosexual arousal or activity.

Many people have the erroneous conviction that gay people are inveterate child molesters and recruit new converts by seduction.

Many gays and straights have been led to believe that there is one stereotypical way to live as a gay person, overlooking the great diversity of gay lifestyles that exist, although often hidden. Others hold the idea that individuals are *either* heterosexual or homosexual, contrary to the fact that sexual behavior and fantasy exist on a continuum.

In a more insidious form, homophobia is also evident when gay people are tolerated only if they keep their sexual orientation secret and do not "flaunt" it. Many gays have also accepted this attitude, without examining what this reveals about their self-worth. Many of them are unaware of the price they have paid for remaining, presumably comfortably, in the closet.

It is no wonder, then, that given the way they are regarded by others and have come to regard themselves, many gay people suffer from low self-esteem, depression, guilt, and self-hatred. They may feel extremely vulnerable because of their "secret" and may fear exposure and blackmail, which may interfere with choosing a career they want. In their social isolation they may become increasingly self-absorbed. They may tend either to deny their homosexuality or to parade it injudiciously.

Many of them lead a compartmentalized existence, in which their personal and professional lives rarely overlap. Because of their "condition," they may feel the need to isolate themselves from their families and colleagues, and may be reluctant to be actively involved in community, religious, or professional groups. They may be trapped in unhappy marriages as a cover. At times their self-disgust and pessimism may be expressed in a compulsive searching for anonymous sexual relationships.

For many people, there is a need to transmit something of themselves to future generations. This may in part be denied to gay people because of society's reluctance to have them function as parents or in other child-care capacities.

## Gay and Lesbian Relationship Styles

There is no one way of living life as a gay man or lesbian woman. There are at least as many ways of being gay as there are of being nongay. There are many false ideas about gay relationships, the most pervasive probably being that they cannot last—especially those involving males.

A comparison of gay, lesbian, and nongay couples is instructive. There are far fewer legal, societal, and institutional supports for homosexual relationships, and cultural guidelines are only rarely available: homosexual relationships are therefore usually more dependent on an extended friendship network. The two partners must establish their own mutual commitment to one another in order to stay together for any length of time. Another factor tending to instability is the usual absence of offspring in most gay households.

Gay, lesbian, and nongay couples can be thought of as being made up of two men, two women, and a man and a woman, respectively. From this standpoint a gay male couple is composed of two individuals, both of whom have been socialized into the male role. This represents a relationship demonstrating the undiluted effect of masculine values in our society. (It should be kept in mind that gay males have been culturally inducted into a predominantly traditional masculine *social* role, even though their *sexual* orientation may be atypical.)

Males in our society are generally expected to be autonomous, sexual beings. For two gay males to attempt to establish a relationship, their autonomous strivings will need to be hemmed in, and their sexual independence does not fit easily into the traditional nongay mold of monogamy. In gay male relationships that have lasted over many years, it has been found that sexual fidelity is usually absent, and, in fact, often appears to interfere with the viability of the relationship. Instead the couple operates on a "best friends" concept, with emotional commitment to each other and to the relationship, together with some type of sexually "open" arrangement.

Gay males, in keeping with their masculine social role, will often seek varied and frequent sexual activity with a variety of partners, without intense personal involvement. Sexual activity will not necessarily be tied to ongoing relationships, and may be short-term or purely physical. This is a style that lesbians and nongay women often find difficult to appreciate.

Analogously, a lesbian couple is composed of two individuals both socialized as females, and represents femininity, as expressed in relationships, in a relatively pure fashion. Traditionally, women in our culture are socialized to be nonsexual "nest-builders." Is it any wonder, then, that when lesbian relationships are studied, it is found that they usually last longer than those of gay males, and are more characterized by sexual fidelity, and, at times, fusion and symbiosis?

The nongay couple represents the blending, blurring, or conflict between the man and the woman, representatives of the two social sex roles. The elements of difference, mystery, and resistance, so common in nongay relationships, are frequently absent in gay couples. In same-sex couples there is a tendency for high rapport between the two partners, because of their similarities. This leads to an easy initiation of sexual relationships, but also to an early onset of either recognition of a mismatch or of boredom when sex is the key factor in the relationship.

## THE LIFE COURSE OF THE GAY AND LESBIAN PHYSICIAN

As we have seen, perhaps 50% of gay and lesbian physicians will have demonstrated atypical gender behavior as children. At least a substantial portion will have been regarded as "sissy boys" and "tomboy girls." The boys may have been more distant from their fathers, and both the boys and girls may have felt some degree of alienation from their same-sexed peers. Some of them may even have been explicitly stigmatized for their atypical interests and behaviors.

With the growing awareness of same-sex interest and arousal in adolescence, coupled with a lack of positive validation or role models, some who might want to be physicians may suffer increasing discomfort, fear, shame, and isolation, together with various types of overcompensation. During the college years, many of the men may have had some gay sexual encounters, and at least a few of them will have begun identifying themselves as "gay." Some will have emerged into a gay subculture, either overtly or covertly. To the extent that they had come to view themselves as "pathological" in some way because of their homosexual interests, they may have lacked motivation for pursuing a medical career, for which they might otherwise have been very well suited. If they have believed, for instance, that gays were child molesters, or were of necessity giddy transvestites, they may not have felt it appropriate to pursue careers as physicians.

Some of the dilemmas at this stage were well described by Dr. Howard Brown, in his autobiography, *Familiar Faces, Hidden Lives.* Dr. Brown was appointed as the first health services administrator in New York City in 1966, and in 1973 announced publicly that he was gay. He wrote:

> I had entered Hiram College on a pre-law scholarship, but in my last year there I decided to become a doctor. I reasoned that I could not become a lawyer because I found it hard to talk to people, a difficulty I attributed to the fact that I had a secret: "something is wrong with me." What exactly was wrong I did not know. I was sexually excited by members of my own sex, yes, but on the other hand I remained unconvinced that I was a queer because I did not find myself sufficiently disgusting.
>
> I applied to Western Reserve Medical School in Cleveland in 1943 and was accepted, but before I could matriculate I was drafted (then discharged a year later to resume my studies). Shortly before I entered the army, in a moment of panic, I took a train up to Cleveland to discuss my sexual dilemma with the aging chairman of the Department of Psychiatry at the medical school. He told me I couldn't possibly be homosexual. I was going to become a doctor, wasn't I?

> Homosexuals didn't become doctors; they became hairdressers, interior decorators, that sort of thing. He explained away my urges as "delayed adolescence."

When applying to medical school, the gay or lesbian applicant has to deal with the issue of whether or not to reveal his homosexual orientation. Most will go out of their way, when filling out the application form and in the face-to-face interview, to avoid giving any hint of their gayness because of their fear of negative consequences. Unfortunately, the attitude in most medical schools is such that this is still probably the wisest course.

Dr. Brown went on to note that in medical school he found a homosexual lover who felt happy with his life, but Brown felt that he himself was neurotic and perverted. When their relationship broke up over this issue,

> I marched off to the new chairman of the Department of Psychiatry and told him that I was a homosexual. This one didn't mention hairdressers. He counseled me to quit medical school at once and go into analysis.

In another example, a woman, on her application to medical school, listed a series of publications on lesbianism, but decided not to be open about her own personal lesbianism during her interviews. The Chairman of the Applications Committee, who had apparently been informed of the extremely favorable impression she had already created, assured her prior to the last of her scheduled interviews that she would be accepted. Her final meeting of the day took place with a faculty member who asked her questions related almost exclusively to her personal and sex life. Her application was later turned down. She subsequently learned from an inside source that the basis for her rejection was that she was a lesbian who did not regard her deviant sexuality as a problem.

What may happen if one does become known in medical school as a homosexual? One medical student revealed recently that after he had become active in various gay activities on his campus, he started getting "Dear Faggot" letters in his mailbox with obscene epithets and suggestions. Also included were photographs depicting sadomasochistic activities. Obviously upset and shaken by the experience, he was uncertain what to do. He wondered what sort of reception he might get were he to go to the Dean of Students with the story.

Because of these issues and others related to the stresses of coming out in medical school, he was feeling increased tension and difficulty concentrating. He decided to go to the Student Mental Health Center to seek psychiatric counseling. There a psychiatrist implied that his problem was due to his homosexuality and that this issue needed to be made the main focus of any future sessions. The student found this point of view unacceptable, decided to terminate his contacts at the Center, and instead sought help from gay-oriented counseling groups in the community.

Continued concealment carries disadvantages, too. In one instance, two lesbian medical students had become lovers and were looking forward to internship. They wanted to arrange to be matched together in the same city, in order to maintain their relationship. However, they were fearful of revealing too much to their internship advisor, who would also be writing letters of recommendation for them. In individual interviews with him, the two women responded to his questions by saying that they were not married and did not currently have any serious romantic involvement with a man. They did not mention their wish to be matched together. Their advisor then told them that, based on their superior performance, they should each apply to the best programs available.

For those medical students who are still "fighting it" or who are not comfortable about "going public" the consequences may be those of having to lead a double life. They often become alienated from other students and faculty who might be potentially supportive. Their perceived need to hide unfortunately serves to perpetuate the vicious cycle: Afraid to go public → no challenge to negative gay stereotypes → no positive gay role models → afraid to go public → and so on.

Thus, one Missouri physician, after learning at a recent American Medical Association meeting that there were gay doctors' groups in several cities, was heard to say that there might well be a few gay doctors in San Francisco or Los Angeles, but he was convinced that there were certainly no gay doctors in Missouri!

During internship and specialty training, physicians concerned about their sexual orientation may find themselves forced to withdraw even further from their colleagues or feign heterosexual interest. By now, more of their peers have either gotten married or are seriously dating, and the homosexual house staff officer may feel out of place if he or she is unable to join in with the usual heterosexual conversation or social activities. This may be the time when they feel secure enough to have come out into the gay world and have begun to establish homosexual and homosocial relationships, which most of them feel they need to keep entirely separate from their professional colleagues. This counterfeit existence and "double-entry bookkeeping," together with the ever-present fear of imminent exposure, can create an atmosphere of tension and fragmentation. Physicians at this stage in their career often already have involvements with the geographic area and the professional colleagues that they will want to maintain in the future. Feeling separated and alone during these years can therefore have serious personal and professional consequences.

After they have started their practice, many gay and lesbian physicians may feel the need to marry in order to hide their homosexual interests. Living with a homosexual lover would be at least awkward in most localities. Such physicians are faced with the choice of marrying, living alone, or moving to a large city in which their professional and social lives could be more easily separated.

Those who do get married may feel able to act on their gay impulses only when they are away from home. One successful orthopedic surgeon, for example, a gay male in his late thirties, lives with his wife, children, and in-laws on a large family estate. His wife, engaged in her family's business, presumably does not know about her husband's surreptitious homosexual activities, which are usually carried out anonymously in gay "cruising" areas. He is charming and successful, and has been maintaining this mode of existence for almost a decade.

In order to avoid detection, gay and lesbian physicians will often not join their medical or specialty societies, not attend their medical school reunions, and not be involved appropriately in community affairs, in contrast with their nongay colleagues. They may avoid these settings because of their fear of calling attention to themselves and having their homosexuality discovered.

Here is part of a letter, written recently by a physician, that exemplifies some of the internal and external problems of being both gay and a doctor:

> Writing this letter is both very difficult and very painful because it forces me to write on paper what I have said only once. I am a gay doctor. I am a physician in a field which is markedly homophobic—I am a pediatrician. Somehow it is all right for a heterosexual doctor to examine a teenage woman, but it is perverted for a homosexual doctor to examine a young boy.
>
> I am frightened of admitting my homosexual nature to my colleagues. I know of no other physicians who are gay. Perhaps if I knew someone who felt the way I do, I could cope better. I once came very close to telling my parents about my feelings. It was during a time when I was seeing a psychiatrist. I could not go through with it and I am no longer seeing this psychiatrist.
>
> I guess what this rambling letter is saying is that I am lonely, scared and in need of companionship. I love being a doctor but not a homosexual doctor.

The childbearing years are often critical ones for the female physician, faced with the painful difficulty of trying to reconcile a career with motherhood. A childless lesbian physician in her thirties had been raised in a stable middle-class family with the expectation that she would some day be a mother. Her lover had previously been married, and was raising her two children. In spite of the fact that the couple had a satisfying relationship together, for the physician there was nevertheless an inescapable sense of urgency and conflict regarding the possibility of artificial insemination, for which she sought counseling.

By mid-career, in their forties and fifties, gay and lesbian physicians may come increasingly to realize that time is beginning to run out. They may regret not having been true to their sexual inclinations. These thoughts about having missed something may be coupled with increasing homosexual urges and a deteriorating heterosexual marriage. At this time some of these physicians may become more actively homosexual and begin to live a more openly gay existence.

This often leads to a divorce from their spouse, often traumatic and costly for the homosexual physician. Lawyers representing a hurt, angry spouse may use the issue of homosexuality not only to secure the divorce itself, but to obtain as much as possible in the settlement. The financial and emotional revenge may lead to a smear campaign, as a result of which the gay or lesbian physician is forced to leave the locality and lose custody of the children.

One young pathologist in his early thirties, for example, found himself increasingly attracted to a homosexual way of life and finally told his wife about his inclinations. She became very upset, and a messy divorce followed, in which the gay physician's homosexuality was used to deprive him of his children as well as much of his savings and property. He was in considerable turmoil for several months, but then decided to leave the town in which he had been living and move to a city with a larger and well established gay community. There he became involved with gay professional groups, got another hospital position, and found a gay male lover with whom he moved in. Within a year he had established a new and successful life for himself.

Children may become the focus of the divorced spouse's resentment. One such case involves a middle-aged female internist with an 8-year-old daughter. She had her first lesbian experience when she was 40, and soon became able to acknowledge her homosexuality. She divorced her husband, but worried that he would vindictively try to gain custody of their child. Taking her daughter along, she moved to a small town across the country with her lesbian lover. All three now live together, and are attempting to protect their anonymity. The woman commutes to her office at a medical center in a large city nearby, and her lover has developed a drinking problem.

In other marriages, the spouse knows about the partner's homosexuality and covertly or overtly acquiesces in it. Although unusual, these marriages can at times remain quite stable for long periods of time. One gay male physician in his late forties told his wife about his homosexuality and about the fact that he had been seeing a much younger man in a nearby city for several years. She, a successful career woman, was able to accept the situation, and the couple moved to the city; there, the wife worked and the husband established a new practice and was closer to his male lover. Several years later this situation continued to appear stable.

These combined midlife and coming-out crises for gay and lesbian physicians can be rewarding, enriching, and renewing. For example, a gay male physician in his midfifties, whose physician-wife had died a few years earlier, began increasingly to accept and live his gay sexual orientation. Over a period of several years, he came out to his teenage children and to his in-laws, as well as to his professional colleagues, and received, overall, a highly positive response. He became very prominent in professional gay rights organizations, offered his expertise on gay issues at the medical school at which he taught, and found himself living an ever more well-integrated and productive personal and professional life.

For others, these combined issues may be fraught with much more difficulty. The outcome will be related to their characteristic coping style and their reaction to their homosexuality. For example, a highly successful gay male surgeon in his late fifties, had been absorbed almost completely in his work, with meager interpersonal relationships and a chronically unhappy marriage. He finally decided to divorce his wife, whom he had told about his homosexual interests. She was furious and used this information against him in her divorce action. The physician, because of his family and his religious background, felt guilty and uncomfortable with his homosexuality, but nevertheless began to pursue avenues of sexual exploration obsessively, as though making up for lost time. He squandered large amounts of money on young male street hustlers with whom he "fell in love," was rejected by his children and his family of origin, and found himself with no friends, gay or otherwise. He had closed his surgical practice because he was embarrassed to be potentially known as a homosexual in his small town and in the hospitals in which he worked. He spent all his time either alone, or in the company of the young boys he picked up, often drinking too much and quite severely depressed, wondering whether he had perhaps been happier previously in his miserable marriage.

With the era of retirement there comes the possibility for the gay or lesbian physician to look back with satisfaction on a productive life in a helping profession. There can be continued involvement with a lover, friends, and relatives, with either covert or overt expression of his or her gayness to all of these people. For others, however, there may be only continued or even increased social isolation, compulsive but unrewarding self-gratification, and little or no sense of investment in future generations in terms of children or other younger relatives, teaching, or creative work. For some there will be major problems with rigidity and loneliness, just as with the nongay or lesbian physician. However the situation may be exacerbated for the gay or lesbian physician because of his or her need to continue to hide.

An example: a gay physician in his seventies, was in poor health, drank too much, and lived alone. In his earlier life when he had been in the Armed Forces, his homosexuality had been discovered, and he had received a dishonorable discharge. Because of this, his future professional career was impaired, and it also led to his becoming estranged from his family. He found himself forced to work at medical positions below his level of training, withdrew from others because of his embarrassment, and started drinking heavily. After his retirement he became actively involved with a gay physicians' organization, which was his one source of outside personal and professional contact. In this setting he proved to be extremely engaging, intelligent, and witty. He died penniless, and had not been in touch with his family for many years. Funeral arrangements were carried out by the gay physicians' group and by a very small handful of other acquaintances.

## Other Specific Stresses

***Breakup.*** During the breakup with a lover, many of the issues and difficulties common to such an experience in nongay couples will also be in evidence; in addition, there will be some factors specifically related to the partner's homosexual identity. For example, the breakup may come to be seen as the inevitable consequence of homosexuality. One of the myths about gay people, as noted above, is that they are unstable, and that their relationships are doomed to failure. In the crisis over separating from a lover, a gay physician may succumb to such beliefs, becoming exceedingly depressed and regretful not only about the breakup per se, but also about his or her identity as a gay person. At such times gay physicians may consider trying to change their sexual orientation in order to avoid further "inevitable" disappointments of similar sorts. Increased distress will occur if the partners believe in the myth that gay male relationships are based on long-standing sexual, rather than emotional, fidelity.

The gay physician's self-hatred for being gay may surface and be turned into an exaggerated and irrational hatred of the ex-lover. This person may be seen as embodying many of the negative characteristics regarding homosexuality, which the gay physician has heretofore utilized in self-castigation. The gay physician may fear exposure of his or her homosexuality, which might result from an ex-lover's suicide attempt. In a recent instance, an unhappy former lover wrote to a hospital where the physician had staff privileges, revealing her ex-partner's sexual orientation. Because of such occurrences, the closeted gay physician may have reason to be concerned about emotional or financial blackmail on the part of an ex-lover.

***Death of a Parent.*** This may evoke some reactions specifically related to homosexuality, to the degree that one has negative feelings about one's own homosexuality and also subscribes to one or another psychological theory as to its cause. If an individual feels bad about his or her homosexual orientation, then at the time of a parent's death that parent may be blamed for having caused the homosexuality. A dead parent's sins of commission or omission may be mentally highlighted, which may interfere with the survivor's ability to deal with his or her grief. There may be guilt feelings at not having lived up to the parent's expectations in regard to marriage and grandchildren; or regrets may persist because one did not openly share one's homosexuality with the deceased parent, thus cutting off a major avenue of communication and intimacy that would have otherwise been possible.

***Vulnerability.*** The additional stress of being continually vulnerable to exposure as a closet homosexual has been alluded to before. Thus divorce actions or separations may be more problematic for gay than for nongay physicians. To the extent that a married gay male physician, for example, engages in various types of anonymous sexual encounters, he may be more prone to arrest, blackmail, exposure, or physical injury. Furthermore, a gay physician may be much more reluctant to seek health care for a possibly gay-related medical or psychological condition because of the fear of exposure.

## UNIQUE OPPORTUNITIES

There can be no doubt that homosexuals are subject to damaging psychological and social pressures because of society's negative attitudes toward them. These pressures often have undesirable consequences, many of which have been alluded to already. However, the challenges that homosexuals face may produce specific positive adaptations as well.

For example, a career in the health professions may be particularly suitable for gay men and lesbians. Being already "outsiders" in terms of society's norms for sexual and social behavior, gay people have greater potential for empathizing with the sufferings of others, particularly those of minority groups, and of ministering to their needs. A career as a physician represents the professional nurturing of others, and thus helps to avoid what might otherwise be excessive narcissistic self-concern. This latter state may result from society's forcing the homosexual into hiding, and from the absence of offspring or of societally sanctioned marriages in most homosexual relationships. Being undistracted by the responsibilities of married life can allow some gay physicians potentially to be of more service to others.

Many homosexuals have learned to "read" the reactions of others in order to protect themselves, and thus may have gained increased sensitivity to others people's negative feelings and attitudes. They may also possess a lively sense of humor, based not only on the self-contempt seen also in other oppressed groups, but also on the incongruity of who and what they know they are compared with what society believes them to be. Their "outsider" status often allows them to be acute observers and critics of society at large, and gives them a vantage point other than that of being totally immersed in their own culture and its values. The gay subculture would appear to be less rigidly stratified, and social class and racial barriers are much more permeable than in the nongay community.

Gay people are generally untraditional with respect to gender and relationship roles. More than nongay people, they tend toward an androgynous mixture of stereotypic male and female ideas, feelings, interests, and behaviors. With traditional gender roles being increasingly questioned in our current society, such a combination of traditional "masculine" and "feminine" attributes may be highly adaptive and desirable.

This discussion has perhaps tended to reinforce the erroneous idea that individuals must necessarily be defined as either gay or nongay. This overlooks the diversity of human sexual orientation, as substantiated by life experience and research data. If categories are needed at all, at least a third one, bisexuality, should be added. As an illustration, there are substantial numbers of "gay" and "lesbian" individuals who want to continue a basically stable and sound heterosexual marriage, as do the spouses. They manage to do that by means of various modifications of the nongay marital ideal.

In their freedom to experiment with a variety of relationship styles, gay people may be doing some of the "spade work" for society at large. Gay relationships are generally nonhierarchical and roles are not assigned according to traditional gender stereotypes. Nongay relationships often give more emphasis and importance to life-long monogamy and to sexual rather than emotional fidelity. These values are not nearly so strongly held by gay people, who may have much more freedom to experiment in constructing a relationship that satisfies their needs.

There is also evidence to suggest that gay partners may have a higher degree of sexual communication and satisfaction, and that there is considerably less fear of sexuality among gays than there is among nongays. In addition, gay sexual availability appears to be less of a problem, and because many gay men are "promiscuous" they usually have a greater interest in maintaining their personal and physical attractiveness.

## THE GAY AND LESBIAN PHYSICIAN AS PATIENTS: UNIQUE NEEDS

When the gay or lesbian physician is in need of medical or psychiatric help, certain factors will need to be kept in mind. One is the need for absolute confidentiality, in most cases, about the fact that the physician-patient is homosexual. Unless the gay physician indicates otherwise, the sexual orientation must be kept secret and not become a subject for gossip with colleagues, office workers, or relatives; nor is it something to be written into the medical record, where a secretary or someone who subpoenas the doctor's records may see it. The physician who discloses his or her gay identity to the treating doctor should not have to risk being discovered by others, with the possibility of disastrous consequences.

The physician may hesitate to reveal his or her homosexuality for fear that colleagues may be alienated by such information, and may then subject that person to moral pronouncements or insensitive care. Of course, not disclosing one's sexual orientation may risk failing to impart information crucial to medical or psychiatric treatment, and thus seriously impair its effectiveness. The treating physician needs to make clear to the patient that he or she is not only aware of the problems regarding confidentiality, but is prepared to deal with them adequately and in conformity with the patient's needs.

It is a truism to state that the treating physician should be professional, rather than judgmental about the patient's lifestyle, and should indicate full acceptance of the patient as a human being.

In any discussion of sensitive topics such as sexual orientation, a good rule is to give the patient permission to discuss these issues without attempting to pry or apply pressure. Awareness of a gay patient's possible fear, shame, and embarrassment will certainly be helpful. Some older persons may refer to themselves as "homosexuals," while often younger, more "liberated" people will refer to themselves as "gay." Most homosexual women prefer to be called "lesbians"; some will reject any such labeling. It is always useful to inquire as to what if any label the patient would care to apply to himself or herself. One will certainly want to avoid the use of such pejorative words as "promiscuous," "perversion," or "abnormal."

A treating physician should not assume that all patients are "Kinsey O" (exclusively heterosexual in arousal and behavior), since large numbers are not. Nor should one assume that because a patient is married he or she does not have extensive or even predominant homosexual interests. As much as possible, questions should be framed without any heterosexist bias. For example, it would be preferable to ask a woman "Do you use birth control?" rather than "What form of birth control do you use?"

A complete social and sexual history is obviously part of an adequate workup of any patient. In gathering a social history one might prefer to ask "Who lives at home with you?" rather than "Are you married?" in order to get at significant relationships, or "If you should become very ill, is there any man or woman particularly important to you whom I should involve in your care?"

One should try to inquire about the extent and types of sexual contacts and practices with the mental assumption that "everyone may have done everything." In bringing up the issue of homosexual behavior with very sensitive patients, one might think of saying, "Homosexuality is becoming quite open now. Many people have such experiences—perhaps you have?" or, "Some types of homosexual activity can cause medical problems. The more I know about what you do the more I'll probably be able to help you." One should also ask about any functional sexual problems, the use of recreational drugs, the use of any implements to enhance sexual activity, and other questions that indicate an awareness of homosexual lifestyles.

In psychiatric counseling, one should avoid expressing the opinion that homosexual behavior or fantasies may be "just a passing phase" unless there is very good evidence to substantiate this. One should be equally cautious about believing that all that is needed to reverse the homosexual interest is some satisfying heterosexual activity. If one subscribes to the idea that homosexuality per se is a sign of pathology, one may be tempted to make "gayness" the issue of counseling, irrespective of what the specific concern of the patient may be. One may also get into the position of promising a "cure" for the homosexuality—a goal which may be both irrelevant and impossible.

In counseling the gay physician, one will be involved in fighting the negative myths and stereotypes related to homophobia, and in carefully evaluating and forcefully counteracting their inroads, including self-contempt and social isolation.

One should try to work towards building a more positive gay identity: this would include exploring the possibility of further progress in the "coming-out" pathway, in appropriately timed stages. One could productively assess both the costs and gains of continuing to remain hidden as contrasted with those of coming out. Gay physicians in crisis will probably need encouragement to join appropriate gay groups in their communities, if such exist, or they can become involved vicariously (by mail, for example) with such organizations as gay physicians' groups located elsewhere. In addition, a gay physician's characteristic intellectual curiosity may be put to use by encouraging such a person to read gay history, research, and biography.

## THE PHYSICIAN'S ROLE IN FIGHTING SOCIETAL PREJUDICE

The American Medical Association has recently issued a report, adopted as A.M.A. policy, advocating better training and increased experience for physicians with respect to the health care needs of homosexuals. In a related A.M.A. publication, the need for physicians to act on a broader social scale to combat anti-homosexual attitudes is stressed:

> Societal attitudes, of course, can play a major role in determining how comfortable a homosexual will be with his orientation and can greatly influence the nature of his self-image. The empathic physician as a practitioner will try to help his homosexual patient achieve a positive sense of well-being and self-worth in the face of social antagonism while he strives as a health educator and community leader to eliminate the prejudice and stigma that cause so much personal anguish and suffering.

## BIBLIOGRAPHY

### GENERAL BACKGROUND

1. Bell AP, Weinberg MS: Homosexualities: A Study of Diversity Among Men and Women. New York, Simon and Schuster, 1978.

2. Marmor J: Homosexual Behavior: A Modern Reappraisal. New York, Basic Books, 1980.

3. Tripp CA: The Homosexual Matrix. New York, McGraw-Hill, 1975; New American Library Signet Books, 1976 (paperback).

4. Vida G: Our Right to Love. New York, Prentice-Hall, 1978.

## COMING OUT

1. Bell AP, Weinberg MS, Hammersmith SK: Sexual Preference—Its Development in Men and Women. Bloomington, Indiana University Press, 1981.

2. Cass VC: Homosexual identity formation: A theoretical model. J Homosex 1979; 4(3):219–235.

3. Coleman E: Developmental stages of the coming out process. J Homosex 1981/82; 7(2/3):31–44.

4. Gartrell N: The lesbian as a "single" woman. Am J Psychother 1981; 35:502–516.

5. Lee JD: Going public: A study in the sociology of homosexual liberation. J Homosex 1977; 3(1):49–78.

6. Troiden RR: Becoming homosexual: A model of gay identity acquisition. *Psychiatry* 1979; 42:362–373.

## HOMOPHOBIA

1. Position statement on homosexuality and civil rights. Am J Psychiatry 1974; 131(4):497.

2. Official Position Statements of the American Psychiatric Association in Precis Form, 1948–1975:46: Homosexuality; 47:Homosexuality & Civil Rights. Washington DC, American Psychiatric Association, pp 13–14.

3. Churchill W: Homosexual Behavior Among Males. New York, Hawthorn Books, 1967.

4. Malyon AK: Psychotherapeutic implications of internalized homophobia in gay men. J Homosex 1981/82; 7(2/3):59–70.

5. Weinberg G: Society and the Healthy Homosexual. New York, Doubleday Anchor Books, 1973.

## RELATIONSHIP STYLES

1. McWhirter DP, Mattison AM: Psychotherapy for gay male couples. J Homosex 1981/82; 7(2/3):79–91.

2. McCandlish BM: Therapeutic issues with lesbian couples. J Homosex 1981/82; 7(2/3):71–79.

3. Krestan J-A, Bepko CS: The problem of fusion in the lesbian relationship. Fam Process 1980; 19:277–289.

4. Peplau LA: What homosexuals want. Psychology Today 1981; (March): 15(3):28–38.

5. Peplau LA, et al.: Loving women: Attachment and autonomy in lesbian relationships. J Soc Issues 1978; 34(3):7–27.

LIFE COURSE

1. Brown H: Familiar Faces, Hidden Lives—The Story of Homosexual Men in America Today. New York, Harcourt, Brace, Jovanovich, 1976.

2. Coleman E: Bisexual and gay men in heterosexual marriage: Conflicts and resolutions in therapy. J Homosex 1981/82; 7(2/3):93–103.

3. Silverstein C: Man to Man: Gay Couples in America. New York, William Morrow & Company, 1981.

UNIQUE OPPORTUNITIES

1. Heilbrun CG: Toward a Recognition of Androgyny. New York, Alfred A. Knopf, 1973.

2. Singer J: Androgyny: Toward a New Theory of Sexuality. New York, Anchor Press/Doubleday, 1976.

3. Pleck JH: The Myth of Masculinity. Cambridge, The MIT Press, 1981.

4. Masters WH, Johnson VE: Homosexuality in Perspective. Boston, Little Brown & Company, 1979, chap 5, 11.

UNIQUE NEEDS

1. Altschuler KZ, Burchell C, Jerome EK, Kessler DR, Manahan WD, Owen WF, Peske ED: Facing homosexuality's medical issues (Parts I–VI). Patient Care 1980; 14 (Sept 15):17–86, 14 (Sept 30):48–93, 14 (Oct 30):68–143.

2. Dardick L, Grady E: Openness between gay persons and health professionals. Ann Int Med (Part I) 1980; 93:115–119.

3. Kessler DR, Owen WF: What a straight doctor should know to treat gays. Med Econ 1979; 6:123–134.

4. Owen WF: The clinical approach to the homosexual patient. Ann Int Med (Part I) 1980; 93:90–92.

5. Moses AE, Hawkins RO Jr: Counseling Lesbian Women and Gay Men. St Louis, The CV Mosby Company, 1982.

FIGHTING SOCIETAL PREJUDICE.

1. American Medical Association: Health Care Needs of Homosexuals. Chicago, IL, AMA, 1981.

2. Gadpaille WJ: Understanding the varieties of homosexual behavior. *In* Sexual Problems in Medical Practice, Lief HI (ed). Chicago, IL, AMA, 1981.

## Resources

ORGANIZATIONS

1. American Association of Physicians for Human Rights, P.O. Box 14366, San Francisco, CA 94114.

This group provides a physician referral service, information, educational programs, and speakers. It has members and branches in many U.S. and Canadian cities.

2. Caucus of Gay, Lesbian and Bisexual Members of the American Psychiatric Association, c/o American Psychiatric Association, 1400 K Street, NW, Washington, D.C. 20009.

This is an organization of psychiatrists that can be useful for information and referral, and also serves an important supportive role in helping gay physicians.

3. National Gay Task Force, 80 Fifth Avenue, New York, New York 10011.

The largest national gay organization, devoted to education and promotion of gay civil rights.

FILMS

1. Word Is Out (Mariposa Films).

In documentary style, traces the lives of a group of gay people. An excellent introduction to gay diversity, challenges, and coping styles.

2. Sunday, Bloody Sunday

A sensitive 1971 film directed by John Schlesinger about human relationships, with Peter Finch, portraying an English doctor, and Glenda Jackson both in love with the same bisexual young man.

# The Foreign Medical Graduate

The earliest physicians in North America, apart from Native American medicine men, were mostly of foreign origin. In the 17th and 18th centuries, European medical schools such as Edinburgh, Scotland attracted many American students who later returned and helped found some of the first medical schools in the United States. By the end of the 17th century Harvard was turning out medical graduates; it may be assumed that, given the tenor of the times, the relationship between foreign medical graduates and American medical graduates was sometimes uneasy. In those days, graduates from American schools not infrequently traveled to Paris, London, Padua, and Vienna to learn the latest surgical and medical techniques before returning home to practice. Many of the doctors who served and ministered on both sides of the lines in the Civil War were educated outside the country.

Thus foreign medical graduates are not a new phenomenon in America. Following World War II, there was a shortage of well trained doctors in the United States and foreign graduates were welcomed with open arms. Once the US government relaxed regulations and made it easy for foreign physicians to obtain preferential visas, many foreign doctors availed of the opportunity to come to America for training or to settle permanently. The Federal government recognized that the training of physicians was expensive: each American graduate had to be subsidized to the tune of $40,000. Foreign graduates saved American taxpayers that amount. This warm welcome of foreign medical graduates to America continued until the mid-1970s. Then, their reception began to grow cooler as the output of physicians from American medical schools climbed to 13,815 in 1978 from 6611 in 1960. In contrast, out of 14,476 new medical licenses issued in 1972, 6661 (46%) were given to graduates of foreign schools. In 1960, 1419 foreign medical graduates were licensed for the first time.

The reasons a physician leaves his or her homeland and

comes to practice in America are perhaps as varied as the number of foreign doctors in America. Some flee political oppression, others seek expanded professional opportunity, and still others search for a higher standard of living. In this chapter, Drs. Moises Gaviria and Ronald Wintrob survey a subgroup of foreign physicians, graduates from Peru, to ascertain the reasons they are working in America.

It is paradoxical, but the first medical school in the New World was founded in Peru, on the heels of the conquistadores, in the first half of the 16th century. The first degree of doctor of medicine in the Americas was granted there in 1551. Though the doctors in this study are Peruvian their responses to questions indicate that they could just as easily have come from medical graduates from Ireland, Israel, or India.

*J.P.C.*

# 18

# The Foreign Medical Graduate*

*Moises Gaviria*
*Ronald Wintrob*

In 1950 the ratio of American medical graduates (AMGs) to foreign medical graduates (FMGs) undertaking postgraduate training in American residency programs was approximately 10:1. By 1975 that same ratio was approximately 2:1, and approximately one of every two newly licensed physicians was an FMG.[1] The ratio of AMGs to FMGs practicing medicine in the United States in 1975 was 5:1 (that is, 366,000 to 78,000).[2] In most years between 1966 and 1975, the number of FMGs obtaining American visas was equal to or greater than the number of graduates of all American medical schools.[1] While these data leave little room for doubt about the importance of the numerical contribution of FMGs to the pool of medical personnel in the United States, there has been extensive and heated debate about the quality of their contribution to the American health care system.[2-6]

Another perspective on the issue of the increasing contribution of FMGs has been the political and ethical one emanating from the fact that, during the same 25-year period (1950–1975), the country of origin of most FMGs has shifted progressively from North America and Europe to Asia; from countries relatively well supplied with physicians to countries with health personnel shortages.[2] Mick has summarized this perspective: "Underdeveloped nations are educating thousands of physicians who ultimately end up practicing in what is perhaps the most developed nation."[1]

---

*Paper presented at the 132nd annual meeting of the American Psychiatric Association, Chicago, May 1979.

Concerning the quality of service provided by FMGs, critics point to (1) their relatively high failure rate on licensing and specialty certification examinations as compared with AMGs; (2) their comparatively high rates of practice in institutional settings, in positions which AMGs tend to regard as professionally inferior; and (3) their comparatively low rates of affiliation with medical schools and teaching hospitals.[1–6] These criticisms, along with the increasing numbers of new medical schools and expanded class size at both new and established medical schools, seem to have influenced the drafting of the Health Professions Educational Assistance Act of (October) 1976.[7] The Act has restricted immigration of FMGs by requiring successful completion of an examination equivalent in standard to Parts I and II of the National Board of Medical Examiners (the Visa-Qualifying Examination or VQE) *before* applying for a visa. Furthermore, the Act restricts the length of time FMGs are permitted to stay in the United States, making it particularly difficult to remain after completion of postgraduate training.

Against this background, we set out to determine the influences on career choices, and the professional and psychosocial adaptation of a subgroup of FMGs—those from Peru—who had completed their postgraduate training during 1964–1973 and had either returned to Peru or decided to remain in the United States to practice. At the time of our study (1974–1975)[8] there were some 600 Peruvian doctors in the United States; two-thirds were engaged in practice and one-third in residency training.[9]

The present report concerns a sample of those who determined to remain in the United States after postgraduate training, 50 of whom were interviewed by the authors in the Northeast, mid-Atlantic, and Great Lakes regions, where the numbers of all FMGs are comparatively high.[1] We focus on the professional, economic, and psychosocial factors that led to their decision to remain in the United States to practice. To understand the context of their decisions, we also include data on reasons for coming to the United States.

***Note:*** In reviewing our data, we must emphasize two caveats limiting generalizability. First, the sample of 50 physicians interviewed for this study comprises only 20–25% of all Peruvian physicians practicing in the United States who had completed their postgraduate training here between 1964 and 1973, and the sample does not include those practicing in the west, south, and southwest of the country. Secondly, the sample may not be representative of all Peruvians practicing medicine in this country in specialty distribution, proportion who are board certified, and proportion primarily involved in medical education. Data on these points were not available for the entire sample of Peruvian physicians in the United States.

## DEMOGRAPHIC CHARACTERISTICS

The age range of these 50 physicians was 26–50 years, with a mean age of 35. All subjects are men.* The study population includes physicians trained in internal medicine, surgery, pathology, psychiatry, obstetrics and gynecology, and pediatrics. Forty-five (90%) of these physicians had graduated from one of the two medical schools in Lima, Peru's capital city.

At the time of interview, 44 subjects (88%) were married, five (10%) were single, and one was divorced. Among the 44 married doctors, half were married to Peruvian women. Of the 22 physicians who married non-Peruvians, 18 had married American women during the course of their postgraduate training in the United States.

Forty-three of the 50 subjects had come to the United States on Exchange Visitor visas; 40 of them ultimately changed their visas to permanent resident status. Only seven of these 50 physicians came to the United States on immigrant visas.

Thirty physicians (60%) were board certified in their specialty. As shown in Table 1, those who were board certified tended to be involved principally in academic medicine, whereas those who were not board certified tended to be engaged primarily in private practice.

## DETERMINANTS OF THE DECISION TO COME TO THE UNITED STATES

Most of the 50 physicians in this study came to the United States primarily to undertake postgraduate training in programs they felt to be superior to those available in Peru at that time. Forty of them (80%) made this decision while they were in medical school or during their internship in Peru. The main factor that influenced their decision was the advice and/or example set by faculty supervisors who had them-

**TABLE 1.** PRINCIPAL PROFESSIONAL ACTIVITY IN THE U.S. OF 50 PERUVIAN PHYSICIANS

| | Academic Medicine | Private Practice | Hospital Staff | Total |
|---|---|---|---|---|
| Board certified | 15 | 11 | 4 | 30 |
| Not board certified | 4 | 15 | 1 | 20 |
| Total | 19 | 26 | 5 | 50 |

*At the time these physicians completed their medical degrees, approximately 90% of the graduates of Peru's medical schools were males.

selves taken postgraduate training in the United States. A second factor was the wish to undertake training in specialty programs not available in Peru; their intention was to return to Peru after specialty training and obtain a faculty appointment at the medical school from which they graduated. A third factor in the decision to go to the United States for postgraduate training was the anticipation that such training would be a valuable asset in terms of social and economic prestige when they returned to Peru to practice.

In only a few cases (12%) was the decision influenced by the physician's inability to obtain a satisfactory position in Peru after internship. The attraction of better-paid positions in the United States was a factor of limited importance.

The attraction of the quality of US postgraduate training programs not available in Peru at that time is further demonstrated by the finding that 70% of these physicians expected to stay in the United States for periods of three to five years: a time sufficient to finish postgraduate training, but not to enter professional practice here. Data correlating stage of professional career at the time of arrival in the United States and expected duration of stay (Table 2) indicate that those who came shortly after internship intended to stay five years or more; however, only three of the 50 physicians intended at the time of their arrival to remain permanently.

The decision to come to the United States for postgraduate training had a profound psychosocial impact on the physician and his family. Issues of separation from the nuclear and extended family were almost universally described as difficult and stressful experiences. Conversely, the wish to get away from turmoil within the physician's family was not a significant factor in the decision to go to the US. Nor was flight from social and/or political turmoil in Peru an important motivat-

**TABLE 2.** TIMING OF THE DECISION TO COME TO THE U.S. AND YEARS EXPECTED TO STAY

| Time of Arrival in US | Anticipated Length of Stay (years) | | | Remain in US | Total |
|---|---|---|---|---|---|
| | 1–2 | 3–5 | >5 | | |
| Immediately after internship | 2 | 13 | 10 | 3 | 28 |
| One year after internship | 0 | 4 | 7 | 0 | 11 |
| During the course of residency training in Peru | 0 | 6 | 0 | 0 | 6 |
| After residency training in Peru | 0 | 4 | 1 | 0 | 5 |
| Total | 2 | 27 | 18 | 3 | 50 |

**TABLE 3.** RELATIVE IMPORTANCE OF FACTORS DETERMINING THE DECISION TO COME TO THE U.S.

| Factor | Major Importance | Minor Importance | Negligible Importance |
|---|---|---|---|
| Superior quality of US training programs | 49 | 1 | 0 |
| Wish to contribute to improvement of medicine in Peru after completing training in US | 33 | 9 | 8 |
| Academic prestige of US training | 16 | 20 | 14 |
| Financial advantages of obtaining training in US rather than Peru | 14 | 13 | 23 |
| Social prestige associated with US postgraduate training | 10 | 18 | 22 |
| Avoidance of stressful situation at home | 2 | 3 | 45 |

ing factor, in contrast to other Latin American FMGs, such as those from Cuba in the 1960s and from Chile and Argentina in the 1970s.

The relative importance of each of the motivating factors is summarized in Table 3.

## DETERMINANTS OF THE DECISION TO STAY IN THE UNITED STATES

### Timing of the Decision

The majority of subjects made the decision to remain in the United States during the last year or two of their postgraduate training; 15 during residency and 17 during postresidency fellowship training (see Table 2). Seven physicians had gone back to Peru with the intention of remaining there, but ultimately decided to return to the United States to practice.

### Factors Influencing the Decision

Factors that influenced the decision to remain in the United States can be categorized for conceptual purposes into those that are primarily professional, economic, and personal.

Although nearly all subjects came to this country with the intention of returning to practice in Peru after their residency and fellowship training, most developed increasing doubts about their ability to have the kind of professionally stimulating life in Peru that they had hoped for. They were troubled by the comparatively disorganized or ne-

**TABLE 4.** PROFESSIONAL FACTORS INFLUENCING THE DECISION TO REMAIN IN THE U.S.

| Factor | Major Importance | Minor Importance | Unimportant |
|---|---|---|---|
| Concern about being unable to practice effectively because of the disorganized/deteriorating condition of the medical services system in Peru | 16 | 11 | 23 |
| Concern that Peruvian universities were in too much turmoil to allow for the development of an academic career | 11 | 14 | 25 |
| Concern about being unable to obtain a faculty appointment at a Peruvian medical school | 12 | 8 | 30 |
| Concern about being unable to do effective research in Peru | 10 | 9 | 31 |

glected state of the public, government-supported hospitals and clinics, and by the diminished level of support for the medical schools and teaching hospitals in Peru. As a consequence, their sense of commitment to contribute to the improvement of publicly supported health services and their wish to be affiliated with medical schools and teaching gradually became undermined. They became increasingly troubled by reports of government policy unfavorable to improvement in publicly financed health services and by reports of turmoil, demoralization, and resignations of highly respected faculty members at the medical schools. Those physicians planning academic careers in Peru became convinced that it would be impossible for them to obtain adequate funds or facilities to develop research programs. Letters from family and friends changed their tone from encouragement to return to Peru to advising caution and consideration of alternatives. As the reported problems of the major hospitals, clinics, and medical schools increased in scope and frequency—confirmed in some cases by visits to Peru and by attempts to establish themselves there professionally—these physicians came to the decision to stop thinking about returning to Peru to practice, and became permanent residents of the United States. The relative importance of each of these factors is summarized in Table 4.

Economic factors proved to be as important as professional ones in determining that these physicians would remain here. A central concern, one that was cited as a determining factor of major importance by half these physicians, was a fear of being unable to provide for the financial security of their families through practice in Peru. Closely linked to that fear was the concern that they would be unable to obtain

**TABLE 5.** ECONOMIC FACTORS INFLUENCING THE DECISION TO REMAIN IN THE U.S.

| Factor | Major Importance | Minor Importance | Unimportant |
|---|---|---|---|
| Fear of being unable to support the family in Peru | 25 | 9 | 16 |
| Concern about being unable to obtain a satisfactory position in Peru | 22 | 7 | 21 |
| Wish to save money before returning to Peru | 17 | 5 | 28 |
| Fears of loss of financial security due to socialization of medical practice in Peru | 13 | 8 | 29 |
| Need to provide financial support for family in Peru | 11 | 6 | 33 |

a position in either the public or private sector of medical practice that could dispel their fears of financial insecurity. To offset those fears, one physician in three indicated that a major factor in deciding to stay in the United States was a wish to save money to be relatively free of financial need at that indefinite, but distantly perceived time when the physician would return to Peru with his family to live—though not necessarily to practice. One physician in four expressed fears about financial security in terms of his anticipation that medical practice in the private sector would be steadily and drastically reduced as a consequence of government policy intended to socialize all medical services. Finally, some physicians decided to remain for reasons related to the need to provide for the financial support of family members in Peru. The relative importance of these factors is summarized in Table 5.

In the category of personal factors influencing the decision to practice in the United States, we found that Peruvian women married to Peruvian physicians were *more* likely than American women to express opposition to returning to Peru to live, as shown in Table 6. In some cases, the issue of what country the couple would live in once the physician had completed specialty training was discussed at length and

**TABLE 6.** PERSONAL FACTORS INFLUENCING THE DECISION TO REMAIN IN THE U.S.

| Factor | Major Importance | Minor Importance | Unimportant |
|---|---|---|---|
| Peruvian wife did not want to go back to Peru | 6 | 8 | 8 |
| Non-Peruvian wife felt she could not adapt to living in Peru | 4 | 6 | 12 |

was an important issue in the decision to get married. However, most physicians' wives in this study, whether Peruvian or American, tended to defer to their husbands' convictions about the professional and economic advantages of practicing and living here. In a few cases, the attitude of the wife in support of staying in the United States was adamant, threatening the stability of the marriage if the physician insisted on returning to Peru.

## THE DECISION-MAKING PROCESS

The decision-making process about whether to remain in the United States or return to Peru was complex, involving both "push" factors (mitigating against returning to Peru) and "pull" factors (encouraging permanent US residence) interacting over a period of several years.

As the process moved toward consolidation of the decision, many physicians reported a specific experience that crystallized or confirmed their decision to remain. The experience most frequently mentioned in this regard was a vacation visit to Peru as the physician neared the point of completing his training. The purposes of those visits home were both professional and personal, and discouraging on both counts. Eighty percent of these physicians had entered into serious negotiations to practice in Peru. However, their expectations that by a visit to Peru they could confirm details of a faculty and/or hospital staff appointment failed to materialize, promised positions turned out to be unavailable, or salary provisions proved to be grossly inadequate. Family, friends, and professional colleagues, though happy to see the visiting physician, could only advise him not to return to practice for the foreseeable future. The following comment was typical:

> When I was chief resident, I went back to Lima for a two-week vacation. My family had been putting pressure on me to come home, and so had my wife's family. I wrote to some of my teachers at the medical school to try to get a faculty appointment. They encouraged me to return to Peru, but couldn't promise a job. When I got to Lima I became convinced of one thing; that there was no way to be sure I could get a job at the medical school or the (major public) hospital. And with the salary they were offering, I knew I wouldn't be able to support my family.

Despite the obstacles, seven of the 50 physicians did go back to Peru to practice; but after a period varying from a few months to several years, they gave up in frustration and returned to the United States. At the time of their return to Peru, these physicians had not taken the Federated Licensing Examination (FLEX) that would have permitted them to practice here and needed to complete that requirement in order to establish themselves in a US practice.

Seventeen physicians indicated that a factor of major importance in their decision to remain here for at least a few years after specialty training was the wish to save enough money to enable them to be financially secure when they returned to Peru. However, having decided to stay on, some of these physicians—and their wives and children—became socially and professionally integrated in their communities, developing a range of commitments that ultimately made them change their mind about returning to Peru to practice, as the following comment illustrates:

> After I finished my residency training, I decided to stay here for five years to save some money and then return to Peru with enough money to buy a house and start a private practice in Lima. But the children have grown up here and my wife is not too enthusiastic about returning. She likes living here now and we have established economic security in this country.

## DISCUSSION

We have indicated that there has been a marked increase in the number of FMGs from Asian countries during the past 20 years, and a proportional decrease in FMGs from Canada, Europe, and Latin America. By the early 1970s, 70% of FMGs arriving in the United States were coming from Asian countries,[10] whereas those from Latin American countries declined to 5% of new entrants in 1974, though still comprising 16% of FMGs enrolled in US internship and residency programs.[10,11] It should also be noted that, by the mid-1970s, the majority of FMGs were choosing to remain here after they had completed postgraduate training. Between 1965 and 1974, the number of immigrant visas issued to physicians who entered this country on Exchange Visitor visas increased from a ratio of 1:30 to a ratio of 1:2.[12] As this trend toward permanent US residence became evident, the debate intensified about the wisdom of US immigration policy regarding FMGs and about the quality of their contribution to the US health care system.

Reviewing the data on the sample of Peruvian FMGs who have decided to remain in the United States, we find the following:

1. They came to the United States to undertake specialty training unavailable or comparatively undeveloped in Peru at that time.

2. They were attracted by the high quality of training programs at US teaching hospitals and were largely uninfluenced by political, financial, and familial problems in Peru.
3. They intended to return to Peru after their postgraduate training.
4. They came here on Exchange Visitor visas even though they could have readily obtained permanent resident visas at that time.
5. They were strongly motivated to contribute to the improvement of medical education and publicly financed health care services in Peru.
6. Most of them made the decision to remain in the United State during the last year of postgraduate training and following frustrated efforts to obtain a professionally satisfying position in Peru.
7. Sixty percent were board certified.
8. Thirty-eight percent were involved in medical education as their primary professional activity.

There was a close correlation between professional and economic "push" factors mitigating against practicing in Peru. Expressed concerns centered around decreased support or deterioration of publicly financed Peruvian medical facilities and medical schools. To understand the sociopolitical context of these concerns, a brief description of the Peruvian health services system is necessary.

There are five separate and largely independent systems providing medical care in Peru:

1. Ministry of Health facilities, which include many of the major hospitals and outpatient clinics in the country;
2. hospitals and clinics run by the Social Security Administration and financed by contributions of nongovernment workers and their employers;
3. the charity hospitals, publicly financed but not government administered, and comprising some of the country's major hospitals and clinics;
4. Armed Forces facilities, each service having its own system of hospitals and clinics; and
5. private sector care, comprising office practice and outpatient and inpatient facilities.[13]

These systems coexist with little coordination at a national planning level. During the past ten years, government spending on Ministry of Health facilities has declined, both proportionally in comparison with the budgets of other Ministries and in gross expenditure. Ministry of Health expenditure for maintenance and improvement of its facilities has been comparatively much less than Social Security, Armed Forces, and private sector expenditure. At the same time, the charity hospitals and clinics have experienced a sharp decline in financial support. Thus the country's main publicly financed medical facilities, its major teaching hospitals affiliated with medical schools, have suffered a deterioration of quality, both in services and in staff morale. Government policy has led to decreased support of universities, causing a similar decline of resources and morale. Despite eroded financial and policy support, enrollment in medical schools, which had been expanded in the 1960s, continued in the 1970s to produce an increased number of medical graduates. In common with their colleagues in other countries, most Peruvian physicians have stayed in the major urban areas where they undertook their medical education. However, the public sector could no longer increase its number of salaried physicians, nor could the salaries provided keep pace with inflation or with comparable salaries in the private sector. Competition for salaried positions at private clinics and hospitals became steadily sharper, while the available pool of people able and willing to support the private practice of medicine began to decline as a consequence of government policy and inflation. More physicians were competing for fewer patients in the private sector, and positions in major hospitals, clinics, and medical schools were fewer as well as poorly paid. The result has been fierce competition among physicians, leading to division, mistrust, and disillusionment within the profession, as well as underemployment and exploitation of many younger physicians trying to establish careers in hospital service, teaching, and private practice. Given these conditions, it is understandable that fears of being unable to obtain a position that is professionally stimulating and that pays enough to support the family have ultimately been dominant in determining the decision of these physicians not to return to Peru to practice. Added to these "push" factors are the "pull" factors of high quality and comparatively well organized (or, as many subjects described it, efficient) US medical facilities, the comparatively unlimited professional opportunities in hospital or office practice and in teaching, and the marked financial advantages of US professional life.

How do these findings compare with reports concerning US migration of physicians from other countries? A number of investigators have emphasized the primacy of the "pull" factors of practice in the United States that we have described for Peruvian physicians.[14–17] For example, Ronaghy and co-workers, surveying Iranian doctors in the United States in the mid-1970s, found that among the 35% ($N$ = 202) of respondents who indicated that they did not intend to return to Iran, reasons most commonly given were (in rank order) better professional facilities available in the United States, better employment opportunities in the physician's specialty, higher salaries, lack of job security in Iran, greater professional satisfaction, and better research opportunities.[16]

Many Peruvian physicians expressed concerns about the diminishing status and prestige of the medical profession in Peru and the declining morale of practitioners, not only because of the financial insecurities of medical practice, but because of the frustrations of trying to practice in conformity with a quality standard that was often not possible because of a lack of facilities, equipment, and trained and dedicated personnel, as well as the constraints of national policy decisions. These concerns, as well as the corollary concerns about increasing governmental control of medical practice leading to even greater erosion of professional gratification, provide an intriguing comparison with recent migration of Canadian physicians to the United States. In the case of Canadian doctors, concern about inadequate or deteriorating medical care facilities is a minor theme, but concern over government policy as it affects the task and satisfactions of medical practice is a major concern. Migrating Canadian physicians express dissatisfaction with the increasing bureaucratization of practice, feeling that there has been a sharp erosion of professional gratification.[18] They contend that national health insurance has increased demand for medical services for medically insignificant problems and that a sense of depersonalization has invaded doctor–patient transactions such that they feel overworked, professionally manipulated, and abused, while arbitrary restrictions are placed on their practice income. They feel that as far as private practice is concerned, professional satisfaction and comfortable standard of living are easier to achieve in the United States. The attitudes of these recent Canadian migrants stand in contrast to those of Canadian doctors who migrated here in the 1960s, for whom a principal attraction of US practice was the greater availability of research facilities and funding.[19]

The timing of the decision to remain in the United States has been the subject of considerable discussion among investigators of physician migration. Most physicians in our sample determined to remain after they had been living in the country for four or five years. Ronaghy et al., in the case of Iranian physicians, found that 65% who had completed specialty training did not intend to return to Iran, compared with 16% of those still in training.[16] Schmiedeck's study indicated that it took seven to nine years after migration before the physician's decision to remain in the host country became consolidated.[15] Schmiedeck contends that a primary motivating factor in physician migration is the stifling of social mobility within the established power and prestige structure of the home country, and that, "the greater the gap between professional aspirations and the opportunities for their fulfillment, the more likely migration (and resettlement) becomes."[15] The findings for Peruvian physicians lead to a similar conclusion.

A number of investigators of physician migration have emphasized the importance of marriage to American women in determining physicians' decisions to remain here.[14,15] By contrast with those reports, the findings of this study are that marriage to an American woman is *not* more likely to lead to such a decision. Neither did we find the converse to be true: that marriage to a Peruvian would influence decision-making in favor of a return to Peru. The women in this study, whether Peruvian or American, were about evenly divided in their preferences to live here or in Peru. Another striking finding, which we recognize could be a distortion reflecting a wish-fulfillment statement of the physicians interviewed, was that wives tended to defer to their husbands' feelings about the professional advantages of US practice.

Finally, the findings of this study bear on the crucially important subject of the quality of the contribution of FMGs to American medical care and medical education. The primary professional activity of half (52%) the physicians in this survey was private practice. In that group of 26 practitioners, 11 were board certified. This figure of 24% is significantly lower than the national average of 50–90% board certification across all specialties.[20] Nationally, 15% of all faculty members in American medical schools hold doctoral degrees (M.D., Ph.D., or equivalent) from foreign universities;[21] the proportion reaches 20% for M.D.s.[21] Nineteen of the 50 physicians (38%) in this study were primarily involved in medical education; 15 of them (79%) were board certified. This group included physicians at all levels of academic rank. Several had achieved distinguished careers in teaching and research. The correlation between board certification and quality of care provided remains an undetermined issue, but the intragroup difference in board certification between those engaged primarily in private practice and those at medical schools is striking. Intragroup differences of this kind have been a subject largely overlooked in studies of FMGs.

Addressing the issue of quality of service provided by FMGs from a somewhat different perspective, Feldstein and Butter have pointed out that of the 60,000 US residency positions in 1974, 54,000 were in hospitals affiliated with medical schools; that is, only 10% of all residency positions were at unaffiliated hospitals.[2] Most (70%) of the subjects of this study undertook residency training in programs that were university-affiliated. In a number of states, including several from which our sample of Peruvian physicians were drawn, more than 50% of house staff positions are filled by FMGs. This is particularly true in inner-city hospitals.[2] The deleterious impact of rapidly reducing the numbers of FMGs in those states and at those hospitals appears obvious, both in terms of the likely withdrawal of medical care from people served by those hospitals, and in terms of the functioning of the hospitals affected. It would be particularly unfortunate (objectionable?) that a reduction in FMGs would impact most directly on the patient population of inner cities already comparatively underserved in medical care.

## REFERENCES


1. Mick SS: The foreign medical graduate, Sci Am 1975; 232:14–21.
2. Feldstein P, Butter J: The foreign medical graduate and public policy: A discussion on the issues and options, Int J Health Serv 1978; 8:541–558.
3. Weiss RJ, Kleinman JC, Brand VC, Feldman JJ, McGuinness AC: Foreign medical graduates and the medical underground, New Engl J Med 1974; 290: 1408–1413.
4. Weiss, RJ, Kleinman JC, Brand VC, Felsenthal DC: The effect of importing physicians—return to a pre-Flexnerian standard, New Engl J Med 1974; 290: 1453–1458.
5. Dublin TD: Foreign physicians: Their impact on U.S. health care, Science 1974; 185:407–414.
6. Lowin A: Foreign medical graduates: An evaluation of policy-related research, Report NSF-C214, INTERSTUDY, Minneapolis, 1975.
7. Health Professions Educational Assistance Act of 1976 (PL 94-484), 94th Congress, Report N 94-887, Washington, DC, Government Printing Office, 1976.
8. Gaviria M, Wintrob R: Foreign medical graduates who return home after U.S. residency training: The Peruvian case, J Med Educ 1975; 50:167–175.
9. Haug JN, Martin BC: *Foreign Medical Graduates in the United States.* AMA Center for Health Services Research and Development, Chicago; 1971.
10. Graduate Medical Education, Annual Report on Graduate Medical Education in the United States, J Am Med Assoc 1973; 226:921–995.
11. Health manpower in the Americas: Basic statistics. *In* American Conference on Health Manpower Planning, Background Documents, Washington, DC; Pan American Health Organization, 1973, vol 3, chap 10.
12. Lockett B, Williams K: Foreign Medical Graduates and Physician Manpower in the United States, US Dept. HEW, Health Resources Administration Publication No. 74-30, Bethesda, Maryland, 1974.
13. Hall, L.T. *Health Manpower in Peru—A Case Study in Planning.* Baltimore, Johns Hopkins University Press, 1969.
14. Belsasso G, Laratapia H, Laratapia L: Determining factors in migration and adaptation of Mexican psychiatrists to the United States. A Mexican viewpoint, Amer J Psychiatry 1970; 126:1318–1321.
15. Schmiedeck RA: The foreign medical graduate and the nature of emigration, Psychiatr Opin 1978; 15:38–40.
16. Ronaghy H, Zeighami E, Farahmand N, Zeighami B: Causes of physician migration: Responses of Iranian physicians in the United States, J Med Educ 1976; 51:305–310.

17. Miller MH: The foreign resident as a disappointed person, Psychiatry 1971; 34:252–256.
18. Korcok M: 'We like it here' say Canadians practising medicine in United States, Can Med Assoc J 1977; 116:1308–1311.
19. Powles WE, Gysbertsen JB, Robertson JF: Migration of Canadian physicians to psychiatry in the United States, Part I: Dimensions and costs of the net brain drain, Can Psychiatr Assoc J 1972; 17:59–64.
20. Levit EJ, Sabshin M, Mueller CB: Trends in graduate medical education and specialty certification, New Engl J Med 1974; 290: 545–549.
21. Datagrams: Foreign-trained full-time faculty in United States medical schools, J Med Educ 1970; 45:185.

# Retirement

A physician faces three major choices in his or her professional career: the first is what specialty to choose, the second is where to locate, and the third is when to retire. Independent practitioners, if they continue to enjoy good health, can continue practice almost indefinitely. Not for them does an arbitrary age of 65 or 70 signify that they shall be active and industrious one day and put out to pasture the next. Physicians have more freedom in this regard than most. Having planned prudently, a physician may choose to retire as early as 50 or work through 80 and beyond. Given such a wide latitude and the current life expectancy, it is even conceivable that a physician may spend more time in retirement than in active practice.

Retirement is a decision that most physicians face sooner or later, and there are many knotty questions regarding it. They agonize over when to quit and how; they wonder if there will still be a place for them in medicine and what will life be like after they have listened to their last cardiac murmur or performed their last surgical procedure. Fiscal well-being is another area of concern, as is the prospect of a limitless ocean of leisure time that has to be filled. A physician who retires without proper planning may have exchanged one set of problems for another.

Life is filled with paradox and medicine is no different in this regard. The narrow confines of active medical practice may be the meat on which a physician thrives while the apparent unfettered freedom of retirement may be the poison that erodes vitality. Our culture values youth highly and looking forward to the future is considered positive. Looking back, like Lot's wife, is negative. What about retirement, the time of life when one may have more inclination to look back than forward? Can retirees continue to look forward and enjoy life? Must they think, like the old man in Zorba the Greek, that they will live forever?

In this chapter on retirement Dr. John Donnelly, a retired physician, addresses these and other issues.

*J.P.C.*

# 19

# The Retired Physician

*John Donnelly*

For most physicians in active practice, retirement is vaguely perceived as a distant time of life in which the busy pace of work will give way to the leisured enjoyment of the rewards of caring for the needs of others. That time is dimly envisaged as a period in which they will relax and enjoy doing the things they have always wanted to do; but unless they have a clear perception of what they want to do, they are likely to be doomed to disappointment. The future, after a few months of "relaxation" or "catching up on things to be done" appears to stretch out indefinitely with little or no stimulation or important objective, accompanied by a sense of loss and a feeling of uselessness.

Such is the experience of most active individuals committed to their occupation prior to retirement. Physicians are no different. When that time comes, the reality is so very different from the cloudy fantasies of the past. For many physicians, retirement, involving a complete break with practice, brings not a more fulfilling life but rather an empty existence with few aims and objectives. The steady routine of attendance at the place of occupation is shattered. The friendships and acquaintances so casually accepted as an integral part of life are rapidly disrupted. They just are no longer there. One's pre-suppositions may be far from reality.

Many physicians never seriously consider that they will retire: they have a sense that they will continue in practice as long as they remain in good health; since years of complete retirement will be few, it is argued, it is useless to prepare before that time ensues.

Not too long ago, there was a popular belief that the life span of doctors was less than the normal for the population. There was a common myth of the hard-pressed, overworked physician dying suddenly from conditions induced by the stress of this occupation. Just as the insurance disability premiums for doctors under 70 years indicate that physicians are a relatively better risk than average for avoiding incapacitating disorders, so the improvement in their life span has increased chances of several incapacitating infirmities in the later years of life. Those are the real years of retirement for many. Whereas most individuals in other fields retire at 65 years, physicians, by and large, continue to work past that age, albeit on a reduced schedule. With the average life span of 73–75 years for men, the average man spends eight or so years in active retirement. While their age of death varies greatly, doctors, on the other hand, probably have on average about four or five years to "enjoy their golden years" before the aging process imposes its limitations.

Like most individuals, then, the vast majority of physicians rarely contemplate or plan what they will do when they cease practice. As long as there is no chronological age of mandatory retirement, such as is customary in business and other occupations, the medical person is not forced to consider in a serious manner what to do when that day comes. It is a fact that most are involuntarily retired, not because of any societally determined chronological milestone, but due to ill health and aging—forces regarded as alien. Their whole lives have been devoted to defeating illnesses when they occur in others. How much more important it is, therefore, for physicians to deny their existence when signs of them appear in themselves.

It is, of course, true that certain external forces compel a reduction in professional activities. The typical medical bylaws of the hospital, which have long provided a workshop for the physician's practice, require a change of status and a reduction of privileges at a certain age, particularly for those in the surgical specialties. This is comparable with the rules of compulsory retirement in other occupations, based on age alone and not on competence; like those rules, it is founded on social values and principles established in decades past when life expectancy was significantly lower and when the preservation of physical health and personality functioning in the elderly were much less evident than they are today. When the average life span was substantially shorter than now, there were psychological factors at work in setting the arbitrary age for mandatory retirement at 65. One was that the working man, with so few years of his life left, should be entitled to enjoy those "declining" years. Another factor, which today operates more with regard to individuals occupying management and executive positions, is that the individual, by the mandatory retirement age (be it 60 or 65 years) has given his or her best and should step down to allow the younger breed the opportunity to make its own unique contributions to the success of the enterprise.

Due partly to an increasing recognition that large numbers of working individuals are as capable of continuing to work after 65 as before that age and partly because of economic and demographic forces foreseen to be operating in the near future (for example, a decline in the number of workers relative to the total population), the Federal government has extended the official age of the onset of vocational uselessness to 70 years.

All physicians recognize that the aging process in others does diminish the intellectual powers and physical capacities of the individual, but they are more conscious than others that this varies widely from one person to another with regard to age of onset, the degree of impairment, and the rate at which the latter progresses. When it becomes a necessity to confront the fact that they themselves are showing signs of such developments, the reaction is one of denial either that such exist or—if the evidence is incontrovertible—that there is any impairment of vocational functioning. By denial is meant that the individual does not allow the undesirable thought or evidence to reach the level of consciousness because of the painful emotion which would accompany it.

For physicians who arrive at the stipulated time of reduction of privileges, the loss is felt as a threat to their life-long pattern of work and to their self-esteem. For them, it is a major loss of status. For those who have not faced up to this coming change in status, acceptance is particularly difficult. Bitterness is frequent because they see the loss as rejection by their peers and deprecation of their expertise. For surgeons, for example, long accustomed to unquestioning compliance by others, to have to accept oversight by a younger colleague can be intensely traumatic.

Because the effects of the aging process are insidious in onset, physicians, as with nonmedical individuals, do not at first recognize their appearance. Not in themselves incapacitating, they carry the implication of greater difficulties down the road. A need to ask a patient to repeat what he has just said, a slippage in memory, forgetting to carry out intended small tasks, a stiffness in the fingers or swelling of the joints, a diminished enthusiasm to go to the office in the morning, and a greater sense of lassitude than hitherto in the evening—all or any one of these are what may be called early warning signs. These are harbingers of future morbidity, if not mortality: the omens of the time approaching when major changes lie only a relatively short way ahead.

How much attention is paid to these phenomena varies remarkably from individual to individual. Personal circumstances, such as economic situation and obligations, present and future, obviously are motivating forces. Personality usually is the determining element. Individuals who are oriented to and have practiced long-term planning for themselves and their families may approach retirement in a more precise and detailed manner. Individuals oriented mainly to dealing "sufficient unto the day" will usually brush the warnings aside, denying the desirability of standing back and taking a long, hard look at the future.

Confronted with these portents, most physicians tend to react not so much by refusing to face the realities of future infirmities but rather by underplaying the speed at which these may progress. Physicians are in a fortunate position compared with that of similarly aged business friends and associates who have been retired at a specified chronological age. Denial of their own mortality is reinforced by the comments of such friends who enviously tell them in casual conversation on social or other occasions, how fortunate physicians are because they can choose to go on working as long as they want and how desirable it is to be in such an independent position.

The ability and opportunity to enjoy a period of transitional part-time retirement is the ideal to anyone in any occupation, especially for individuals who preserve the capacity for activity, be this physical or intellectual or a combination of both. Such a transitional period provides a time in which to ease the harsh psychological readjustment from a fully scheduled pattern of daily activities to one of professional inactivity.

For doctors in private practice, especially those in solo practices, a gradual scaling down in the work load serves greatly to making the transition to full retirement a more acceptable process. When a working relationship with a younger practitioner is possible, the phasing out of professional activities is more easily accomplished. Time is gained for making an adjustment to retirement and the gradual rather than sudden establishment of a new structure of living. Similarly, those in group practice have the same opportunity to withdraw over a space of time.

A sad picture is presented by physicians who develop clear signs of the aging process and who continue, for whatever the reasons, to practice as though still in their prime. Even on a reduced schedule, they find their appointment hours become less and less filled. Old faithfuls still seek their attention but new patients and new referrals become increasingly less frequent and the issue of whether to continue to maintain an office becomes a significant economic reality. As reality is forced upon them the stress may be intolerable and result in severe clinical depression.

When progress to complete retirement is foreseen by physicians as likely to be a slow process, the desirability or advisability for planning a rearranged schedule of living is not so evident or of such immediate urgency. Since the readjustment from active work to none at all is usually a very stressful experience, this might seem particularly true for those who pursue a medical career in salaried positions. Such physicians are in the identical position as nonmedical individuals in business and industry. However, persons in employed occupations at least know (or, as the lawyers say, should have known) the specific time at which the change will have to be effected. Successful adaptation to retirement is made by most such physicians. Retirement for them may impose less stress because, by and large, they have been accustomed by the nature of their employment to separate themselves from their work at the end of each day and each weekend.

The degree of involvement in the care of patients, the pleasantness and compatibility of the work situation, and the psychological rewards from the work vary greatly and, accordingly, influence the ease of changing one's life patterns. At a recent medical school class reunion in England, the range of attitudes toward retirement was revealing. Approximately 60–70% of the class were gathered, not only from the United Kingdom but quite a number from such far away countries as Canada, Spain, South Africa, Malaysia, and the United States. All the physicians practicing in the British Isles either had retired within the previous year or would retire within the following one. Of those practicing outside the United Kingdom, all except one were still in active practice and fully intended to continue working. None of the retired UK practitioners regretted retirement; in fact, they were happy about it. Those about to do so expressed the general feeling that "they could not wait to put up their feet."

The contrast in attitudes toward retirement was striking. With regard to financial security in old age, none of the UK physicians had concerns of a financial nature because government pensions in the National Health Service are both generous and annually adjusted with the consumer price index. On the other hand, dissatisfactions with the conditions under which they worked or had worked were freely vented.

In the United States, for physicians in nonsalaried positions, financial security, especially in inflationary times (such as recently) is a significant source of concern. Unless they have laid out a long-term plan and foresee the means of maintaining the standard of living they feel appropriate in retirement, the motive to continue work is strong. Correspondingly strong is the motive to delay and postpone decisive planning for the time it will cease. An inflationary economy reinforces this still further because not only the cost of necessities climbs: the costs of avocational pursuits (e.g., country club dues, golf carts, theater tickets) also rise, often at a far greater pace than is compensated by increases in income from investments.

Dynamically oriented psychiatrists hold that individuals with obsessive-compulsive traits tend to translate anxiety about their security into acquisition and accumulation of economic assets. Of these, the most common, in addition to cash, have traditionally been in the area of stocks and bonds, real estate, and so-called "tangibles," such as gold and precious stones. It is generally assumed that physicians as a group are in the category of "asset-rich persons." Though varying with the vagaries of the national economy, stocks have been a favorite investment tool of physicians who perhaps are attracted to such instruments because they are the hallmark of the entrepreneur. Moreover, stocks are clearly defined entities with relatively precise attributes, such as price and earnings, information about which is readily available in the business section of newspapers. The interest of many physicians in the stock market is therefore founded on a number of psychological factors which, coming together, provide an avocational interest well-suited to them professionally, economically, and psychologically.

Following the market, periodic and frequent review of their holdings, and even some trading activity comprise a constant and continuing avocational pursuit for a segment of both active and retired physicians. In addition to keeping them abreast of their financial situation, this has another advantage: it keeps them "alive," in that the market is itself a fluctuating animal, the movements of which are closely associated with the physician's own economic and personal security, on a daily or monthly basis, and certainly on a longer-term framework.

The concept of personal financial security extends beyond the individual; also included are dependents, particularly the spouse. The welfare of adult children who are not yet firmly established in careers sometimes falls within the psychological ambit of causes of insecurity. Retirement for many physicians, therefore, does not always conform to the fantasy of a ripe old age in which responsibilities of the working years have been met and eliminated.

Periodic review of each existing will throughout adulthood is advisable in the light of changes in economic and physical health and in the situation of spouse and children. Regular review is also indicated by ongoing changes in the State and Federal statutes governing the disposition of the properties of a decedant. In retirement, periodic examination is equally important: many retired individuals have moved their principal residence to other states whose laws governing the taxation of estates are more favorable to the beneficiaries than those of the state in which they lived and worked.

Retirement also calls for careful review and reappraisal of the principles which have governed the management of one's assets. For example, a long-held investment philosophy based on long-term growth which was appropriate during income-producing years may well cease to be appropriate for providing maximal income plus security. Alternatively, earlier disposition of property by gifts, both appreciated stocks or other real property, to those who would otherwise ultimately receive it may be indicated. Estate planning during the period of retirement may call for reevaluation of one's long-standing convictions and biases—a psychological readjustment as sweeping and as difficult as stepping from full-time active practice to no practice at all.

For many retired physicians there is a kind of disposition other than a will to be considered. Doctors more than anyone else are very aware of the liabilities associated with maintaining life at a vegetative level, such as occurs with a lingering terminal illness in postcatastrophic conditions. Many physicians hold firm beliefs that the distress and purposelessness of mechanical maintenance of life is not for them and their relatives. They do not want to be needlessly kept alive by heroic measures or the use of modern technological advances. However, for reasons not difficult to understand, many who feel this way fail to undertake the making of a living will giving precise instructions to surviving kin specifying his wishes in the event such a condition should occur.

It is appropriate that such an instrument should be drawn when the individual is in a sound state of health, preferably even before retirement. If not drawn earlier and if the intention continues, action should be taken early in retirement. There are a number of good reasons for so doing. To make such a will requires confrontation with one's own demise, a confrontation easier to manage when the reasons for it seem far distant in time. The nearer the potential event, the greater the motivation, both conscious and unconscious, to avoid facing it. Further, the more evident that the individual was in a sound state of mind when giving the instructions the less stress is placed on the person having the burden of ordering the "pulling of the plug." Morbid as it may sound, consideration of future calamity and of its effects on loved ones is a wise concern of the retired physician from both humanitarian and economic standpoints.

Although the reasons for delaying retirement are often attributed to economic factors, such as loss of income and financial insecurity, other psychological mechanisms are more powerful, arising out of the role work has played in one's emotional well-being. The majority of physicians are dedicated to their occupation. For most, the practice of medicine is by far the most rewarding aspect of their lives; all other interests take a secondary place. Family life for physicians is well recognized as yielding priority to the needs of patients.

This devotion to work is not, of course, confined to physicians. Individuals in executive and management positions have responsibilities which they hold all important as physicians do theirs. Among them, it is not uncommon to find the so-called "workaholic" who spends all waking hours involved in work. Neither is it uncommon to find in the medical profession those whose sole purpose in living and whose source of gratification is the care of patients. For these physicians, no other significant interests or activities exist.

The majority of physicians manifest some aspects of the workaholic. Over the past many years, attempts have been made to elucidate personality characteristics to explain why different individuals select particular vocations, leading to the postulation of numerous theories, none of which is completely convincing. Nevertheless, some revealing information has emerged.

Perhaps up to 80% of physicians fall into the category of personalities who manifest obsessive-compulsive traits. This is not to be interpreted in a pejorative but rather a positive sense. All successful individuals whose work necessitates paying close attention to fine details require the attributes present in that kind of personality. These qualities include not only attention to detail but also conscientiousness, orderliness and the elimination of disorder, an ability to see relationships between objective phenomena, and a commitment to as near perfection as possible. Almost always these are accompanied by an abundance of energy and the drive to complete the task at hand. Clearly, these are attributes to be highly prized in physicians and no doubt are correlated with the reasons why doctors as a body are not only economically successful but highly regarded by their patients.

As with all personality types, however, this one has some not-so-positive aspects; for example, close attention to matters at hand is frequently associated with the postponement of decisions which do not have to be made immediately. One area in which this tendency towards procrastination appears most prominently in physicians is in the management of their own personal affairs. To these they pay far less attention then they do their patients, tending to delegate these responsibilities to others, as many a doctor's spouse will testify.

Humans are social animals due to the long period of dependency from birth to maturity. In adult life, they become creatures of habit, at least in a modern, highly organized society. The patterns of routine behavior become themselves almost the purpose of living, their underlying reasons obscured. The expectations of today are based on the experience of yesterday.

Relationships with others of similar interests provide for a structure and purpose for living. Physicians find such fellowship with individuals of comparable social status and educational and vocational achievements. Equally important, interpersonal relationships are more easily formed and maintained in the workshop. The physician's day is customarily a highly scheduled one. It is highly structured from morning to night, with visits to hospitalized patients, office hours seeing patients, and possibly home calls and emergency situations. This pattern is a continuous one.

A physician's personal identity, self-image, and self-esteem are largely derived from professional work as, indeed, is his or her social status. Feelings of personal security are intimately linked to the structure of the working day; when retired, the accustomed sources of major gratification are removed. Whereas each day was largely patterned by others (patients and responsibilities), retirement may bring endless empty hours, unless he or she has prepared for that time. Disruption (or cessation) of long-established behavioral patterns sometimes places chronic stress on the adaptive resources of the individual. This phenomenon occurs in adults at all ages but especially in middle age and beyond—for example, following loss of long-held employment with no prospect of replacement.

The life of a physician more than any other professional is a running series of relationships, each varying in intensity, with patients and their relatives, office assistants, hospital personnel, and other physicians. With retirement, therefore, there is not only an absence of the usual sources of self-esteem and personal identity, but also a destruction of the relatively fixed behavioral patterns which formerly organized daily routine.

Amongst the most persistent discomforts of retirement after an active working life are the endless unfilled hours, a condition more actively experienced by individuals whose energy levels remain relatively high. Sleep patterns do not change suddenly with retirement. Nor is the individual as fatigued at the end of the day. Waking tends to occur at the same hour as previously but, after the initial "honeymoon" of the luxury of lying abed is over, the absence of purpose for arising begins to impinge on awareness. Restlessness and boredom can be devastating in some persons, resulting in pervasive, chronic depressive feelings. These are manifested as a gradual loss of interest and initiative regarding any activity requiring effort, with an increasing disinclination to leave the home—and an increasing irritability in response to small frustrations. This irritability becomes a source of grave distress to the spouse.

Among other potential causes of emotional distress arising in retirement is one of "personal distance." This is a frequently recurring problem for retirees in general and one to which physicians are as vulnerable as others. Each person has a need to maintain his or her own unique identity. This includes maintaining a personal psychological space separating one from all other persons—a kind of envelope or barrier. This personal distance varies from individual to individual, but also varies in each individual with regard to the degree of intimacy with each other person—it is usually least with one's spouse. When this space is intruded upon by a second person, a sense of discomfort may be produced, and frequent discomfort leads to irritation. Thus, a very private individual requires considerably more distance than a backslapping extrovert.

The degree of personal distance also varies from time to time with each individual, sometimes depending on how engrossed one is with a task or activity. Even with another to whom one is devoted, intrusion by that individual is liable to occur when much time is spent together.

The significance of this in retirement lies in the inescapable situation of two people who have previously led lives during which the greatest proportion of waking hours has been spent apart from each other. Withdrawal from active practice inevitably results in great amounts of time together being added to that which was customary and routine. Among the spouses of retired persons, there is the old saw "for better or for worse, for breakfast and for dinner, but not for lunch!" This epitomizes the occasions for minor frictions which, previously relatively spread out in terms of frequency, become greatly increased in number, as the intervals between the occasions during which irritations subside become shorter in length. This is especially so when the physician whose work kept him absent during the day now spends long stretches of time at home.

With some physicians, this may be an even greater problem than for the average retiree; or perhaps one should say that it is a greater problem for the spouse of the physician who has not enough to occupy the new free hours. Spouses of physicians, by and large, are a very patient group of individuals. Whether because of personality development from infancy or whether from having learned to adjust to the demands of the work of a doctor, they accept infringements on their lives as the price to be paid for their lot in life. Physicians, on the other hand, are long accustomed—at least until recently—to having their demands accepted by others as though this were the natural law. Their occupational responsibilities require conformity with their orders and requests by those who work with them.

For the physician's spouse, retirement carries the implication of major changes in that those priorities which were all important now become secondary to coping with the physician–mate. Most spouses believe that retirement will bring greater personal equality. The physician, at least at first, may find it difficult to adapt to this change. Partly because of increasing rigidity in dealing with situations, which is the accompaniment of the aging process, the physician may be prone to react in a negative fashion to infringement on the usual way of doing things. The spouse, on the other hand, has in a manner of speaking postponed gratification of many needs for so many years and anticipated fulfillment of them at this stage in life; not infrequently, the envisaged El Dorado is as far away as ever.

This situation is particularly likely to arise in the case of individuals whose range of interests other than work is nil and whose satisfactions have been derived almost completely from it. In retirement, they have no alternative for the satisfaction of emotional needs other than to turn to their spouses, manifested by constant demands with behavior such as following them around the home and leaving little time for them to be alone. For the spouse who has survived because of an ability to accept the physician's absence, this can be a frequent source of considerable stress. It is not as though physicians are always totally passive and dependent on their spouses; other times, they expect their other needs to be gratified even if the occasion does not fit in with their spouses' immediate commitments.

The reverse side of this situation arises when retirees have a totally absorbing interest which they pursue with all their concentration and energies: spouses who have developed routines to make their lives acceptable, find their interests are not taken as important, and react in frustration. For example, the wife of a retired male physician may derive a satisfaction in her creative efforts in such simple routines as preparing meals. Failure of the husband to come promptly to the table while the food is warm and (especially after repeated calls) turns potential gratification into irritation. A frequent adaptive pattern to repeated experiences of this kind is to develop an isolation within oneself, inevitably creating an emotional self-protective barrier which extends into other areas of the relationship.

The enjoyment of the years of retirement determine one's feelings of personal security to which good health and sufficient financial resources contribute. However, these in themselves do not provide satisfaction of the psychological needs created by withdrawal from medical practice; if anything, they accentuate those needs.

Retirement for physicians brings fundamentally the same options as those for individuals in executive and comparable positions. Whether or not the path of gradual retirement may be taken by doctors, there arises suddenly or gradually a great number of hours in the average day during which he or she must find a suitable and satisfying occupation in which to engage. Many retired business executives have found rewarding activity in acting as volunteer consultants to small or new businesses. Volunteering direct patient medical services by physicians is limited for several reasons: one may well be the feelings of loss of professional status in most situations where volunteering might be possible. Further, in the litigous climate of today, there is the ever-present and discouraging possibility of a malpractice suit. Even when there are no grounds for an action, the fact that the physician is retired places him or her in a vulnerable position.

Opportunities for part-time work do arise, however, especially in metropolitan areas. Many of these call for medical expertise and are without the limitations indicated above. When available, they are of inestimable value to the physician who needs to maintain a medical identity. Those individuals who have established and maintained broad interests throughout their lives are well situated to enjoy retirement, for these provide opportunities to make use of their abilities in a purposeful and gratifying way. With regard to physicians, when these activities involve benefiting other individuals, the satisfaction is doubly rewarding. For the individual, they provide an emotional continuum of gratifying action, bridging the disruption of the patterns of adaptation which occur on cessation of practice. Thus, those practitioners who are able to achieve gratification through teaching or medical writing often are able to pursue such activities with a rewarding sense of continuity in their contributions to medical science. For others, frequent or regular attendance at medical society meetings offers a sense of professional continuity, as well as a source of maintaining professional and social relationships; unless these activities have been followed prior to retirement, they are not likely to be very satisfying.

For the physically preserved, foreign travel has increasingly provided stimulation for those no longer confined by heavy duty schedules. One opportunity for travel, which has increased rapidly in the recent years, combines medical seminars with trips to foreign lands. County and state medical societies and auxiliaries are now undertaking sponsorships of such ventures. For many retired and semiretired physicians, they have filled a void, providing stimulation in ways not otherwise easily achieved. Foreign travel, especially in congenial groups, appeals to individuals endowed with a sense of curiosity, an inquiring mind, and abundant energy, attributes shared by many physicians. Organized in parallel with medical meetings, they offer opportunities for professional contacts and keeping up with progress in the field. However, for a variety of reasons including economic, even when there is interest, travel is not a sufficient answer: such trips rarely are greater in length than two or three weeks.

For most retired physicians, success comes from structuring life to involve intellectual and physical activity, to replace the patterns of medical practice. The level of content depends to the greatest degree on the pursuit of interests that are meaningful to the individual. The physician who has long established extramedical interests has an incomparable advantage over those whose dedication to medical practice excluded such pursuits: avocational interests rarely spring spontaneously from the ashes of an otherwise successful career.

These interests appear to be derived from success at utilizing innate skills of which there are probably a limited number, and which vary from individual to individual. Each of these may be applied in a range of different activities. These skills include manual, verbal, linguistic, artistic, and athletic abilities. The level of each skill appears to be distributed, populationwise, on the bell curve. Often chance determines in what area individuals will find pursuits from which they derive life-long gratification. To expect to find them once the aging process has set in, when the physical capacity to implement them is waning and when resources of energy are diminishing, is asking for the improbable.

Golf, perhaps the most popular outdoor sport of physicians, is an example of this. With few exceptions, all of the retired physicians one finds on the course commenced playing at a much younger age. It is a sport purely personal in terms of ability and challenge to mastery of the player, yet it also involves competitiveness and provides the opportunity for personal relationships with others.

To become gratifying, an avocational pursuit involves emotional investment of one's energies over long periods of time; it must create an internal challenge to mastery by the use of one's talent and knowledge; and there must be evidence of success or progress from time to time. For these reasons, retired persons seldom take up physical sports for the first time. Thus, golf, which is not infrequently seen by the young and uninitiated as a futile and purposeless game, is tried in the early and middle adult years, becoming a major interest and for retired individuals continues as great a challenge as when they were younger. Statistics gathered by the National Golf Foundation indicated that players over 65 years of age played 62,800,000 rounds of golf in 1980. This figure is surely evidence that golfers who are retired gained incalculable satisfaction—even when particular shots, games, or scores can be the sources of temporary despair!

Pursuits that are creative are emotionally rewarding—painting, photography, and construction of decorative or utilitarian objects, are examples. The concept of creativity is, perhaps erroneously, customarily thought of only as applicable to a limited number of activities. Most avocational pursuits contain an element of creativity combined with a personal challenge to the individual. Creativity is largely the successful utilization of any skill. Gardeners are aware that their efforts, including continuous weeding, have a creative objective. Even when they know that all is as they desire, tomorrow will bring a repetition of seemingly never-completed tasks. Gardening, indeed, may be viewed as calling for motivations akin to nurturing on the one hand, and as a continuing contest with nature on the other.

Most outdoor activities require a degree of physical fitness which will generally diminish with advancing age, limiting and eventually necessitating withdrawal from them. Ideally, greater gratification will be achieved by involvement in activities of both outdoor and indoor kinds which may be followed according to the seasons of the year. That way, when outdoor activity becomes limited, an alternative is already established.

Avocational pursuits serve many purposes, not least of which are the opportunities to develop relationships with other persons of mutual interests and social and educational status. Such acquaintances and friendships in many circumstances replace those which dissipated on retirement. Of course, these other individuals are most likely to have established their avocational pursuits long before retirement, so their level of expertise is also most likely to have advanced beyond the beginning retiree's stage.

Contentment in retirement is thus far from being an automatic reward for a life of working for the benefit of humanity. It is largely the outcome of preparation in earlier years and depends on what the individual brings when entering it. Many retired physicians appear to find that time of life a relatively pleasant existence because they have engaged in extramedical activities appealing to their interests and challenging their innate skills. Retirement is, for them, a smooth continuation of their more active years. Acceptance of other changes in the structure of their lives is made so much easier—a shifting of emphasis rather than an abrupt change in direction.

Recognizing that each physician is an individual differing psychologically from every other, only general principles can be suggested with regard to planning for retirement. Physicians should begin to think about what they will be doing when they retire by the time they are firmly established in an area of medical practice. This is not to suggest that they become preoccupied with their "golden years," but rather that they contemplate, on occasion, what their current days would be like if the hours spent practicing medicine were to be filled with enjoyable alternatives. Do they have other pursuits which engage them in meaningful and rewarding experiences? Do these offer the potential for developing social relationships? Do they have deep interests that they would pursue when the frailties and accompaniments of age limit their physical activities? To confront such questions in a serious fashion sets the stage for planning for retirement.

Psychological preparation must begin in early adult years. Examination of the causes of unhappiness in later life bring to light certain general factors. With regard to physical comfort and the quality of life desired, financial considerations are a major concern. Economic security calls for developing assets which will provide the level desired. An overall view of real and potential financial resources and how they will contribute to living costs is necessary to provide a realistic picture of the future. Economic reality does not conform solely to hopes and fantasies that everything will continue as is. Pensions and annuities, for example, often turn out to be worth a lot less in real value than they seemed at one time because of inflation. If it is necessary to begin additional accumulation of assets, the sooner this is recognized and commenced, the better. It may even be advisable to modify the present lifestyle in some degree.

The physical health of the retired person is something that cannot be planned or foreseen. Nevertheless, recognition of the costs associated with illness, including senility, over and above those covered by insurance, is advisable in the evaluation of future financial outlays. For example, the possibility of ending one's days in a nursing home should be considered in financial planning. Just as drawing up a will is an essential part of estate planning, so some thought might be given to drawing up a "living will" to cover certain eventualities.

While financial planning is conducive to peace of mind in the future, the actual time spent on this during retirement years is minor. Real enjoyment comes from a structured life which provides constant and repetitive satisfactions. These are psychological in nature and are closely linked to the satisfactions and gratifications achieved throughout one's adult years. Preparation for retirement includes sound evaluation of pleasures experienced and their sources outside the practice of medicine. Seeking out activities that are emotionally rewarding to the individual is the key. Decisions to devote time to them on a regular basis have to be made and kept. Most individuals have some knowledge of pursuits that interest them and these provide the basis for further development. Those which provoke a challenge to the individual are the ones most likely to become the source of keeping the spirit alive, as well as laying the groundwork for the structure of otherwise empty days and weeks: humans are creatures of habit as much in retirement as in their more active years.

Most important in all planning is the necessity to include the spouse. Often retirement raises large questions such as a change in residence. The offspring have usually left the family home which is now larger than needed, costly to maintain, and unnecessarily demanding of personal energies. Whether to move, or more usually, where to move, is clearly a joint consideration. A move, for example, to the Sun Belt may be attractive in many ways, but close examination reveals some of the problems which may be encountered. This inevitably results in severing or abandoning the social links, friendships, and activities of the spouse which have provided gratifications through the years. For both, it may require establishing a new life, new friendships, and new social relationships without a ready-made foundation of a working situation. For some, affiliating with their church or temple offers a new start.

For physicians and their spouses who wish to explore planning for retirement, the Department of Practice Management of the American Medical Association offers seminars in association with medical societies, as well as at its headquarters.

Physicians, like others, have an obligation to their dependents, the natural objects of their bounty, to draw up wills to ease the burden of their passing. Equally, it may be argued that, for their own future well-being, they have an obligation to prepare for the time when their professional work will cease.

# Index